BRAIN INJURY REHABILITATION:
Clinical Considerations

*This volume is one of the series,
Rehabilitation Medicine Library,
edited by John V. Basmajian.*

* Originally published as part of the Physical Medicine Library, edited
by Sidney Licht.

BRAIN INJURY REHABILITATION:
Clinical Considerations

Edited by

M. Alan J. Finlayson, Ph.D., C. Psych.

Department of Psychology
Chedoke-McMaster Hospitals
Professor, Department of Psychiatry
McMaster University
Hamilton, Ontario, Canada

Scott H. Garner, MD, FRCP (C)

Director, Acquired Brain Injury Program
Chedoke-McMaster Hospitals
Associate Professor, Medicine
McMaster University
Hamilton, Ontario, Canada

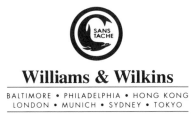

Williams & Wilkins

BALTIMORE • PHILADELPHIA • HONG KONG
LONDON • MUNICH • SYDNEY • TOKYO

A WAVERLY COMPANY

Editor: JOHN P. BUTLER
Managing Editor: LINDA S. NAPORA
Copy Editor: RICHARD H. ADIN
Designer: DAN PFISTERER
Illustration Planner: WAYNE HUBBEL
Production Coordinator: ANNE STEWART SEITZ

Copyright (c) 1994
Williams & Wilkins
428 East Preston Street
Baltimore, Maryland 21202, USA

RC387.5
B74
1994

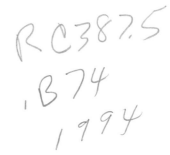

Accurate indications, adverse reactions, and dosage schedules for drugs are provided in this book, but it is possible that they may change. The reader is urged to review the package information data of the manufacturers of the medications mentioned.

Printed in the United States of America

Library of Congress Cataloging in Publication Data

Brain injury rehabilitation : clinical considerations / edited by M.
  Alan J. Finlayson, Scott H. Garner.
      p.   cm. — (Rehabilitation medicine library)
   Includes index.
   ISBN 0-683-03224-0
   1. Brain damage. 2. Brain damage—Patients—Rehabilitation.
  I. Finlayson, M. Alan J. II. Garner, Scott H. III. Series.
   [DNLM: 1. Brain Injuries—rehabilitation. WL 354 B8139 1994]
RC387.5.B74 1994
617.4'81044—dc20
DNLM/DLC
for Library of Congress   92-48433
                                                                      CIP

                                                   93 94 95 96 97
                               1   2   3   4   5   6   7   8   9   10

For Margaret and Alistair
who lit the flame
and Anita who has nurtured
and protected it.
To Mary Kay Lane, Byron Rourke,
and Ralph Reitan,
my heartfelt gratitude.
(MAJF)

Thanks to Iris, Herb, and Margaret
for their support and love.
(SHG)

Series Editor's Foreword

In this past decade, many serious scholars and clinicians have plunged into the frightening epidemic of head injuries. They have managed the problems of neuropsychologic rehabilitation pragmatically and almost by instinct. To address them about *Brain Injury Rehabilitation: Clinical Considerations* is unnecessary. They will recognize its wisdom and value, its important contribution to the rather panic-driven literature on the subject.

Having assumed that group's early acceptance, we conceived and planned this volume to be a pivotal one for the many thousands of clinicians, support personnel, administrators, and families who deal with the multitudinous problems at all levels of recovery and apparent failure. *Brain Injury Rehabilitation* is state of the art for all who have a large or small involvement in the treatment of individuals with brain injury.

The editors, Drs. Finlayson and Garner, are affiliated with a superb rehabilitation system in Ontario, Canada, where the team effort has reached a level of sophistication rarely seen even in the most worthy clinics. The editors, in turn, gathered international and interdisciplinary authors of both eminence and common sense to cover the field scientifically and clinically.

The field of knowledge is growing and simultaneously decaying rapidly. Even the best informed writers may in time regret words written today about brain injury rehabilitation. Nevertheless, the analyses, recommendations, and opinions of our authors will serve the last decade of the 20th Century well. I predict that *Brain Injury Rehabilitation* will be a much used resource as the authoritative book about optimal rehabilitation of human beings with head injury.

JOHN V. BASMAJIAN
O. Ont. MD, FRCPC, FACA, FSBM
FABMR, FACRM (Australia)

Preface

Increasingly, acquired brain injury is being recognized as a major health/ social problem. Trauma produces a myriad of injuries, impairments, and disabilities, which result in a variety of handicaps. The diffuse nature of brain trauma results in a complex mixture of physical, behavioral, cognitive, and emotional problems that have an impact upon the individual, his/her family, and society at large.

In *Brain Injury Rehabilitation: Clinical Considerations,* the authors present a multidisciplinary approach to the management of clinical problems exhibited by individuals with head injury. The delivery of care to this population in many ways parallels the natural recovery process. Thus, different needs are present at acute stages of injury than at more advanced stages. In the early stage, medical and physical problems are more critical; in later stages, psychologic and social factors predominate.

Since treatment of brain injury is a developing field of rehabilitation, state-of-the-art clinical technology is presented from a variety of disciplines' perspectives. However, the focus of this book is on the clinical needs of the patient, and there is less emphasis on discipline-specific objectives. Furthermore, every effort has been made to ensure that the research base underlying each methodology has been critically reviewed and documented for the clinician who wishes to pursue an in-depth study of a topic. The role of family and consumer groups as partners with rehabilitation specialists in the development of services has been emphasized. In short, this volume addresses the principles and practices of rehabilitation for individuals with brain injury.

Finally, the editors recently were awarded a major grant for brain injury rehabilitation based upon a continuum of care model. The spirit of this model permeates the text.

M.A.J.F.
S.H.G.

Acknowledgments

We wish to acknowledge the help and contributions of our colleagues at Chedoke-McMaster and Hamilton General Hospitals. Thanks to Maureen Tomalty assisted with the clerical work. A very special thank you goes to Sandy Shannon who worked tirelessly to see this project through to completion. We would like to thank Dr. John Basmajian for his encouragement and guidance throughout this project. The staff at Williams and Wilkins have been very helpful, particularly Linda Napora and Anne Stewart-Seitz.

(MAJF & SHG)

Contributors

Dennis P. Alfano, Ph.D.
Associate Professor
Departments of Psychology and Biology
University of Regina
Regina, Saskatchewan, Canada

Karen Allen, Ph.D.
Director of Training
Rehabilitation Research and Training Center
SUNY at Buffalo
Buffalo, New York

John R. Davis, Ph.D.
Psychologist
Schneider Dvali
Department of Psychiatry
McMaster University
Hamilton, Ontario, Canada

Kenneth W. Dunn, Ph.D., C.Psych.
Assistant Clinical Professor
Department of Psychiatry
McMaster University
Psychologist
Chedoke-McMaster Hospitals
Hamilton, Ontario, Canada

M. Alan J. Finlayson, Ph.D., C.Psych.
Department of Psychology
Chedoke-McMaster Hospitals
Professor
Department of Psychiatry
McMaster University
Hamilton, Ontario, Canada

David J. Fordyce, Ph.D.
Section of Physical Medicine and Rehabilitation
Virginia Mason Medical Center
Seattle, Washington

Cynthia A. Gambarotto, B.Sc. (PT), M.C.P.A.
Senior Physiotherapist
Acquired Brain Injury Program
Chedoke-McMaster Hospitals
Hamilton, Ontario, Canada

Scott H. Garner, MD, FRCP(C)
Director, Acquired Brain Injury Program
Associate Professor of Medicine
Chedoke-McMaster Hospitals
Hamilton, Ontario, Canada

Gordon Muir Giles, Dip.CTO OTR
Director of Occupational Therapy
Guardian Foundation
Berkeley, California

Daryl Gill, Ph.D., C.Psych.
Director
Rehabilitation Psychology and Neuropsychology
Assistant Professor
Departments of Psychiatry and Internal Medicine
Principal Investigator
Neuropsychology Research Unit
University of Manitoba
Winnipeg, Manitoba, Canada

Gerald Goldstein, Ph.D.
Research Career Scientist
Highland Drive
Veterans Administration Medical Center
Pittsburgh, Pennsylvania

Carolyn Kelley Gowland, MHSC., P.T.
Assistant Professor
School of Occupational Therapy and Physiotherapy
Faculty of Health Sciences
McMaster University

Research Manager
Pediatrics, Neurology and Long-Term Care
Physiotherapy Department
Chedoke-McMaster Hospitals
Hamilton, Ontario, Canada

C. Thomas Gualtieri, MD
North Carolina Neuropsychiatry
Chapel Hill, North Carolina

Richard Linn, Ph.D.
Director of Research
Rehabilitation Research and Training Center on Brain Injury
SUNY at Buffalo
Buffalo, New York

Elaine MacNiven, Ph.D.
Douglas Hospital
Research Centre
McGill University
Verdun, Quebec, Canada

Louis Malenfant, Ph.D.
Universite de Moncton
Moncton, New Brunswick, Canada

Steffen Malik-Høegh
Neuropsykologisk AFD
Sønderborg Sygehus
Sønderborg, Denmark

Catherine A. Mateer, Ph.D.
Department of Psychology
Good Samaritan Hospital
Puyallup, Washington
and
Departments of Speech and Hearing Sciences
Neurological Surgery
University of Washington
Washington, DC

Allan D. Moore, M.A.
Departments of Psychiatry, Psychology and Medicine

University of Manitoba
Neuropsychology Research Unit
Health Sciences Clinical Research Centre and
Society for Manitobians with Disabilities, Inc.
Manitoba, Canada

Lois C. Peters, Ph.D., C.Psych.
Departments of Psychiatry, Psychology and Medicine
University of Manitoba
Investigator
Neuropsychology Research Unit
Health Sciences Clinical Research Centre and
Society for Manitobians with Disabilities, Inc.
Manitoba, Canada

John T. Povlishock, Ph.D.
Professor of Anatomy
Virginia Commonwealth University
Richmond, Virginia

Ray G. Rempel, M.Sc.
Director
Ontario Head Injury Association
St. Catharine, Ontario, Canada

Ahmos Rolider, Ph.D., C.Psych.
Professional Rehabilitation
Opportunities (PRO)
Hamilton, Ontario, Canada

M.M. Sohlberg
Department of Speech
Good Samaritan Hospital
Puyallup, Washington

Michael Stambrook, Ph.D., C.Psych.
Associate Professor
Department of Psychiatry
University of Manitoba
Principal Investigator
Neuropsychology Research Unit
Health Sciences Clinical Research Centre

Director, Clinical Services Society for Manitobians with Disabilities, Inc.
Winnipeg, Manitoba, Canada

Donald T. Stuss, Ph.D.
Director of Research
Rotman Research Institute of Baycrest Centre
Professor of Psychology and Medicine (Neurology)
University of Toronto
Toronto, Ontario, Canada

Beth Urbanczyk, M.S.
Clinical Coordinator
Speech Language Pathology
New Medico Rehabilitation Center of the Capital District
Schenectady, New York

Alex B. Valadka, M.D.
Division of Neurological Surgery
Medical College of Virginia
Virginia Commonwealth University
Richmond, Virginia

Joy Van Houten, Ph.D.
University of Kansas
Lawrence, Kansas

Ron Van Houten, Ph.D.
Mount Saint Vincent University
Halifax, Nova Scotia, Canada

Barry Willer, Ph.D.
Associate Professor in Psychiatry and Rehabilitation Medicine
SUNY at Buffalo
Director
Rehabilitation Research and Training Center on Brain Injury
Buffalo, New York

Mark Ylvisaker, Ph.D.
Assistant Professor
Department of Communication Disorders
College of St. Rose
Albany, New York

Contents

SECTION III Community Integration

MECHANISMS OF INJURY AND RECOVERY

1

Challenges in Rehabilitation of Individuals with Acquired Brain Injury

M. ALAN J. FINLAYSON
SCOTT H. GARNER

The nature of acquired brain injury (ABI) results is a range of complex physical, cognitive, behavioral, and emotional problems. The scope and magnitude of these problems varies for each individual. The impact of ABI on family, friends, and the community at large is considerable and only just now being realized.

EPIDEMIOLOGY

The incidence of head injury is difficult to ascertain as bumps on the head are ubiquitous in human activity. Mild head injury, which can result in diffuse axonal injury, can occur in the context of sport, work, and community activities. An acquired brain injury is often correlated with violence in society, so the epidemiology of violence is of concern to clinicians and public health planners, but the most significant, single cause is as a result of motor vehicle accidents (see Chapter 19).

The incidence of hospitalization has been the most common way of identifying the frequency of head injury and has consistently been around 200 per 100,000 per year. It has been difficult to identify the prevalence of people living with the sequelae of ABI as many readapt to their social roles and they become part of the silent epidemic with handicaps which are truly hidden. Prevalence data is hard to obtain and very little exists in the literature. Information on disability was collected as part of a recent Canadian census. Preliminary analysis of that data suggests that acquired brain injury has a prevalence estimate of 74 per 100,000 aged 15 years or older. Approximately 16% of that population is institutionalized. However, as the population ages the rate of institutionalization is much higher (31% of those over 65). The prevalence rate for male/female is approximately that of the incident data, 1.7:1. These data are summarized in a recent review (Willer, Abosch and Dahmer, 1991).

Generally, the focus in ABI is on young adults with head injury. However, examining the age distribution in the population at large, it would seem that head injury has a trimodal distribution. Infants and toddlers are vulnerable as are the elderly. However, the highest incidence per age group is found among young adults (aged 15–24) (e.g., Willer et al., 1990; Cohadon, Richer, and Castel, 1991).

REHABILITATION

"Rehabilitation is defined as the development of the person to the fullest physical, psychological, social, vocational, avocational, and educational potential consistent with his or her physiological or anatomical impairment and environmental limitations" (Whyte and Rosenthal, 1988). Clearly, brain injury rehabilitation is a broad field, encompassing a range of problems that require a variety of solutions. The common goal, however, is to reduce handicap by optimizing an individual's functioning through either the enhancement of the individual's skill repertoire or the modification of the environment in which she/he must function. Inherent in this definition is a dichotomy between medical and social models of head injury rehabilitation. This can be encapsulated in the succinct definition of head injury rehabilitation: SAVE A LIFE—GET A LIFE.

Traditionally, professional attitudes and available resources have been directed to trauma support systems and early medical management in order literally to *save a life*. However, once the patient has healed, there are fewer resources available to assist the individual with brain injury in his/her successful reintegration into the community. The ability to *"get a life"* is significantly limited and the individual experiences post-coma abandonment (Rempel, 1992).

We have found it helpful to conceptualize rehabilitation in the context of the classification of the consequences of disease proposed by the World Health Organization (WHO, 1980). The consequences of disorder or disease are viewed on three levels: Impairment, Disability, and Handicap. An impairment is "any loss or abnormality of psychological, physiological, or anatomical structure or function" (WHO, 1980, p. 27). Disability represents "any restriction or lack (resulting from impairment) of ability to perform an activity in the manner or within the range considered normal for a human being" (WHO, 1980, p. 28). Handicap is "a disadvantage, for a given individual, resulting from an impairment or a disability, that limits or prevents the fulfillment of a role that is normal (depending on age, sex, and social and cultural factors) for that individual" (WHO, 1980, p. 29).

The WHO lists 7 categories of handicap: Orientation, physical independence, mobility, occupation, social integration, economic self-sufficiency, and other. These can be distilled to the fundamental aspects of life: Living, Loving, and Doing. In our own lives we wish for the ability and the means to sustain life; the capacity to love oneself and others; and an opportunity to participate in purposeful, productive, and pleasurable activities. Individuals with disabilities should have the same opportunity for housing and support in daily living; opportunity to relate socially, sexually and spiritually; and access to vocational and avocational pursuits. Reduction of handicap then allows the individual with the disability literally to *get a life*.

Reduction of handicap and the enhancement of the quality of these aspects of living can arise from a modification of impairment, disability, or handicap. Acquired brain injury is not a curable disease (although it can be prevented). Instead it is a neverending process of recovery requiring different levels of rehabilitation and program needs. Individuals who would have died 10 years ago, now struggle to find solutions for their problems in lifelong living. The ultimate test of rehabilitation success is the functioning of individuals with ABI within the community. Thus, a major focus of rehabilitation must be on community interventions. However, we cannot then abandon our ongoing efforts at physical/medical interventions because in order to *get a life*, we must first *save the life*. Maintaining an appropriate balance between these seeming tensions is one of the major challenges facing rehabilitation professionals.

MISSION STATEMENT

The impairment/disability/handicap paradigm forces clinicians to identify what domain they are addressing. It is imperative in rehabilitation to consider all ways to help an individual suffering from the sequelae of ABI. This means remediating impairments where possible by fostering functional abilities to the utmost; but, ultimately, it is our belief that most clinicians value the re-establishment of meaningful social roles (i.e., handicap dimension) and/or successful reintegration back into community living.

To date most text books, and the rehabilitation literature in general, address impairment and disability issues but recently other recent books have tackled the issue of community reintegration (e.g., Ylvisaker, 1988; Kreutzer and Wehman, 1990). In this volume we also have felt it necessary to give considerable attention to issues of community reintegration and to identify the skills relevant to the patient's ultimate designated living environment in a functional manner. However, there are chapters which are more oriented to impairment issues and their remediation (i.e., Chapters 6, 8). Other chapters focus on very practical functional skills (i.e., Chapter 7), and the issue of ultimate community reintegration (Chapter 16).

CONFLICTS AND CHALLENGES

Different approaches tend to favor different aspects of the individual's recovery. Prioritization of needs may vary depending upon the site of treatment (i.e., general hospital vs. rehabilitation center vs. community setting). While this may be appropriate, there is a danger that certain approaches may be fostered by the culture of the environment rather then the needs of the individual with ABI. For example, one of the basic conflicts to overcome is that of the medical model which fosters an attitude of identifying the "problem" with the patient so that something can be "done" to the patient (Condolucci, 1991).

This is in contrast to a rehabilitation approach which employs a holistic view to identify a hierarchy of functional deficits which interact directly with the environment and acknowledges an interdependence of influence. When done in this manner rehabilitation fosters an attitude of working *with* the patient and cannot be done successfully unless the patient, their family, and others in their environment participate in the rehabilitation process. The parallels between this tension and historical discussions of nature/nurture (Anastasi, 1955) or mind/body (Freedman, 1992) are striking. In fact, Freedman (1992) reminds us that "the tension between the socially conditioned purposive self and impersonal biological processes is an inescapable intrinsic tension" (p. 858).

This dichotomy in approach has other counterparts in rehabilitation which reflect different perspectives which may be legitimate but lead to different ways of dealing with similar problems. It is much like the parable of the elephant and the 10 blind men. The elephant may appear very different depending on where any of the blind men touch the elephant, whether that be the trunk, the tusk, the side, or the tail, even though each is part and parcel of the elephant.

Other dichotomous tensions exist in the field. One can be identified as the impairment-handicap tension which is best illustrated by the apparent difference between cognitive and functional behaviorist views (see Chapter 5). Wood (1990a) has described this conflict as the difference between an approach emphasizing declarative knowledge vs. procedural knowledge. The cognitive perspective tends to address inherent abilities and will often infer actual behavior on the basis of hypotheses identified by knowing in great detail the nature of existing impairments. On the other hand the behaviorist view downplays knowledge about aptitudes and potential performance in favor of identifying actual performance or function.

Similar examples could be given for physical deficits. For example, if no attention were paid to gait but instead was devoted to the enhancement of muscle strength, range of motion, and coordination, then a similar gap in measurement of impairments and the actual functional ability to walk in a community environment would exist. In most cases, actual physical function is more clearly generalizable, but, as task complexity increases, more effort needs to be applied to understanding the utilization of these skills in a given community environment.

The professional squeeze represents a significant tension experienced by service providers. In our Province, health care is administered by the provincial government in a socialist context, while below the 49th parallel an entrepreneurial model currently holds sway. However, regardless of the philosophical model, professionals are caught between the wants and needs of patients/clients and families and the guidelines or laws of the funding source. The elimination of the middle person will not solve this problem.

Tensions also exist for the advocates of survivors living with the sequelae of ABI. The anger and frustration of advocates can be directly related to two different issues: First is the need for society to create environments which support community living even in the face of significant disability (see Chapter 17). Proponents of this perspective attempt to change society's view of individuals with disabilities so that there is greater acceptance of people who appear to move, talk, or act outside of accepted norms (see Chapter 16). This requires the creation of not only appropriate domiciliary environments but also appropriate activity environments which allow work, play, loving relationships, and an appropriate "circle of friends".

Secondly, advocates recognize the need to foster rehabilitation environments and also ask for the development of rehabilitation resources which provide an opportunity for skill development and behavioral change.

The most suitable option would be to have appropriate care immediately after injury as this can prevent the development of maladaptive behaviors and optimize functional skills. Unfortunately for many individuals early intervention is lacking and they end up living in the community or in other settings suffering as a result of significant maladaptive behavioral patterns or other preventable complications.

While there is a need for society to change and become more accepting of persons who do not fit the common mold, it is always going to be hard to "fit in" when challenged by behaviors that are disruptive and aggressive. These behavioral episodes often result in "crises" and immediate decisions must be made to deal with these very difficult problems. Unfortunately, the common result is relegation to a prison or an inappropriate psychiatric environment, as comprehensive rehabilitation environments which facilitate adaptive change are still lacking in most communities. These "crises" points are often opportunities, as they may help some clients to see the reality of their life as it is and may help them face the difficult process of change, rather than face the consequences of family breakdown or other inappropriate placements such as jail. However, positive options have to be available at these turning points or these opportunities will be lost.

As opportunities are developed, the conflict between the sharing of existing resources with other groups of disadvantaged persons and the development of head injury "ghettos" will have to be faced. Bush (1992) reminds us of the need to unite our efforts to secure appropriate opportunities for all. There is little advantage to competition among groups for limited resources. Furthermore, the "disease of the month" or telethon approach to funding can be dehumanizing.

A further tension exists between institutions and community. Patients, their families, and many professionals working in the community tend to view health care facilities dealing with the early phases of rehabilitation as institutions. However, the many professionals working in these centers view themselves very much as a part of the community. One's perspective is, thus, important in defining community. We remember a colleague, with a strong religious conviction who chose to enter a community. From another point of view, it could be argued that it was an institution being entered.

Achieving the aims of head injury rehabilitation requires creative problem solving. In many cases we have developed community based programs and transitional living centers that are merely an outward extension of traditional rehabilitation values and practices; that is, impairment and disability focused. Impairment and disability treatment paradigms have been extended to the community without necessarily considering the context in which they occur nor recognizing that they may not necessarily lead to efficient reduction of handicap. Perhaps a better approach would be to consider institutions without walls. That is, resources would be deployed where they are most needed—in the patient's own environment. For example, coaching could be provided in a job situation; supportive independent living could be provided by a trainer or assistant on an as needed basis; and direct assistance with the establishment of interpersonal relationships where they occur could be implemented. In so doing, rehabilitation could be delivered in an individualized manner providing the necessary support for "living, loving, and doing" in the patient's own community.

It is important to remember, however, that a community is not just institutions without walls; it is also institutions. The concept of community needs to be re-examined as a continuum of opportunity and our goal as rehabilitation professionals should be to maximize these opportunities for our clients in the environment that best accommodates their needs. In particular we must reconsider the concept of asylum.

A review of community mental health (Caplan, 1967) reveals that throughout history the pendulum has swung between the creation of structured environments for individuals who cannot cope in society (building an institution) and movements that free people from these rigid structures and allow them to live in the community. Thus, the tension between community and institution is in reality a conflict of individual needs and accompanying freedom of choice vs. programmatically determined needs and lack of choice.

Such a continuum of opportunities, however, is essential for individuals with ABI because of their unique cognitive and behavioral limitations. In developing options for lifelong living, consideration is given to such roles as case manager, meta cognitive prosthetic device (Michenbaum, 1989), or surrogate frontal lobes. These are not intended as pejorative terms by their users. Instead, they recognize the protective role that cognitive and behavioral limitations command for the well-being of the individual. In many ways such functions are reminiscent of the original concept of an asylum as a place of "refuge and recuperation" (Wing, 1990). As ABI rehabilitation rediscovers the community and evolves into lifelong living, it will be important to examine the history of the community mental health movement and reconsider the concept of asylum—asylums not necessarily as structures but as a process that can occur anywhere in the environment (Wing, 1990).

Such a review should also consider the parallels between head injury rehabilitation and the adolescent years. The turmoil and anguish of parents and teenagers, as they struggle with protection versus independence while the child becomes his/her own person, is similar to the tension of caregivers wishing to safeguard their charges and the desire of victims for autonomy. No clear prescription is available for either dilemma.

The ultimate challenge for rehabilitation clinicians and investigators will be to reduce handicap and provide opportunities for satisfactory living, loving, and doing. The relative efficacy of interventions focused on impairment, disability, or handicap dimensions will have to be determined. Many efforts (including those described in this volume) will be tested and found wanting or discovered to be highly appropriate. We believe that a balance of the tensions described will be found and we trust that this volume will facilitate that harmony.

References

Anastasi, A. (1958). Heredity, environment, and the question "how"? Psychological Review, 65, 197–208.

Bush, G.W. (1990). Self-esteem: the first step to empowerment: toward a conceptual ase for rehabilitation and advocacy. Building a lifetime of growth conference report. St. Catherines, Ontario: Ontario Head Injury Association.

Caplan, R.B. (1969). Psychiatry and the community in nineteenth century America. London: Basic Books.

Cohadon, F., Richer, E., and Castel, J.P. (1991). Head injuries: Incidence and outcome. Journal of the Neurological Sciences, 103, S27–S31.

Condolucci, A. (1991). Interdependence: The route to community. Orlando: Paul M. Deutsch Press, Inc.

Freedman, D.X. (1992). The search: Body, mind, and human purpose. American Journal of Psychiatry, 149, 858–66.

Kreutzer, J.S., and Wehman, P. (1990). Community reintegration following traumatic brain injury, Toronto: Paul H. Brooks.

Meichenbaum, D. and Perrin, L. (1989). Cognitive-behavioural interventions for persons with head injury. York County Hospital presentation.

Rempel, R.G. (1992). A report on postcoma abandonment in Ontario. St. Catharines, Ontario: Ontario Head Injury Association.

Whyte, J. and Rosenthal, M. (1988). Rehabilitation of the patient with head injury. In: DeLisa, J.A. (ed). Rehabilitation: Principles and practice. Philadelphia: J.P. Lippincott.

Willer, B., Abosch, S., Dahmer, E. (1990). Epidemiology of disability for traumatic brain injury. In Wood, R.H. (ed). Neurobehavioral sequelae of traumatic brain injury. New York: Taylor and Francis, Inc.

Wing, J.K. (1990). The functions of asylum. British Journal of Psychiatry, 157, 822–27.

Wood, R.L. (1990a). Neurobehavioral paradigm for brain injury rehabilitation. In: Wood, R.L. (ed). Neurobehavioral sequelae of traumatic brain Injury. New York: Taylor and Francis, Inc.

World Health Organization. (1980). International classification of impairment, disabilities, and handicaps. Geneva: Author.

Ylvisaker, M., Gobble, E.M. (eds) (1988). Community Re-entry for head injured adults. Boston: Little, Brown and Company.

2

Pathobiology of Traumatic Brain Injury

JOHN T. POVLISHOCK
ALEX B. VALADKA

In any consideration of the multiplicity of traumatic insults that can be brought to bear upon the brain parenchyma, it soon becomes obvious that the effect of these upon the brain may be varied and thus may translate into different patterns of morbidity and recovery. When speaking of traumatic brain injury, one typically divides such injuries into either a missile or nonmissile type. In general, penetrating missile injuries create localized, focal lesions which result in morbidity directly related to the primary site of injury. In such patients, mortality is usually high; yet in those who survive, recovery is sometimes surprisingly good because of the highly focal nature of the primary insult. Unfortunately, as our cities are fast being transformed into urban war zones, this type of injury is becoming increasingly common. Despite this fact, however, no substantive effort has been made to investigate the pathobiologic consequences of missile injury. Other than the obvious destructive forces of the missile penetration, little else is appreciated regarding the pathobiology triggered by such injury.

Like penetrating missile injuries, nonmissile injury to the brain is also a feature common to modern society. Such events as falls, sporting-related accidents, assaults, and motor vehicle accidents subject the brain to shear and tensile forces that involve both local as well as diffuse brain abnormalities. With assaults or falls, it is typical to see more focal damage related to the area of primary contact. Additionally, with fracture of the cranial vault, there may be damage to the superficial epidural vessels and, particularly, in the case of falls, rupture of the bridging vessels can occur. In contrast to the situation seen with assault and falls, motor vehicle accidents, involving both passengers and pedestrians, cause much more complex and devastating injury to the brain. In such cases, due in part to the differential acceleration of the brain, both focal as well as diffusely localized damage can occur. Because of this, pathologists have long characterized nonmissile head injuries in terms of focal vs. diffuse abnormalities. Focal abnormalities traditionally include contusion and hematoma formation, while diffuse injuries include diffuse axonal injury, hypoxic/ischemic change, diffuse brain swelling, and, rarely, diffuse petechial hemorrhage (Adams, et al., 1985). With most vehicular accidents, the brain sustains translational forces that move the brain in a sagittal plane in the cranial vault. This causes the frontal and temporal poles to move over the bony, rough cranial vault, with focal contusions occurring as the consequence of this movement. During motor vehicle accidents, the brain is also subjected to rotational/angular acceleration, which causes more diffuse CNS (central nervous system) involvement. In this case, it is believed that the rotational/angular forces of injury bring shear and tensile forces to bear on the brain, thereby damaging fibers and microvessels scattered throughout the brain parenchyma (Strich, 1956, 1961; Adams, et al., 1982).

This concept was elegantly tested in a subhuman primate model developed at the University of Pennsylvania. In these laboratories, it was demonstrated that when baboons were subjected to movement in the sagittal plain, only focal contusion and/or subdural hematoma were created. Although damaging, these changes did not contribute to prolonged unconsciousness (Adams, et al., 1985; Gennarelli, et al., 1982). However, when rotational/angular forces were applied to these animals, it was noted that significant morbidity followed despite the fact that mass lesions were not a consequence of such injuries. In fact, with increasing degrees of angular acceleration, prolonged posttraumatic unconsciousness and coma occurred (Gennarelli, et al., 1982). When the brains of these animals were examined by traditional light microscopic methods, it was noted that, with increasing rotational force, proportionally greater numbers of damaged axons could be seen throughout the injured brain (Gennarelli, et al., 1982). As a direct correlation appeared to exist between the number of damaged axons and the subsequent morbidity, this led Gennarelli and his colleagues to hypothesize that the larger the number of axons damaged, the greater the degree of neuronal disconnection and subsequent neural failure and morbidity (Gennarelli, et al., 1982). Findings similar to those observed in subhuman primate models of traumatic brain injury have also been noted in autopsy material from humans involved in motor vehicle accidents. In such cases, head-injured humans can show significant morbidity without concomitant mass lesions or significant contusion (Adams, et al., 1982). When the brains of such patients have been studied, widespread or diffuse axonal damage has been recognized, thereby suggesting that the widespread axonal injury was the anatomical correlate of the observed morbidity.

In the above passages, we have attempted to provide a brief introduction to some of the more common changes occurring with traumatic brain injury of both the missile and nonmissile type. Having provided this basic template of the pathobiology of various forms of traumatic brain injury, we will now focus on the more unique features of injuries of the nonmissile type. Emphasis will be placed upon nonmissile injuries because, unlike primary missile-induced injury, much of the pathobiology of nonmissile injury is known, allowing for a more complete consideration of those factors contributing to morbidity and recovery. In this regard, we will systematically review both the vascular and brain parenchymal changes typically associated with such injuries. The preferential vulnerability of neural vs. vascular elements will be fully developed in the context of mild, moderate, and severe traumatic brain injury, with a consideration of how these changes contribute to both morbidity and recovery. The potentially adverse consequences of secondary posttraumatic insults, such as hypoxia and hypotension, will also be considered, and their roles in the genesis of continued morbidity and dysfunction will be evaluated. Lastly, various management strategies will be considered, ranging from those routinely employed in the medical/surgical setting to those undergoing evaluation in ongoing clinical trials.

BRAIN'S RESPONSE TO TRAUMA

Vascular Change

As noted above, nonmissile traumatic injury to the brain typically involves both focal and diffuse changes. In falls, assaults, or motor vehicle accidents, contusions are a common manifestation of focal injury to the brain. Again, generally related to the nature and site of impact, contusions can be found in multiple cortical sites. Most commonly, they are seen on the tips of the frontal and temporal lobes, where these cortical regions normally cross the relatively rough surfaces of the anterior and middle cranial fossae, respectively. Typically, contusion manifests itself as a wedge-shaped lesion with its apex directed away from the cortical surface. It originates as a hemorrhage resulting from vascular damage sustained at the moment of impact, typically first recognized at the gray/white interface. Such hemorrhage leads to infarction within the related cortical gray, and, thus, the contusion resembles a hemorrhagic infarction confined to the cortical surface. With time, reactive glial elements encapsulate the infarction, ultimately creating a residual cystic cavity. The pattern of contusional development appears similar in both animals and man and generally requires many days to evolve from a discrete hemorrhagic site into an area of ischemic change and, ultimately, infarction.

In addition to contusion seen within the superficial cortices, traumatic brain injury can also be associated with other forms of vascular change. As is well recognized, assaults, falls, and motor vehicle accidents can be associated with tearing of the epidural vessels. This results in bleeding into the epidural compartment, creating a mass effect that can displace the brain, elevate intracranial pressure, and generate life-threatening physiologic changes. Similarly, the shear and tensile forces of traumatic injury can also disrupt the bridging veins, causing the development of a subdural hematoma, which over a more prolonged posttraumatic course can result in a mass lesion with its damaging consequences.

In addition to these intra- or extradural vascular abnormalities, traumatic brain injury is almost invariably associated with some degree of subarachnoid hemorrhage, caused by the rupture of pial vessels within the subarachnoid space. While little is known about the long-range consequences of such subarachnoid blood, recent evidence suggests that such blood can contribute to the onset of vasospasm which, in turn, could result in reduced regional cerebral blood flow, with devastating consequences to the injured brain (Doberstein, et al., 1990). Traumatic brain injury can also give rise to intraparenchymal vascular injury. Foci of hematoma can be identified within subcortical white matter, basal ganglia, and brainstem sites, which, dependent upon their localization, may also contribute to significant morbidity. Diffuse petechial hemorrhage can also be associated with head injury; however, when recognized, it is almost invariably associated with severe morbidity or mortality (Adams, et al., 1985).

In concert with the above described structural vascular changes, it is also well known that various forms of functional vascular change can also occur following traumatic brain injury. Depending upon the severity of the initial traumatic brain insult, such functional vascular change can include the impairment or loss of autoregulation (Lewelt, et al., 1980, 1982; Enevoldsen and Jensen, 1978), impaired physiologic cerebral vascular responsiveness to changes in arterial blood gases (Wei, et al., 1980; Marion, et al., 1991), altered cerebral blood flow (Bouma, et al., 1991; Dewitt, et al., 1986; Yamamaki and McIntosh, 1989; Marion, et al., 1991; Muizelaar, et al., 1989; Obrist, et al., 1979, 1984; Overgaard and Jewell, 1974), and altered blood-brain barrier status (Povlishock, et al., 1978). With the most severe traumatic brain injuries in both animals and man, autoregulation may be significantly impaired or lost (Lewelt, et al., 1980, 1982; Enevoldsen and Jensen, 1978), allowing flow to the brain to become dependent upon the systemic arterial pressure. In this context, elevated blood pressure would result in hyperemia, whereas decreased blood pressure would result in hypoperfusion. Traumatically induced shifts in the autoregulatory curve or range could be of particular significance in those patients sustaining secondary insults (vida supra). As noted, these autoregulatory abnormalities appear most pronounced in severe injury, however, less dramatic autoregulatory changes have also been described with more moderate injuries.

Impaired vascular responsiveness to blood gas change has also been described in both animals and man sustaining severe traumatic brain injury. In animals, impaired vascular responsiveness to hypocapnia has been described (Wei, et al., 1980), and in man, CO_2 vasomotor responsiveness can also be impaired following severe traumatic brain injury. Normally, hyperventilation will reduce pCO_2, causing arteriolar vasoconstriction. With injury, this pCO_2-related vasoconstriction can be impaired, with the degree of impairment reflecting, to some extent, the type of injury (Marion, et al., 1991). In addition to these abnormalities in autoregulation and in CO_2 responsiveness, laboratory studies have also shown other forms of impaired cerebral vascular function following traumatic brain injury. Perhaps one of the most intriguing findings concerns endothelial-dependent relaxation in traumatically brain-injured animals. Normally, agents such as acetylcholine induce dilation through the release of endothelium-derived relaxing factor (EDRF) which, in turn, acts on the vascular smooth muscle. In the traumatic condition, however, the normal vasodilatory endothelial-dependent response is converted to vasoconstriction (Ellison, et al., 1989). In fact, in the early posttraumatic period, the topical application of acetylcholine to traumatically brain-injured animals results in sustained vasoconstriction which appears to lessen over a prolonged posttraumatic course (Ellison, et al., 1989). Although the overall relevance of these endothelial-dependent phenomena to brain-injured man is at the moment unclear, it is our impression that the impaired endothelial-dependent relaxation, coupled with changes in autoregulation and in CO_2 vasoresponsiveness, suggests that the cerebral blood vessels may not be well equipped to maintain homeostasis in the face of declining blood pressure and/or changed blood gas composition. Conceivably, all these factors can explain the brain's vulnerability to secondary posttraumatic insult, and this will be discussed in a later section of this chapter.

Paralleling the above described vascular changes that occur with traumatic brain injury, other functional changes, particularly those involving cerebral blood flow, can also occur. Although primary traumatically induced ischemia has been suggested on the basis of the postmortem analyses of severely brain-injured patients (Graham and Adams, 1971; Graham, et al., 1978), the recognition of posttraumatic ischemia in patients has not been a common event. In fact, most blood flow studies have provided a rather confusing picture of those cerebral blood flow (CBF) changes occurring after severe traumatic injury. Some investigators, such as Barclay, et al. (1985), have noted global CBF reduction in head-injured patients in comparison to age matched controls. Further, they found an association between low regional cerebral blood flow and focal brain injury, while observing that increased regional CBF correlated with improved cognition. In contrast, however, other investigators have reported that increased blood flow is a finding common to traumatically brain-injured patients (Muizelaar, et al., 1989a, b; Obrist, et al., 1979, 1984). Recently, however, new information has emerged which suggests that these discrepant findings may relate to the timing of the posttraumatic blood flow studies. Specifically, in patients without surgical mass lesions, Marion, et al. (1991), reported that, in the first hours of injury, global CBF is low, followed over time by a hyperemic phase that peaks within 24 hours. Further, these same investigators demonstrated that global CBF values varied to some extent with the type of traumatic brain injury. These important studies have been extended recently in our own institution, where new evidence has emerged that the above described reduced CBF values can reach ischemic levels early in the posttraumatic course of some severely injured patients (Bouma, et al., 1991). Importantly, these new CBF studies demonstrate that only when the blood flow studies are performed within the first hours postinjury can reduced or ischemic blood flows be recognized. Typically, reduced flows seen in the early posttraumatic phase tend to normalize or reach increased levels over time. Thus, based upon these recent studies, one may conclude that the blood flow abnormalities seen postinjury most likely reflect the timing of the flow studies.

Concomitant with the above described overt structural, functional, and flow changes, traumatic brain injury also elicits perturbations of the blood-brain barrier. As has long been recognized, the blood-brain barrier resides in the cerebral vascular endothelium which serves as an interface to regulate the movement of various solutes from the blood to brain front, thereby allowing for the maintenance of a stable brain microenvironment. With traumatic brain injury, however, overt, as well as subtle, endothelial change allows for the passage of normally excluded substances into the brain parenchyma (Povlishock, et al., 1978). In some cases, normally excluded serum proteins can enter the brain together with a host of other substances normally confined to the blood front. In this regard, it has long been assumed that, with disruption of the barrier, the passage of serum proteins contributes to an osmotic gradient which, in turn, translates into a temporally delayed increase in brain water, termed edema. In this scenario, it has been assumed that the edema, in turn, contributes elevated intracranial pressure with the damaging consequences associated with this. Within the scope of this review, it is impossible to consider all issues relevant to traumatically related induced edema and attendant ICP change, and in this matter, the reader is referred to one of several reviews in this area (Thornheim, 1985). Suffice to say, that contemporary thought on the role of the barrier perturbation in the generation of edema has become much more complex. Blood-brain barrier perturbation in itself is an acute event, whereas the genesis of edema with attendant ICP rise is a more delayed phenomenon in both animals and man. Further, although the passage of serum proteins may be important for the concept of brain edema, there is now compelling evidence that the passage of other blood borne factors may be equally or perhaps more significant in the pathobiology of traumatic brain injury. In this regard, the passage of blood borne neurotransmitters as well as other related solutes may directly contribute to some of the cellular dysfunction seen with injury (Hayes, et al., 1991).

In regards to the myriad of vascular abnormalities described above in relation to traumatic brain injury, many factors have been postulated to contribute to their genesis. Clearly, the shear and tensile strains of trauma may act directly upon the cerebral vessels and elicit both structural and functional change. Similarly, the pressor responses associated with traumatic injury may also be contributing factors. Recent studies have begun to appreciate that both the traumatic event and its accompanying hypertensive episode result in the accelerated metabolism of arachidonate with the increased production of prostaglandins (Wei, et al., 1980; Kontos, et al., 1980; Wei, et al., 1981; Kontos, et al., 1981; Kontos, Wei, and Povlishock, 1981; Povlishock and Kontos, 1985). With the increased production of prostaglandins, there is a concomitant production of oxygen radicals of which the superoxide anion figures prominently (Kontos, et al., 1983, 1984; Wei, et al., 1985). To date, the superoxide anion has been clearly linked to many of the vascular abnormalities described in the previous section. As can be seen in Figure 2.1, the superoxide anion has been shown to have direct effects upon both the cerebral vascular endothelium and the arteriolar smooth muscle wall. In the context of the endothelium, the associated radical production has been linked to altered endothelial-dependent responses (Ellison, et al., 1989), alterations in blood-brain barrier status (Wei, et al., 1986), overt endothelial change (Kontos and Povlishock, 1986), and the potential for enhanced platelet aggregation. Similarly, this same superoxide anion surge has also been associated with change in vascular diameter as well as abnormal vasoreactivity. Collectively, then, it appears that the superoxide anion, in particular, may be responsible for many of the vascular abnormalities associated with traumatic injury which, as such, may contribute to morbidity and mortality. In the experimental setting, the use of superoxide anion scavengers, such as superoxide dismutase, has blunted virtually all of the above described abnormalities, and this compelling evidence has led to the use of superoxide dismutase in clinical trials. Although the trials to assess this in the clinical population are currently underway, the long-range hope is that the early use of such drugs postinjury will lead to a significant improvement in the morbidity and mortality associated with this devastating condition.

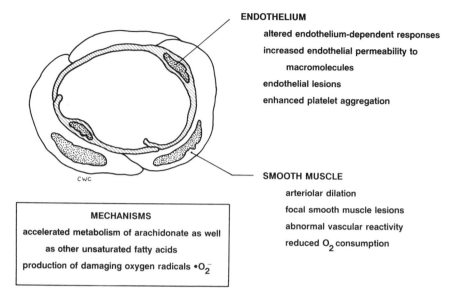

Figure 2.1. Characteristic endothelial and smooth muscle damage seen following traumatic brain injury. The endothelial damage includes altered endothelial-dependent responses, increased permeability to macromolecules which reflects blood-brain barrier damage, endothelial lesions, and the potential for increased platelet aggregation, should a secondary insult ensue. Within the smooth muscle, it can also be seen that the traumatic episode is associated with sustained arteriolar dilation, focal smooth muscle damage, abnormal vascular reactivity, and other functional impairments. Collectively, both the endothelial and smooth muscle change appear related to the accelerated metabolism of arachidonate and, perhaps, other unsaturated fatty acids with the production of damaging oxygen radicals. In this context, the superoxide anion appears to be the most damaging species, and a major contributor to the above described vascular sequelae of traumatic injury.

Brain Parenchymal Change

In addition to the above described vascular events, it is well known that traumatic brain injury can result in primary brain parenchymal change, as alluded to previously. Axonal injury is a consistent feature of the traumatic event, and it has been assumed that such axonal damage results in widespread neural disconnection and ensuing morbidity (Gennarelli, et al., 1982; Povlishock, 1985). Traditionally, traumatically induced axonal damage has been associated, in the early posttraumatic course, with the presence of reactive axonal swellings and retraction balls (Strich, 1956, 1961; Adams, et al., 1982, 1985). With more prolonged posttraumatic survival, the finding of Wallerian degeneration and microglial scarring has also been considered evidence of the traumatically induced axonal damage (Adams, et al., 1985). Historically, it has been assumed that shear and tensile forces of traumatic brain injury tear the axons at the moment of impact, causing them to retract and expel the ball of axoplasm, thereby forming the reactive swelling or retraction ball of classical description (Strich, 1956, 1961) (Fig. 2.2). Laboratory studies of traumatic brain injury have failed to confirm the correctness of this assumption. Multiple animal studies, evaluating minor, moderate, and severe traumatic brain injuries, have been unable to confirm the immediate, traumatically induced tearing of axons. Rather, they suggest that the shear and tensile forces of injury most likely disrupt the axolemma, causing focal cytoskeletal change, which, in turn, impairs anterograde axoplasmic transport (Povlishock, et al., 1983; Erb and Povlishock 1988; Cheng and Povlishock, 1988) (Fig. 2.3). With impaired transport, local axonal swelling ensues. With continued swelling, detachment occurs at the focus of injury, causing the formation of an enlarged, focally swollen proximal axonal segment in continuity with the sustaining cell soma (Fig. 2.4). The more distal axonal segment, now detached from the sustaining soma, degenerates and undergoes Wallerian change (Povlishock, et al., 1983; Povlishock and Kontos, 1985; Povlishock and Becker, 1985). In laboratory investigations, this sequence of reactive axonal change has been recognized to evolve over a 2–24 hour postinjury period, suggesting that considerable time must elapse before axons are frankly disconnected following injury. That a comparable sequence of events occurs in head-injured man has been convincingly shown in several neuropathologic studies, where it was recognized that reactive axonal swellings (retraction balls) are not seen unless the head-injured patient survives the traumatic event by at least 12 hours (Pilz, 1983; Adams, et al., 1989; Blumbers, et al., 1989). This, then, suggests that, even in man, damaged reactive axons cannot be seen immediately following trauma, and instead must evolve over the progressive course described in experimental animals. Although the precise subcellular changes involved in the above described sequence of events have not yet been clearly defined, they obviously merit considerable attention. Conceivably, once identified, experimental strategies could be employed to stop this damaging progression of axonal change.

The above described sequence of axonal damage associated with traumatic brain injury is typically seen to occur throughout the brain in a relatively diffuse fashion. Although, historically, many have focused on axonal injury within the corpus callosum and the dorsal lateral quadrant of the brainstem as the major foci of axonal injury (Adams, et al., 1985; Adams, et al., 1989), it is now commonly accepted that more widespread axonal damage is the more likely consequence of injury (Pilz, 1983; Adams, et al., 1989; Blumbers, et al., 1989). Of importance in the above described sequence of traumatically induced axonal change is the fact

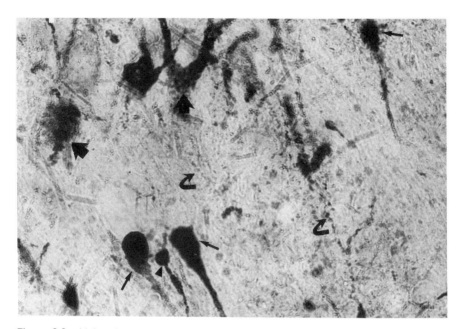

Figure 2.2. Light micrograph reveals traumatically induced axonal damage in an experimental animal. Through the use of anterogradely transported tracers, damaged axons are recognized as enlarged tracer-containing swellings (*arrows and arrowhead*) which occur at the site of axonal disconnection. Note that despite the presence of these reactive axonal swellings, other intact axons (*curved arrows*) can also be seen in the field. *Block arrows* demarcate the appendages of neurons in the field which have been retrogradely labeled with various tracers. ×1,000

that such axonal responses can occur within brain parenchyma revealing no other abnormality. In both human and animal studies, damaged axons can be seen in brain loci where related cells and fibers show no evidence of abnormality (Povlishock, et al., 1983; Povlishock and Kontos, 1985; Povlishock, 1986; Gennarelli, et al., 1989). Further, in the experimental setting, damaged axons can also be seen in brain regions demonstrating no altered cerebral blood flow or metabolism (Povlishock, 1990). Thus, these findings suggest that the axonal response to injury is a primary event and is not necessarily associated with a concomitant brain parenchymal or vascular change. This seems particularly so in the case of mild and moderate traumatic injury and most likely is the situation in many cases of severe traumatic injury.

Although, to date, much attention has focused on the concept of diffuse axonal injury and its overall implications for the morbidity seen in head-injured man, there has been little thought regarding the actual biological consequences of such axonal injury. As noted, with axonal injury, one sees

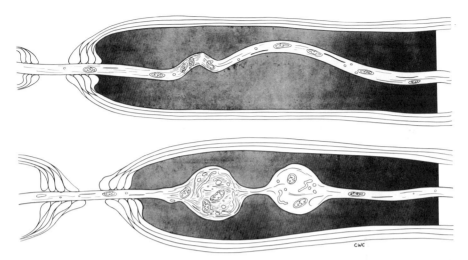

Figure 2.3. Sequence of events ongoing with the initiation of traumatically induced axonal change. Note in the *top panel* that the traumatic injury does not directly tear the axon but rather appears to stretch it, causing its axolemma to become highly infolded. Over time, this perturbation of the axolemma triggers, as is illustrated in the *bottom panel*, a reactive change leading to local axonal swelling, organelle accumulation, and lobulation which sets the stage for frank axonal disconnection, occurring within several hours of the traumatic insult.

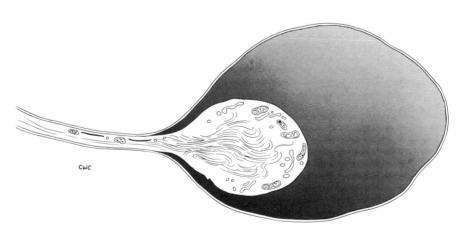

Figure 2.4. Continuation of events shown in Figure 2.3. Here, an enlarged swelling, lacking continuity with its distal axonal segment, has been formed after the progression of those events shown in Figure 2.3. The enlarged swelling is laden with organelles delivered by anterograde transport and is surrounded by an expanded and thinned myelin sheath. This reactive swelling constitutes the retraction ball of classical description.

the swelling of the proximal injured segment followed by degeneration of the distal axonal appendage. When the distal axon degenerates, the axonal terminals associated with the degenerating axon similarly degenerate. Thus, diffuse axonal injury is associated with diffuse nerve terminal loss, which is recognized several days postinjury. Typically, within hours of injury, changes in synaptic terminal morphology can be detected, and by the second day postinjury, the damaged terminals show degenerative changes involving either increased electron density or neurofilamentous hyperplasia (Erb and Povlishock, 1991). These changes precede frank degeneration of the terminal and its phagocytosis by related glial and phagocytic elements (Erb and Povlishock, 1991). Typically, with diffuse axonal injury, the ensuing diffuse deafferentation results in scattered terminal loss (deafferentation) with the retention of related undamaged synaptic input in the respective target field (Erb and Povlishock, 1991) (Fig. 2.5). This situation, as seen with traumatic brain injury, is quite dissimilar from that seen with more focal lesions such as stroke and tumor, which are associated with more concentrated and, therefore, more complete local

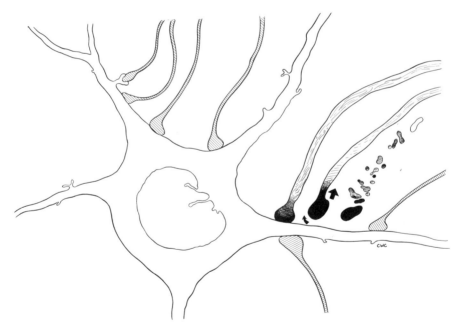

Figure 2.5. Degenerative change typically occurring with diffuse axonal injury. Note that as the axonal injury is diffuse, so, too, is its attended deafferentation. Note also that an electron dense and dying terminal is removed from the neuron while other intact terminal populations remain unaltered. It is its diffuse deafferentation which is believed to constitute the bases for potential adaptive neuroplasticity.

deafferentation. Although incompletely validated, new evidence exists to suggest that the diffuse deafferentation triggered by diffuse injury may create an ideal situation for potential recovery of the injured brain, particularly in those patients sustaining mild or moderate injury (Steward, 1989; Erb and Povlishock, 1991). In this situation, intact undamaged fibers adjacent to deafferented sites may be capable of sprouting and reoccupying the traumatically deafferented target. In the case of minor and moderate traumatic brain injury, in which deafferentation is certainly limited, the return of synaptic input to target nuclei may occur in a quite adaptive fashion (Steward, 1989; Erb and Povlishock, 1991). Conversely, with more severe injuries in which massive widespread deafferentation occurs, the magnitude of the deafferentation may preclude successful or adaptive synaptic recovery and, indeed, may be associated with maladaptive change. Although all these issues require further investigation, they clearly suggest the brain's potential for recovery after injury. These concepts are more fully addressed in other sections of this volume (see Chapter 3).

While much attention has been placed upon axonal injury and its attendant deafferentation, new information is also beginning to emerge on primary traumatically induced synaptic change, which, independent of any axonal-related event, may trigger structural and functional alterations following traumatic brain injury. Although experimental findings have not been directly confirmed in head-injured humans, recent studies conducted in various animal models of mild, moderate, and severe traumatic brain injury have shown that the typical traumatic event is associated with a net phase of excitation (Katayama, et al., 1991). Typically, with the traumatic episode, a massive extracellular elevation of potassium occurs, which directly correlates with massive depolarization of the injured brain (Katayama, et al., 1991; Hubschmann, 1983). Many have hypothesized that this depolarization is associated with a storm of neurotransmitter release, causing abnormal agonist-receptor interactions which, in turn, translate into morbidity (Faden, et al., 1989; Hayes, et al., 1989; Jenkins, et al., 1989). Although many have attempted to focus on the deleterious role of the excitatory amino acids in the damaging sequelae of traumatic brain injury, it has become apparent that the situation is much more complex. Most likely, excitatory amino acids, together with other transmitter systems, are activated following trauma. Perhaps, through interactive mechanisms, multiple transmitter systems influence postsynaptic sites, causing changes in second messenger systems (Hayes, et al., 1991). These changes, in turn, may alter cell function and responsiveness to further synaptic input and thereby lead to abnormal cellular responses. The basic tenets of this concept have been confirmed in various animal model systems, in which antagonists to the glutamate-NMDA receptor, in concert with cholinergic receptor antagonists, have shown significant protective effects (Jenkins, et al., 1988). In animals receiving both scopolamine and phencyclidine prior to traumatic brain injury, a marked improvement in behavioral recovery was observed postinjury. Moreover, in the same animal population subjected to a secondary insult, there has been a marked preservation of those neuronal elements normally lost after secondary injury (Jenkins, et al., 1988). Clearly, these abnormal agonist-receptor interactions do contribute to morbidity in rodent models of traumatic brain injury. It remains to be seen, however, if these events are operant in higher order animals and man.

In the above passages, considerable emphasis has been placed upon traumatically induced axonal injury and the synaptic abnormalities which ensue, with little consideration of the neuronal somatic changes that may occur in response to traumatic injury. This is due largely to the fact that the literature on primary traumatically induced neuronal somal change is limited. Other than the overt neuronal somal damage caused by contusion or secondary ischemia, primary neuronal somal damage is not consistently identified with traumatic brain injury (Povlishock, 1985). Some have identified damaged neurons undergoing chromatolysis; however, there is little evidence to support the assumption that these are primarily traumatically induced changes. Rather, most concur that the neuronal chromatolytic response seen postinjury is merely a direct result of damage to the axon that arises from the involved neuronal soma. Some metabolic studies performed on the injured brain have shown various phases of hyper- and hypometabolism following traumatic brain injury (Hayes, et al., 1984; Katayama, et al., 1991). Some studies utilizing 2-deoxyglucose have also attempted to demonstrate a mismatch between flow and metabolism and thereby suggest a phase of relative ischemia following traumatic head injury. Unfortunately, such correlations have been difficult to prove, and it appears that the various changes in cerebral metabolism most likely reflect regional differences in phases of cellular activation and depression. Obviously, much additional effort is required in this area.

SPECTRUM OF INJURY

In the previous passages, an attempt has been made to explicate some of the common brain parenchymal and vascular sequelae of traumatic brain injury of the nonmissile type. Clearly, all the vascular and neural events described in the preceding passages do not occur in all cases of traumatic brain injury. Unfortunately, to date, most of the information obtained from head-injured man is derived from those severely head-injured patients who are aggressively managed and monitored prior to routine postmortem analyses. As moderate and mild traumatic brain injuries are not routinely associated with mortality, both clinical monitoring and postmortem data on such patients are limited. Thus, no clear consensus exists regarding the actual pathobiology of mild and moderate traumatic brain injury in man. Fortunately, because of the large number of studies conducted in various laboratory models of mild and moderate head injury, coupled with limited information found in the human setting, a general impression has emerged regarding the possible spectrum of neural and vascular change that occurs in mild and moderate traumatic brain injury. In the following passages, we will attempt to detail the pathobiology of mild, moderate, and severe injury, drawing upon both laboratory and clinical findings. In doing so, in regards to man, we will try to equate all comments regarding mild, moderate, and severe traumatic brain injury to the Glasgow Coma Scale (GCS).

As originally described in 1974, the GCS was developed in order to standardize assessment of impaired consciousness and coma. The scale as used today has a 13-point span, ranging from 3-15. It is an additive assessment of 3 aspects of behavior:motor response, eye opening, and verbal response. The spectrum of motor responses varies from the ability to follow commands to the loss of response to pain, with scores ranging from 1-6. Eye opening is a graded response of activity ranging from spontaneous opening (score of 4) to responsive opening (usually in response to speech or pain) to absence of opening (score of 1). Lastly, verbal response ranges from normal speech and orientation to inappropriate words to no response. Scores range from 1-5.

A normal cumulative score in all three categories is 15 points. To date, head injuries have been routinely divided into three categories of severity based upon the GCS score. Severe head injuries include those with scores between 3 and 8, moderate injuries between 9 and 12, and mild injuries 13 or greater. Although the boundaries between those patients with GCS scores of 8 and 9 and between those with scores of 12 and 13 are not entirely clear, the distinction and scale as standardized above appear the most reasonable means for categorizing patients in terms of their response and accompanying pathobiology.

With mild head injury, that is to say patients with GCS scores of 13 or greater, the actual pathobiology is not completely appreciated. As noted above, for obvious reasons, humans sustaining mild traumatic brain injury do not come to routine postmortem analyses, and thus, the literature on this area is limited. In isolated cases of patients sustaining mild traumatic brain injury and then succumbing to nonrelated causes, postmortem analysis shows damaged axons scattered throughout the brain (Oppenheimer, 1968; Peerless and Rewcastle, 1967; Pilz, 1983). In subhuman primates sustaining minor traumatic brain injury, diffuse axonal injury is also suggested by the presence of diffuse degeneration primarily confined to the brainstem (Jane, et al., 1985). Similarly, in various other animal models of minor traumatic brain injury, comparable axonal change and degeneration have been described (Povlishock, et al., 1983). Thus, based upon these limited findings in man, coupled with the parallel observations made in subhuman primates and in other animal species, there is compelling evidence that even with the most trivial insult, axons are damaged throughout the brain and that the diffuse degeneration triggered by such axonal damage most likely contributes to morbidity. To date, numerous studies have associated various forms of morbidity with minor traumatic brain injury (Levin, et al., 1987b), and it is reasonable to speculate that the axonal injury and deafferentation discussed above are the pathobiologic correlates of this morbidity. Interestingly, as patients sustaining minor head injury show significant improvement in function over a 3–6 month posttraumatic course (Levin, et al., 1987b), it is likely that the neuroplasticity, described in the previous section also occurs in head-injured man. Such adaptive neuroplasticity most likely explains the anatomical substrates of the recovery seen in mildly head-injured humans; however, this does not rule out the interaction of other possible anatomical substrates of reorganization (see Chapter 3). In some humans sustaining mild traumatic brain injury, MRI has also revealed lesions within the frontal and temporal lobes which appear to show a direct correlation with both frontal and temporal lobe dysfunction (Levin, et al., 1987a). Interestingly, as these lesions resolve, so do the related neurological abnormalities, suggesting a causal interrelation. Thus, as in moderate head injury to be discussed below, it is possible that mild head injury involves both diffuse axonal injury together with focal parenchymal change, which together contribute to and ultimate influence the ensuing morbidity and subsequent recovery.

With more moderate brain injuries (GCS score of 9–12), many of the events described in the preceding passages again occur. However, now, in many cases, proportionally more axons are damaged, and these contribute to more widespread deafferentation. Also, with moderate injuries, focal lesions are more commonly seen, and, therefore, the damaging consequences of local contusion as well as intraparenchymal hemorrhage may superimpose their effects upon the changes caused by the diffuse axonal injury and deafferentation (Eisenberg and Levin, 1989). In this context, damage to the frontal and temporal lobes correlate with motor and memory disturbances, respectively (Levin, et al., 1987a). MRI typically reveals temporal and frontal lobe lesions following moderate traumatic brain injury, and, again, there is a suggestion that, like mild traumatic injury, the resolution of these MRI changes bears a direct temporal correlation to the resolution of related neurological abnormalities (Levin, et al., 1987a). The recovery seen following moderate traumatic brain injury is most likely multifactorial. In terms of the diffuse deafferentation triggered by moderate injury, adaptive plasticity may allow for significant recovery, and similarly, the resolution of MRI detected change may also account for some recovery. In the case of overt focal lesions such as contusion and/or intraparenchymal hemorrhage, neither neuroplastic changes nor the resolution of an MRI image can allow for complete recovery. Thus, in some cases of moderate traumatic brain injury, persisting focal lesions most likely explain some of the enduring morbidity associated with this condition.

With severe head injury, all of the changes described above occur. However, now overt disruption of the brain parenchyma and its vascular elements also occurs. As noted previously, severe traumatic brain injury is often associated with either epidural or subdural hematomata or with intraparenchymal hematoma formation. Again, these lesions occur concomitant with contusion and perhaps laceration, as well as diffuse axonal injury. Lastly, in some cases, there may be primary ischemia independent of overt vascular damage.

In those severely injured patients whose traumatic course is not complicated by mass lesion or secondary insult, the most likely determinant of morbidity is the overall magnitude of diffuse axonal injury, coupled with the extent of contusional damage. Obviously, when mass lesions occur, other destructive factors superimpose their influence upon the evolving diffuse axonal injury and related brain parenchymal change. The occurrence of focal lesions diffuse axotomy contributes to long-standing and significant morbidity. As noted in the previous passages, areas of significant focal damage cannot recover from traumatic injury. Further, in the case of extensive axonal injury and deafferentation, it is unlikely that adaptive rewiring can occur. In this context, it is conceivable that an ingrowth of nonhomologous fiber connections occurs and, as such, contributes to the persistence of enduring morbidity. Obviously, some of the information presented in the above passages is speculative. Nonetheless, with their basis in both human and experimental animal data, the above hypotheses appear to provide the most likely explanation of both the morbidity and potential recovery seen following traumatic brain injury of varying severity.

SECONDARY INSULTS

In the previous passages, much detail has focused on the spectrum of brain parenchymal and vascular change occurring with severe, mild, and moderate head injury. Although these changes are the most likely determinants of both morbidity and recovery, it is important to bear in mind that the damaging consequences of mild, moderate, and severe injury can be significantly exacerbated by the superimposition of a secondary posttraumatic insult. As alluded to in our previous section, the injured brain is quite susceptible to moderate secondary insults that the normal brain would tolerate well. Typically, because trauma involves damage to multiple organ systems, traumatic brain injury may be complicated by hypotension due to blood loss or by hypoxia secondary to pulmonary obstruction/dysfunction hypoventilation. In cases in which the traumatic event is complicated by a concomitant hypoxic or hypotensive insult, there is evidence emerging from the clinical setting that the outcome of such patients is significantly worse than anticipated on the basis of brain injuries alone. This clinical impression has been more than confirmed in the laboratory setting, where various investigators have subjected head-injured animals to secondary insults, such as modest hypoxia (Ishige, et al., 1987; Jenkins, et al., 1989). In this setting, hypoxic challenges that are normally well tolerated become devastating and can contribute to severe morbidity and mortality in the head-injured animal population. Although the actual pathobiologic consequences of such secondary insults are not entirely known, it has been widely speculated that the impaired vascular function occurring with traumatic brain injury provides inadequate vasomotor responsiveness to the injured brain in the face of a secondary challenge. Although this argument appears quite credible, other laboratory evidence suggests that the damaging consequences of secondary insult may be much more complex. In fact, in animals subjected to traumatic brain injury followed by a sublethal ischemic challenge, there is compelling evidence that blood flow may not be the major factor in determining severe morbidity and mortality (Jenkins, et al., 1989b). In these studies, it appears that the secondary ischemic insult is capable of triggering additional abnormal agonist/receptor interactions which impact upon the previously injured or perturbed brain parenchyma (Jenkins, et al., 1989a and b). In this setting, if the secondary insults are imposed, the pretreatment of animals with antagonists targeted to specific receptor systems has shown not only significant protection of the brain parenchyma but also significant functional recovery (Jenkins, et al. 1988). Thus, in man, the damaging consequences of secondary insults most likely reflect a summation of events mediated by the brain vasculature as well as by the brain parenchyma.

SUMMARY

In the above passages, we have attempted to provide a focused overview of the relevant pathobiology of traumatic brain injury and management strategies employed to blunt or prevent damaging consequences are reviewed in Chapter 4. As can be readily gleaned from this review, traumatic brain injury involves an avalanche of reactive change involving both structural and functional consequences in the brain parenchyma and its related vasculature. In the case of severe traumatic brain injury, neural and vascular dysfunction appear to be co-contributors to morbidity and mortality, and as such, most of the contemporary clinical approaches are targeted to address these, in the best fashion possible (see Chapter 14).

References

Adams, J., Doyle, D., Ford, I., Graham, D., and McLennan, D. (1989) Diffuse axonal injury in head injury: Definition, diagnosis and grading. Histopathology, 15:49–59.

Adams, J., Graham, D., and Gennarelli, T. (1985). Contemporary neuropathological considerations regarding brain damage in head injury. In: Becker, D.P., and Povlishock, J. (eds). Central nervous system status report. Richmond: Byrd Press, 65–77.

Adams, J., Graham, D., Murray, L., and Scott, G. (1982). Diffuse axonal injury due to nonmissile head injury in humans: An analysis of 45 cases. Annal. Neurol., 12:557–63.

Barclay, L., Zemcov, A., Reichert, W., et al. (1985). Cerebral blood flow decrements in chronic head injury syndrome. Biol. Psychiatry, 20:146–57.

Blumbers, P., Jones, H., and North, J. (1989). Diffuse axonal injury in head trauma. J. Neurol. Neurosurg. Psychiatry, 52:838–41.

Bouma, G.J., Muizelaar, J.P., Choi, S.C., Newlon, P.G., and Young, H.F. (In Press.) Cerebral circulation and metabolism after severe traumatic brain injury; the elusive role of ischemia. J. Neurosurg.

Bruce, D.A., Langfitt, T.W., Miller, J.D., et al. (1973). Regional cerebral blood flow, intracranial pressure, and brain metabolism in comatose patients. J. Neurosurg., 38:131–44.

Cheng, C.L.Y., and Povlishock, J.T. (1988). The effect of traumatic brain injury on the visual system: A morphologic characteristic of reactive axonal change. J. Neurotrauma, 5:47–60.

DeWitt, D.S., Jenkins, L.W., Wei, E.P., et al. (1986). Effects of fluid-percussion brain injury on regional cerebral blood flow and pial arteriolar diameter. J. Neurosurg., 64(5):787–94.

DeWitt, D.S., Yuan, X.Q., Becker, D.P., and Hayes, R.L. (1988). Simultaneous, quantitative measurement of local blood flow and glucose utilization in tissue samples in normal and injured feline brain. Brain Inj., 2(4):291–303.

Doberstin, C., Martin, N.A., Caron, M.J., Zane, C., Johnson, J.P., Kathleen, T., and Becker, D.P. (1990). Detection of posttraumatic arterial spasm using transcranial doppler and Xenon-133 rCBF monitoring. Proceedings for the Society for Neurotrauma Society, St. Louis, 1990.

Eisenberg, H.M., and Levin, H.S. (1989). Computed tomography and magnetic resonance imaging in mild to moderate head injury. In: Levin, H.S., Eisenberg, H.M., and Benton, A.L. (eds). Moderate head injury. New York: Oxford University Press, 133–41.

Ellison, M.D., Erb, D.E., Kontos, H.A., and Povlishock, J.T. (1989). Recovery of impaired endothelium-dependent relaxation after fluid-percussion brain injury in cats. Stroke, 20:911–17.

Enevoldsen, E.M., Cold, G., Jensen, F.T., and Malmros, R. (1976). Dynamic changes in regional CBF, intraventricular pressure, CSF pH and lactate levels during the acute phase of head injury. J. Neurosurg., 44:191–213.

Enevoldsen, E.M., and Jensen, F.T. (1978). Autoregulation and CO_2 responses of cerebral blood flow in patients with acute severe head injury. J. Neurosurg., 48:689–703.

Erb, D.E., and Povlishock, J.T. (1988). Axonal damage in severe traumatic brain injury: An experimental study in the cat. Acta Neuropathol., 76:347–58.

Erb, D.E., and Povlishock, J.T. (1991). Neuroplasticity following traumatic brain injury: A study of GABAergic terminal loss and recovery in the cat dorsal lateral vestibular nucleus. Exp. Brain Res., 83:253–67.

Faden, A.I., Demediuk, P., Panter, S.S., and Vink, R. (1989). The role of excitatory amino acids and NMDA receptors in traumatic brain injury. Science, 244:798-800.

Gennarelli, T.A., Thibault, L.E., Adams, J.H., Graham, D.I., Thompson, C.J., and Marcionin, R.P. (1982). Diffuse axonal injury and traumatic coma in the primate. Ann. Neurol., 12:564-74.

Gennarelli, T.A., Thibault, L.E., Tipperman, R., et al. (1989). Axonal injury in the optic nerve: A model stimulating diffuse axonal injury in the brain. J. Neurosurg., 71:244-53.

Graham, D.I., Adams, J.H., and Doyle, D. (1978). Ischemic brain damage in fatal nonmissile head injuries. J. Neuro. Sci., 39:213-34.

Hayes, R.L., Jenkins, L.W., Lyeth, B.G., Balster, R.L., Robinson, S.E., Miller, L.P., Clifton, G.L., and Young, H.F. (1988). Pretreatment with phencyclidine, an N-methyl-D-aspartate receptor antagonist, attenuates long-term behavioral deficits in the rat produced by traumatic brain injury. J. Neurotrauma, 5(4):287-302.

Hayes, R.L., Lyeth, B.G., and Jenkins, L.W. (1989). Neurochemical mechanisms of mild and moderate head injury: Implications for treatment. In: Levin, H.S., Eisenberg, H.M., and Benton, A.L. (eds). Mild head injury. New York: Oxford University Press, 54-79.

Hayes, R.L., Pechura, C.M., Katayama, Y., Povlishock, J.T., Giebel, M.L., and Becker, D.P. (1984). Activation of pontine cholinergic sites implicated in unconsciousness following cerebral concussion in cats. Science, 223:301-03.

Hubschmann, O.R., and Kornhauser, D. (1983). Effects of intraparenchymal hemorrhage on extracellular cortical potassium in experimental head trauma. J. Neurosurgery, 59:289-93.

Ishige, N., Pitts, L.H., Carlson, S., et al. (1987). Effects of hypoxia on rat brain with traumatic injury. J. Cereb. Blood Flow and Metabol., 7(1):s638.

Ishige, N., Pitts, L.H., Pogliani, L., Hashimoto, T., Nishimjura, B.S., Bartkowski, H.M., and James, T.L. (1987). Effect of hypoxia on traumatic brain injury in rats: Part 2. Changes in high energy phosphate metabolism. Neurosurgery, 20:854-58.

Jaggi, J.L., Obrist, W.D., Gennarelli, T.A., and Langfitt, T.W. (1990). Relationship of early cerebral blood flow and metabolism to outcome in acute head injury. J. Neurosurg., 72:176-82.

Jane, J.A., Steward, O., and Gennarelli, T. (1985). Axonal degeneration induced by experimental noninvasive minor head injury. J. Neurosurg., 62:96-100.

Jenkins, L.W., Lyeth, B., DeWitt, D., Hamm, R., Phillips, L., Young, H., and Hayes, R. (1989). Muscarinic and NMDA receptor blockade reduces postischemic EEG spike frequency following TBI and acute secondary ischemia. Society for Neuroscience Abstracts, 15(2):1113.

Jenkins, L.W., Lyeth, B.G., LeWelt, W., Moszynski, K., DeWitt, D.S., Balster, R.L., Miller, L.P., Clifton, G.L., Young, H.F., and Hayes, R.L. (1988). Combined pretrauma scopolamine and phencyclidine attenuates posttraumatic increased sensitivity to delayed secondary ischemia. J. Neurotrauma, 5(4):303-15.

Jenkins, L.W., Marmarou, A., Lewelt, W., and Becker, D.P. (1986). Increased vulnerability of the traumatized brain to early ischemia. In: Baethmann, A., Go, K.G., and Unterberg, A. (eds). Mechanisms of Secondary Brain Damage. New York: Plenum, 273-81.

Jenkins, L.W., Moszynski, K., Lyeth, B.G., Lewelt, W., DeWitt, D.S., Allen, A., Dixon, C.E., Povlishock, J.T., Majewski, W., Clifton, G.L., Young, H.F., Becker, D.P., and Hayes, R.L. (1989). Increased vulnerability of the mildly traumatized rat brain to cerebral ischemia: The use of a controlled secondary ischemia as a research tool to identify common or different mechanisms contributing to mechanical and ischemic brain injury. Brain Res., 477:211-24.

Jenkins, L.W., Povlishock, J.T., Lewelt, W., Miller, J.D., and Becker, D.P. (1981). The role of postischemic recirculation in the development of ischemic neuronal injury following complete cerebral ischemia. Acta Neuropathol., 55:205-20.

Katayama, Y., Becker, D.P., Tamura, T., and Hovda, D.A. (In Press.) Massive increases in extracellular potassium and the indiscriminate release of glutamate following concussive brain injury. J. Neurosurgery.

Kontos, H.A., and Povlishock, J.T. (1986). Oxygen radicals in brain injury. Cen. Nerv. Sys. Trauma, 3:257-63.

Kontos, H.A., Wei, E.P., Christman, C.W., Povlishock, J.T., and Ellis, E.F. (1983). Free oxygen radicals in cerebral vascular response. The Physiologist, 26:265-69.

Kontos, H.A., Wei, E.P., Ellis, E.F., Dietrich, W.D., and Povlishock, J.T. (1981). Prostaglandins in physiological and in certain pathological responses of the cerebral circulation. Fed. Proc., 40:2326-30.

Kontos, H.A., Wei, E.P., Ellis, E.F., Jenkins, L.W., Povlishock, J.T., Rowe, G.T., and Hess, M.L. (1985). Appearance of superoxide anion radical in cerebral extracellular space during increased prostaglandin synthesis in cats. Cir. Res., 57:142-51.

Kontos, H.A., Wei, E.P., and Povlishock, J.T. (1981). Pathophysiology of vascular consequences of experimental concussive brain injury. Trans. Am. Clin. Climatol. Assoc., 30:111-21.

Kontos, H.A., Wei, E.P., Povlishock, J.T., and Christman, C.W. (1984). Oxygen radicals mediate the cerebral arteriolar dilation from arachidonate and bradykinin in cats. Circ. Res., 55:295-303.

Kontos, H.A., Wei, E.P., Povlishock, J.T., Dietrich, W.D., Ellis, E.F., and Magiera, C.J. (1980). Cerebral arteriolar damage by arachidonic acid and prostaglandin G. Sci., 209:1242-45.

Langfitt, T.W., and Obrist, W.D. (1981). Cerebral blood flow and metabolism after intracranial trauma. Prog. Neurol. Surg., 10:14-48.

Levin, H.A., Amparo, E., Eisenberg, H.M., Williams, D.H., High, W.M., McArdle, C.B., and Weiner, R.L. (1987a). Magnetic resonance imaging and computerized tomography in relation to the neurobehavioral sequelae of mild and moderate head injuries. J. Neurosurg., 66:706-13.

Levin, H.S., Mattis, S., Ruff, R.M., Eisenberg, H.M., Marshall, L.F., Tabaddor, K., High, W.M., and Frankowski, R.F. (1987b). Neurobehavioral outcome following minor head injury: A three-center study. J. Neurosurg., 66:234-43.

Lewelt, W., Jenkins, L.W., and Miller, J.D. (1980). Autoregulation of cerebral blood flow after experimental fluid percussion injury. J. Neurosurg., 53:500-11.

Lewelt, W., Jenkins, L.W., and Miller, J.D. (1982). Effects of experimental fluid-percussion injury of the brain on cerebrovascular reactivity to hypoxia and to hypercapnia. J. Neurosurg., 56:332-38.

Lyeth, B.G., Dixon, C.E., Jenkins, L.W., Hamm, R.J., Alberico, A., Young, H.F., Stonnington, H.H., and Hayes, R.L. (1988). Effects of scopolamine treatment on long-term behavioral deficits following concussive brain injury to the rat. Brain Res., 452:39-48.

Marion, D.W., Darby, J., and Yonas, H. (1991). Acute regional/cerebral blood flow changes caused by severe head injuries. N. Neurosurg., 74:407-14.

Maxwell, W.L., Irvine, A., Strang, R.H.C., Graham, D.I., Adams, J.H., and Gennarelli, T.A. (1990). Glycogen accumulation in axons after stretch injury. J. Neurocytology, 19:235-41.

Maxwell, W.L., Kansayra, A.M., Graham, D.I., Adams, J.H., and Gennarelli, T.A. (1988). Freeze-fracture studies of reactive myelinated nerve fibers after diffuse axonal injury. Acta Neuropath., 76:395-406.

McIntosh, T.K., Vink, R., Soares, H., Hayes, R.L., and Simon, R. (1989b). Effects of N-Methyl-D-Aspartate receptor blocker MK-801 on neurologic function after experimental brain injury. J. Neurotrauma, 6:247-59.

McIntosh, T.K., Vink, R., Soares, H., Hayes, R.L., and Simon, R. (1990). Effect of noncompetitive blockade of N-Methyl-D-Aspartate receptors on neurochemical sequelae of experimental brain injury. J. Neurochemistry, 55:1170-79.

Meyer, J.S., et al. (1983). Cerebral hemodynamics and metabolism following experimental head injury. J. Neurosurg., 32:304-19.

Muizelaar, J.P., Marmarou, A., DeSalles, A.A.F., et al. (1989). Cerebral blood flow and metabolism in severely head-injured children. Part 1: Relationship with GCS score, outcome, ICP, and PVI. J. Neurosurg., 71:63-71.

Muizelaar, J.P., Ward, J.D., Marmarou, A., Newlon, P.G., and Wachi, A. (1989). Cerebral blood flow and metabolism in severely head-injured children. Part 2: Autoregulation. J. Neurosurg., 71:72-766.

Obrist, W.D., Gennarelli, T.A., Segawa, H., et al. (1979). Relation of cerebral blood flow to neurological status and outcome in head-injured patients. J. Neurosurg., 51:292-300.

Obrist, W.D., Langfitt, T.W., Jaggi, J.L., et al. (1984). Cerebral blood flow and metabolism in comatose patients with acute head injury. Relationship to intracranial hypertension. J. Neurosurg., 61:241-53.

Oppenheimer, D.R. (1968). Microscopic lesion in the brain following head injury. J. Neurol. Neurosurg. Psychiatry, 31:299-306.

Overgaard, J., Mosdal, C., and Tweed, W.A. (1981). Cerebral circulation after head injury. Part 3: Does reduced regional cerebral blood flow determine recovery of brain function after blunt head injury? J. Neurosurg., 55:63-74.

Overgaard, J., and Tweed, W. (1974). Cerebral circulation after head injury. Part I: Cerebral blood flow and its regulation after head injury with emphasis on clinical correlations. J. Neurosurg., 41:531-41.

Peerless, S., and Rewcastle, N. (1967). Shear injuries of the brain. Can. Assoc. J., 96:577-82.

Pilz, P. (1983). Axonal injury in head injury. Acta Neurochir., 32:119-26.

Povlishock, J. (1985). The morphopathologic responses to experimental head injuries of varying severity. In: Becker D., and Povlishock, J. (eds). Central nervous system status report. Richmond:Byrd Press, 443-52.

Povlishock, J. (1986). Traumatically induced axonal damage without concomitant change in focally related neuronal somata and dendrites. Acta Neuropathol., 70:53-79.

Povlishock, J. (1990). Diffuse deafferentation as the major determinant of morbidity and recovery following traumatic brain injury. Advances in Neurotrauma Research, 2:1-11.

Povlishock, J., and Becker, D. (1985). Fate of reactive axonal swellings induced by head injury. Lab Investigation, 52:540-52.

Povlishock, J.T., Becker, D.P., Cheng, C., and Vaughn, G. (1983). Axonal change in minor head injury. J. Neuropathol. Exp. Neurol., 222-42.

Povlishock, J.T., Becker, D.P., Sullivan, H.G., and Miller, J.D. (1978). Vascular permeability alternations to horseradish peroxidase in experimental brain injury. Brain Res., 153:223-39.

Povlishock, J., and Kontos, H. (1985). Continuing axonal and vascular change following experimental brain trauma. Central Nervous System Trauma, 2:285-97.

Steward, O. (1989). Reorganization of neural connections following CNS trauma: Principles and experimental paradigms. J. Neurotrauma, 6:99-152.

Strich, S. (1961). Shearing of nerve fibers as a cause of brain damage due to head injury. Lancet, 2:443-48.

Strich, S. (1965). Diffuse degeneration of the cerebral white matter in severe dementia following head injury. J. Neurol. Neurosurg. Psychiatry, 19:163-85.

Tornheim, P.A. (1985). Traumatic edema in head injury. In: Becker, D.P. and Povlishock, J.T. (eds). Central nervous system trauma status report. Richmond:Byrd Press, 431-39.

Wei, E.P., Christman, C.W., Kontos, H.A., and Povlishock, J.T. (1985). Effects of oxygen radicals on cerebral arterioles. Am. J. Physiol., 248:157-62.

Wei, E.P., Dietrich, W.D., Povlishock, J.T., and Kontos, H.A. (1980). Functional, morphologic, metabolic abnormalities of the cerebral microcirculation after concussive brain injury in cats. Circ. Res., 46(1):37–47.

Wei, E.P., Kontos, H.A., Dietrich, W.D., Povlishock, J.T., and Ellis, E.F. (1981). Inhibition by free radical scavengers and by cyclooxygenase inhibitors of pial arteriolar abnormalities from concussive brain injury in cats. Circ. Res., 48:95–103.

Wei, E.P., Kontos, H.A., Ellison, M.D., and Povlishock, J.T. (1986). Oxygen radicals in arachidonate-induced increased blood-brain barrier permeability to proteins. Am. J. Physiol., 251:H693–99.

Yamakami, I., and McIntosh, T.K. (1989). Effects of traumatic brain injury on regional cerebral blood flow in rats as measured with radiolabeled microspheres. J. Cereb. Blood Flow Metab., 9(1):117–24.

Yuan, X.Q., Prough, D.S., Smith, T.L., and DeWitt, D.S. (1988). The effects of traumatic brain injury on regional blood flow in rats. J. Neurotrauma, 5(4):289–301.

3

Recovery of Function Following Brain Injury

DENNIS P. ALFANO

In recent years, considerable and growing interest regarding the issue of acquired brain injury and recovery of function has been evident in a number of areas. The various avenues of research and study on this topic have included, amongst others, basic neurobiologic (Cotman and Nieto-Sampedro, 1985) and behavioral approaches utilizing animal models (Chappell and LeVere, 1988), examination of clinical features (Levin, Benton, and Grossman, 1982), delineation of the nature and course of recovery (Dikmen, Machamer, Temkin, and McLean, 1990), examination of factors associated with the quality of long-term outcome (Alfano, Paniak, and Finlayson, 1991; Levin, Grafman, and Eisenberg, 1987), as well as strategies for rehabilitation (Diller and Gordon, 1981; Finlayson, Alfano, and Sullivan, 1987; Sohlberg and Mateer, 1989).

The diversity evident in the avenues of study of acquired brain injury and recovery is undoubtedly a reflection of the complexity of the brain and behavior. This diversity may also reflect, however, fairly widespread concern over the enormity and scope of the very real and practical problems such injuries present. For example, traumatic brain injury (TBI) represents the leading cause of acquired neurologic disability in persons under the age of 50 (Adams and Victor, 1989), and the literature concerning the neuropsychologic and psychosocial sequelae of TBI is replete with studies documenting the extensive and frequently persistent nature of the disorder (e.g., Levin, et al., 1982; Stambrook, Moore, Peters, Deviaene, and Hawryluk, 1990). The costs of TBI in terms of human and economic factors alone are enormous (Miller, 1986), and this disorder ranks as one of the major sociohealth problems facing western society today (Kalsbeek, McLaurin, Harris, and Miller, 1980). As a result, the challenges facing researchers and health care professionals working in this area are numerous and unquestionable (Meier, Benton, and Diller, 1987).

In this chapter, a broad overview of theory, research, and mechanisms concerning acquired brain injury and recovery of function is presented.

Several implications regarding the emerging field of neuropsychologic rehabilitation are briefly discussed against this backdrop.

PRINCIPAL FEATURES OF BRAIN INJURY AND RECOVERY

Brain injury can produce changes in behavior anywhere along the spectrum of attentional, perceptual, cognitive, emotive, and executive aspects of functioning, often affecting more than one domain, and to varying relative degrees (Lezak, 1983). The pattern of recovery of different areas of behavioral dysfunction may also vary considerably (Ogden, 1987; Tabaddor, Mattis, and Zazula, 1984). Variables commonly associated with the degree of recovery and outcome following brain injury can be grouped generally into three principal classifications: 1) preinjury related variables (e.g., age, sex, socioeconomic status); 2) injury related variables (e.g., nature, location and extent of brain injury, duration and depth of coma), and 3) postinjury related variables (e.g., social support, emotional adjustment; Alfano, et al., 1991; Bach-y-Rita and Bach-y-Rita, 1990; Dikmen and Reitan, 1977; Diller and Ben-Yishay, 1988; Fordyce, Roueche, and Prigatano, 1983; Meier, Strauman, and Thompson, 1987; Miller, 1984; Miller, 1986).

Recovery from brain injury can be further characterized in terms of three principal features, namely, the prolonged nature of its course, the persistence of changes in behavior, and the pervasiveness of the consequences of injury. For example, acquired brain injury, particularly in a moderate or severe form, typically involves some significant degree of change in behavior (Mandleberg and Brooks, 1975; Tabaddor, et al., 1984). Further, it is not uncommon for individuals suffering from an injury to the brain to demonstrate temporal changes in behavior spanning years, with residual deficits persisting, to some degree, indefinitely (Bond, 1979; Bond and Brooks, 1976; Dikmen, Reitan, and Temkin, 1983; Dikmen, et al., 1990; Jennett and Teasdale, 1981; Levin, Grossman, Rose, and Teasdale, 1979; Oddy, Humphrey, and Uttley, 1978; Oddy and Humphrey, 1980; Oddy, Coughlan, Tyerman, and Jenkins, 1985; van Zomeren and van den Burg, 1985; Weddell, Oddy, and Jenkins, 1980). There is also evidence that considerable stresses are placed on the family in many cases of acquired brain injury (Brooks, 1991; Lezak, 1988; Neilson, Alfano, and Fink, 1991). As such, the consequences of brain injury are most appropriately viewed within a broad systems framework that encompasses the patient, the family, and the community (see Chapter 15). It is thus clear that the sequelae of brain injury are diverse and that recovery is a relatively long, complex, and pervasive process that can be influenced by a multitude of factors (McClelland, 1988).

CONCEPT OF PLASTICITY

Plasticity refers to modifications in the nervous system that occur in response to either internal or external environmental circumstances or demands (Jacobson, 1978). The principal underlying assumption regarding such modifications is that they are fundamentally adaptive and confer on the organism the ability to survive under the changed conditions. As such, the concept essentially refers to the intrinsic capacity of the nervous system to respond to demands in a functionally adaptive way (Bach-y-Rita, 1980). A considerable literature exists documenting modifications in neuronal chemistry, morphology, and physiology that occur in tandem with normal development, experience, or learning (e.g., Cotman, 1978; Jacobson, 1978; Lund, 1978; Klein, Sullivan, Skorupa, and Aguilar, 1989; Kolb, 1989).

It is interesting that the idea of plasticity or adaptive capability at the neurobiologic level is analogous to the idea of cognitive adaptive ability as described in some theories of biological intelligence (e.g., Halstead, 1947). A general loss of adaptive ability following an injury to the brain has also been suggested as representing a loss of neuropsychologic ability at the highest level of cerebral cortical function (Reitan, 1988).

The inherent plasticity of the central nervous system (CNS) has also received considerable attention in the context of attempts to understand possible mechanisms of, and potential environmental influences on, recovery of function following brain injury (Kaplan, 1988; Stein, Rosen, and Butters, 1974). It is only in recent years, however, that the phenomenon of neural plasticity has been appreciated and emphasized as a basis for the development of rehabilitation procedures (Bach-y-Rita, 1988; Caplan, 1982).

DEFINITIONS AND THEORIES OF RECOVERY OF FUNCTION

Central to the issue of recovery of function following brain injury is the idea that neuropsychologic deficits or other changes in behavior demonstrate a temporal course and move toward resolution as a function of time. Beyond this basic idea, controversy otherwise exists with regard to the manner in which recovery should be defined and measured (Almli and Finger, 1988; Marshall, 1984).

Laurence and Stein (1978) discussed the issue of defining recovery of function following brain injury and offered two major perspectives. The first defines recovery of function in terms of whether or not a behavioral goal is achieved. In this context, an injury to the brain might be conceptualized as eliminating perhaps one or more, but not all, potential strategies or means by which to achieve a behavioral goal. Recovery of function is thus viewed (and measured) according to this definition exclusively in terms of the level of performance attained (i.e., whether the goal is achieved) in some aspect of behavior, regardless of the strategy or process used in doing so. It is interesting that this idea parallels certain research findings of Tolman (e.g., Tolman, 1938) demonstrating that when rats performing a maze learning task are blocked from using a previously successful route, they default to the next most efficient route by which to solve it. Adaptive behavior of this nature may be a reflection of the fundamental adaptive function that brain plasticity subserves. The second perspective offered by Laurence and Stein (1978) also involves the idea of goal achievement, but defines recovery in terms of whether or not goals are achieved through strategies similar, if not identical, to those utilized before the injury. This perspective views recovery in terms of the reinstatement of the specific behaviors or strategies that were lost as a result of the injury to the brain (Levere, 1988). As pointed out by Almli and Finger (1988), recovery of function following brain injury is a relatively frequent finding when the criteria for recovery is defined simply as goal achievement. From a clinical point of view, such criteria might be exemplified by the use of neuropsychologic tests to define and measure recovery of function. The distinction between the idea of the reemergence of the original strategy through which a goal is achieved versus the idea of goal achievement only represents a fundamental theoretical difference between theories of recovery involving some form of restitution of function versus those involving some form of substitution or compensation for a performance related deficit (see below).

Goldberger (1974), and more recently Kolb and Whishaw (1990), summarized the major contemporary theories regarding the basis of recovery of function following brain injury. Essentially, three principal theories have been suggested in the literature: resolution of diaschisis, reorganization of functional systems, and behavioral substitution or compensation for a performance related deficit. The first two of these theories advance the idea that some form of neurologically based process underlies reemergence of behavior disrupted by brain injury through ways or mechanisms similar, if not identical, to those utilized before the injury (Almli and Finger, 1988); they may also fall under the general rubric of the familiar and often used concept of spontaneous recovery of function.

Diaschisis

Diaschisis involves von Monakow's (1911) theory that a brain injury produces functional disturbances (e.g., suppression or inhibition, or possibly even release from inhibition) in the activity of undamaged regions that are functionally (and anatomically) related to, but remote from, the area of injury (Boyeson and Bach-y-Rita, 1990; Smith, 1974). Diaschisis causes behavioral deficits that resolve over time as the functional activity of the intact regions approaches preinjury levels. A related theory includes the idea of some form of generalized brain trauma or shock following injury, which is also thought to dissipate over time (Rosner, 1970). This latter idea might be conceptualized as diaschisis involving disturbance of function in regions of the brain that are not necessarily functionally (or anatomically) related to the area of injury. According to these theories, recovery of function following brain injury might be explained as an artifact of a suppression of behavior that resolves with time, particularly as the acute physiologic effects of the injury to the brain, such as edema or hemorrage, subside.

Functional Reorganization

The theory of functional reorganization centers around the idea that portions of the nervous system that are not permanently injured are actively altered in some way to subserve functions previously carried out by the damaged regions. The specific theories historically associated with the idea of functional reorganization include: 1) equipotentiality and mass action, which are basically Lashley's (1938) notions that the extent of behavioral recovery potentially attainable following brain injury is directly related to the amount of undamaged tissue (mass action), and that the remaining tissue within a defined functional system is able to take over the function of the damaged tissue (equipotentiality), and 2) vicariation, which involves the idea that an undamaged region of the brain, not originally part of the lost functional system, takes over the function of the injured area (Slavin, Laurence, and Stein, 1988).

The general idea behind a concept such as equipotentiality as a possible basis for recovery of function is most relevant to the case of a subtotal injury to a functional region of the brain (Levere, 1988). Consistent with the idea of mass action, the extent of residual (intact) tissue in such a case may be a potentially more critical determinant of the degree of functional recovery that might be expected than extent of damage per se (Lashley, 1938; Reitan, 1966; LeVere, 1988). Theories of functional reorganization may necessarily involve some form of latent redundancy of functional capacity in the nervous system (Marshall, 1984). The idea of the reorganization of brain function following injury is also antithetic to a localizationist view of brain-behavior relationships (Woodruff and Baisden, 1986). For these reasons, as well as others, the continued utility of equipotentiality as a theoretical basis for recovery of function has been questioned (e.g., Kolb and Whishaw, 1988).

Behavioral Substitution

Substitution involves the development and/or utilization of alternate means or compensatory strategies by which to achieve a behavioral goal. Substitution may also involve some element of environmental (re)structuring (Diller and Gordon, 1981). A common example of substitution is the use of a memory book to minimize the impact of a memory deficit. Substitution is also illustrated through the use of imagery as a therapeutic tool to improve verbal memory (Malec and Questad, 1983). In a recent study, Goodale, Milner, Jakobson, and Carey (1990), conducted detailed digitized kinematic analyses of visually guided limb movements in individuals with right hemisphere lesions. Their findings indicated subtle, but persisting, problems with visuospatial control despite apparent recovery of this ability as assessed using conventional paper and pencil neuropsychologic tests. Based on this pattern of findings, Goodale, et al., reasoned that the apparent recovery of visuospatial control as assessed conventionally may reflect more the use of some form of compensatory strategy, rather than true recovery of the function. As such, these observations conform more to the first definition of recovery of function offered by Laurence and Stein (1978), and are consistent with the views of Almli and Finger (1988) mentioned earlier. The theory of substitution as a basis for recovery of function thus involves some form of compensatory adjustment to loss and, as such, differs conceptually from those theories of recovery that purport some form of neurologically based restitution of function (Slavin, et al., 1988).

MECHANISMS OF RECOVERY OF FUNCTION

Following an injury to the brain, an important aspect of neurologically based recovery involves the resolution of the secondary mechanisms of injury (e.g., hemorrage, edema, swelling; see Chapter 2). The minimization of other forms of secondary mechanisms of injury, such as transsynaptic degeneration and other neurotoxic events, may also potentially contribute to recovery of function (Schallert and Lindner, 1990). Additional intriguing bases for recovery are that other specific neuronal responses to injury, such as certain structural and biochemical modifications involving axons, dendrites, or other postsynaptic elements, may occur. The principal mechanisms that have, thus far, been suggested in this context, include collateral sprouting of intact axons, increased dendritic arborization, denervation supersensitivity, and unmasking of so-called silent synapses.

Axonal Modifications

Destruction of axonal fibers represents one of the most consistent neuropathologic features of closed head injury (Levin, et al., 1982). Injured axons in the CNS, however, have an extremely poor capacity for regeneration (Kiernan, 1979; Marshall, 1984). Collateral sprouts arising from uninjured axons, however, have been shown to be a frequent, and fairly consistent, neuronal response to localized injury in the CNS of animals (Cotman, 1978; Cotman, Matthews, Taylor, and Lynch, 1973; Lynch and Cotman, 1975). The growth of collateral axonal sprouts has also been observed to be accompanied by the formation of new synapses (reactive synaptogenesis; Cotman and Nadler, 1978) that have been found, in some instances, to be physiologically functional (Wilson, Levey, and Steward, 1979). The sprouting of new axon collaterals to replace injured axons, the possible reinnervation of regions of the brain that have lost afferents, and the possible formation of new and functional synapses, represents the idea of axonal sprouting as a possible mechanism of recovery of function. Povlishock and Coburn (1989) reviewed compelling electron microscopic evidence, based on an animal model, for the growth of new axonal sprouts following injury to the brain.

Dendritic Modifications

Dendrites provide the major receptive surface for most neurons in the CNS (Kandel, 1981). The amount of dendritic surface available thus represents an important determinant of the amount of information a neuron is able to receive and process (Lux and Schubert, 1975). Kolb (1989) reviewed evidence for increases in dendritic arborization in animals suffering from early brain lesions that were correlated with improvements in behavior. Coleman and Flood (1988) reviewed the idea of dendritic proliferation in surviving neurons as a possible compensatory response to a loss of neighboring neurons in the aging brain. It is still undetermined whether such dendritic modifications are also characteristic of lesion-induced plasticity in adult animal models. Given the axonal modifications described above, however, concomitant reactive dendritic modifications are not inconceivable.

Denervation Supersensitivity

Denervation supersensitivity occurs when following decreased synaptic input (e.g., the destruction of afferent fibers) to a brain region, postsynaptic neuronal responsivity increases. An increase in the physiologic responsivity of postsynaptic receptors, or an actual increase in their number, may underlie this phenomenon (Schwartz and Kellar, 1983). Denervation supersensitivity has been observed at neuromuscular junctions following deafferentation (Levitt-Gilmour and Salpeter, 1986) and in animal models of brain dopamine depletion (Thornburg and Moore, 1975). As a possible mechanism of recovery of function, denervation supersensitivity is the idea that partial deafferentation of an area of the brain, such as that which might occur following axonal injury, may be compensated for by an increase in responsivity of postsynaptic elements to reduced neurotransmitter supply, and thereby mediate functional recovery (Glick, 1974).

Unmasking

Unmasking involves the notion that an already established synapse may be functionally inhibited in the normal state (Kalat, 1988). The functional activity of such a synapse becomes expressed only following some disruption to the system (Kolb and Whishaw, 1990). The idea of unmasking as a possible mechanism underlying recovery of function is still largely hypothetical.

ENVIRONMENTAL ENRICHMENT, PLASTICITY, AND RECOVERY

Environmental enrichment has frequently been used to demonstrate the plasticity of the brain and behavior (Rosenzweig, 1984). The typical paradigm consists of randomly assigning rats that have been raised in the same litter to one of two experimental conditions: enrichment or impoverishment. The enriched environment consists of a number of rats being housed together in a large cage. This environment also contains such things as running wheels, ladders, slides, and other such objects, that the animals are free to explore and manipulate. Frequent changes in these objects insure continued novelty and experience for the enriched animals (Carlson, 1986). The impoverished environment consists essentially of the rats being housed individually under standard laboratory conditions. More recently, some researchers have utilized a larger and more elaborate form of enrichment, modeled directly after a natural environment (e.g., Whishaw, Zaborowski, and Kolb, 1984).

Following exposure to environmental enrichment, significant neuroanatomic and neurochemical changes in the brain have been found. Major reported neuroanatomic changes include increased neocortical weight and thickness (Rosenzweig, Krech, Bennett, and Diamond, 1962), increased dendritic branching (Greenough and Volkmar, 1973; Holloway, 1966; Volkmar and Greenough, 1972), increased numbers of dendritic spines (Globus, Rosenzweig, Bennett, and Diamond, 1973), increased numbers of neocortical synapses (Mollgaard, Diamond, Bennett, Rosenzweig, and Lindner, 1971; West and Greenough, 1972), and an increase in synaptic contact area (Diamond, Lindner, Johnson, Bennett, and Rosenzweig, 1975). Neurochemically, a significantly greater amount of acetylcholinesterase has been measured, presumably reflecting enhancement of central cholinergic function (Krech, Rosenzweig, and Bennett, 1960). At the be-

havioral level, superior maze learning and enhanced performance on numerous other behavioral tasks has been consistently demonstrated in rats
exposed to an enriched environment (Dennenberg, Woodcock, and
Rosenberg, 1968; Smith, 1972). Although the original impetus behind the
work of Rosenzweig and others was to examine possible changes in the
brain associated with learning and memory (Rosenzweig, 1984), the environmental enrichment literature clearly demonstrates that the brain is an
extremely responsive organ, capable of considerable modification as a result of experience (Bakker, 1984).

Environmental enrichment has also been utilized as a potential therapy
in the treatment of neurobehavioral dysfunction in animal models (Davenport and Greenough, 1976; Rosenzweig, 1980). For example, Petit and
Alfano (1979) studied the potential of environmental enrichment to ameliorate the neurobehavioral deficits found in rats exposed to inorganic lead
(Pb). Two levels of Pb exposure were utilized. The higher level of Pb was
sufficient to produce an acute encephalopathy characterized by hind limb
paraplegia and urinary incontinence; the lower level of Pb produced no
overt neurologic signs. Animals exposed to these levels of Pb demonstrated dramatic changes in behavior across a wide range of commonly
used behavioral testing situations (Alfano and Petit, 1981; Petit, Alfano,
and LeBoutillier, 1983). Subsequent studies further delineated a number
of distinct neuroanatomic alterations, particularly involving the hippocampus, in the brains of rats exposed to these levels of Pb (Alfano and
Petit, 1982; Alfano, LeBoutillier, and Petit, 1982; Petit and LeBoutillier,
1979). Following the placement of similarly Pb exposed rats in an enriched environment, Petit and Alfano (1979) found an interaction between
the degree of Pb exposure, environmental enrichment, and the nature of
improved behavior. Environmental enrichment significantly enhanced
maze learning behavior in both Pb groups, did not produce normalization
of locomotor activity in either group, but significantly improved impaired
avoidance behavior of the rats exposed to the low level of Pb only.

To date, environmental enrichment paradigms have been used extensively in studies with animals suffering from a variety of neurologic insults or injuries, including early and adult brain lesions (Schwartz, 1964;
Whishaw, et al., 1984; Will, Rosenzweig, and Bennett, 1976; Will,
Rosenzweig, Bennett, Hebert, and Morimoto, 1977), and hypothyroidism
(Davenport, 1976). The vast majority of the studies in this area have reported considerable improvement in the behavioral capacities of brain
damaged animals following enrichment. The overall pattern of findings
that emerges in reviewing these studies, however, is that behavioral improvement under these circumstances also depends on a number of factors, including the task being used to assess behavior and recovery, the
degree of brain damage being treated, and age at injury or insult. Never-

theless, there is clear and strong support from this literature for the idea of experience-dependent improvement in behavior following brain injury.

INTEGRATION OF THEORY, RESEARCH, AND MECHANISMS

Neuropsychologic and associated performance related deficits clearly improve over time in many patients suffering from acquired brain injury (Bach-y-Rita, 1980; Levin, et al., 1987; Skilbeck, Wade, Hewer, and Wood, 1983). When utilizing animal models, recovery of function following brain damage has also been observed in many instances (Finger, 1978; Finger and Stein, 1982; Finger, LeVere, Almli, and Stein, 1988). Recovery of behavioral function in experimental animals has also been significantly enhanced by environmental enrichment (Davenport and Greenough, 1976). The neurobiologic evidence further indicates substantial modification of intact neural tissue following brain injury (Cotman, 1978; Finger and Stein, 1982; Marshal, 1984). These observations support the following conclusions: 1) That the brain is a dynamic organ, capable of extensive neurologic reorganization following injury; 2) that neuropsychologic abilities in certain acquired disorders, such as TBI and stroke, can, and frequently do, improve over time; 3) that associated performance related deficits also improve with time; 4) that recovery is generally prolonged; 5) that the sequelae of brain injury may persist to some degree; and 6) that enhanced recovery of neurobehavioral function might be possible with environmental stimulation.

In recent years, the various approaches to studying brain injury and recovery have converged to the point where meaningful integration of the neurobiologic and neurobehavioral data have appeared (Boyeson and Bach-y-Rita, 1990; Cotman and Nieto-Sampedro, 1985; Finger, 1978; Finger and Stein, 1982; Marshall, 1984; Finger, et al., 1988). An integration of basic research and theory in this area raises several intriguing prospects. In particular, the possibility exists that neuronal responses to brain injury, such as collateral sprouting of intact axons, reactive synaptogenesis, and/or denervation supersensitivity, may underlie recovery in ways that parallel theoretical notions of functional reorganization. A certain degree of recovery of function might thus conceivably occur via one or more of the above mechanisms, particularly if there is an adequate amount of the functional system left intact, or if another intact functional system of the brain assumes the function of the damaged one. Such an argument might be cogent in instances where the injury to a functional region of the brain is relatively localized and subtotal, and where the overall extent of brain injury is not massive (LeVere, 1988). In the specific case of closed head injury, the possible sprouting of intact axons and/or denervation supersensitivity may represent injury induced neuronal responses that correspond directly to the generally widespread destruction of axonal fibers that is characteristic of the disorder.

The results of numerous environmental enrichment studies clearly demonstrate that the brain is capable of considerable experience-dependent plasticity. It is tempting to conclude that the behavioral improvement observed when environmental enrichment has been applied in animal models of neurobehavioral dysfunction reflects modifications of intact neuronal systems. Based on the known effects of environmental enrichment on brain structure and function, such modifications might include both dendritic and synaptic, as well as neurochemical, changes in the brain. The direct clinical parallel to this idea would be that behavioral changes resulting from brain injury are amenable to direct rehabilitative input, and that associated improvements in behavior may directly involve modifications at the neuronal level. For example, Bakker, Moerland, and Goekoop-Hoefkens (1981), and Bakker and Vinke (1985), observed specific environmental stimulation to alter certain neurophysiologic parameters, and to correspondingly influence functional ability in children with dyslexia. More recently, Jenkins, Merzenich, Ochs, Allard, and Guic-Robles (1990), reported the results of an elegant study demonstrating functional (electrophysiologic) reorganization of primary somatosensory cortex in adult monkeys following intensive and controlled tactile stimulation.

At present, however, the idea of neuronal plasticity as a basis for understanding recovery of function, as well as the corresponding implications for rehabilitation, should be viewed in a fairly broad sense. For example, Cotman and Nieto-Sampedro (1985) pointed out that the relatively short time-course of lesion induced plasticity in animal models may not be a viable basis for the long-term changes in recovery frequently observed clinically. Alfano and Petit (1983) also provided observations suggesting that there are limitations on the degree of lesion induced axonal sprouting potentially attainable following significant neurologic insult. Jacobson (1978) has further questioned the application of the term plasticity to those reactions of the nervous system that occur in response to injury, emphasizing that the term neuronal plasticity is better reserved for adaptive modifications of neurons within the normal physiologic range. For example, the sprouting of intact axons following injury produces neuronal connections that are, by definition, anomalous. As such, the extent to which such neuronal responses to injury may underlie the (re)emergence of behavior that is adaptive has been questioned (e.g., Finger, 1989).

Thus, it is critical that any neurologically based theory, or proposed mechanism of recovery of function following brain injury, take into account the fundamental idea of nervous system plasticity as a basis for beneficial (re)adaptation at the behavioral level. Recent research on the efficacy of brain grafting in reversing neurobehavioral deficits (Becker, Curran, and Freed, 1990; Dunnett, 1990; Stein, 1988a), and neurochemically based approaches to both improving neurobehavioral deficits (Alfano and Petit, 1985; Hayes, Lyeth, and Jenkins, 1989; Levin, et al., 1986; see also Chapter 12) and enhancing recovery following brain injury (Feeney and Westerberg, 1990), should be viewed as exciting innovations that may provide more direct insight into neurobiologic factors and mechanisms underlying recovery of function, as well as provide suggestions for further enhancing it.

NEUROPSYCHOLOGIC REHABILITATION

Traditionally, the focus of clinical neuropsychology has been largely a diagnostic one (Reitan, 1966; Walsh, 1978). Other work in the field has centered on the development of models of brain-behavior relationships (Rourke, 1982). More recently, the field has been undergoing considerable evolution and there is a growing literature that reflects the attention being paid by many neuropsychologists to issues concerning the everyday functioning of patients (Chelune and Moehle, 1986; McSweeney, Grant, Heaton, Prigatano, and Adams, 1985), and to the development of therapeutic strategies for patients with acquired brain injury (Diller and Gordon, 1981; Bach-y-Rita and Bach-y-Rita, 1990). These more recent developments in clinical neuropsychology represent pursuits that are ideally suited to the neurorehabilitation setting (Alfano and Finlayson, 1987).

Historically, there existed the view that damage to the adult brain was irreversible (Bach-y-Rita, 1980; Stein, 1988b). Adherence to this belief typically resulted in clinical approaches emphasizing adjustment to loss (Grzesiak, 1981), rather than attention to the development of therapeutic strategies through which to rehabilitate individuals suffering from neuropsychologically based disorders. The principal rationale for contemporary neuropsychologic notions regarding the rehabilitation of individuals suffering from brain injury draws heavily on the broad base of conceptual and empirical information, reviewed above, concerning brain injury, neural plasticity, and recovery of function. From a rehabilitative point of view, the relevance of neuropsychologic variables as correlates of recovery and outcome following brain injury is also high. For example, a brief survey of the available predictive studies indicates that psychologic factors are key determinants of the degree of recovery that can be expected of patients suffering from stroke (Alfano and Finlayson, 1987). The frequently persistent nature of neuropsychologically based deficits following brain injury further underscores the need to focus rehabilitation efforts on cognitive and behavioral areas of functioning. Intensive neuropsychologic rehabilitation might provide a means through which to capitalize on experience-dependent neural plasticity and, as a result, push recovery of function a step beyond spontaneous recovery alone. In the last decade, neuropsychologic rehabilitation has proven to be a frequently valuable clinical endeavor, and the literature concerning its application and potential efficacy is growing (e.g., Ben-Yishay, 1981; Bracy, 1983; Christensen and Uzzell, 1988; Diller and Gordon, 1981; Finlayson, et al., 1987; Gouvier, Webster, and Blanton, 1986; Mateer and Sohlberg, 1988; Meier, et al., 1987; Miller, 1980; Miller, 1984; Prigatano, 1986; Rao and Bieliauskas, 1983; Reitan and Wolfson, 1988; Sena, 1986). The refining of this important and relatively new area of neuropsychology to the point of delineating theory driven applications (e.g., Mateer and Sohlberg, 1988; Reitan, 1988) founded on a strong empirical base, and which ultimately contribute to the overall rehabilitation of the patient, represents a fundamental and exciting challenge.

References

Adams, R.D., and Victor, M. (1989). Principles of neurology (4th ed). New York: McGraw-Hill.

Alfano, D.P., and Finlayson, M.A.J. (1987). Clinical neuropsychology in rehabilitation. The Clinical Neuropsychologist, 1:105-23.

Alfano, D.P., LeBoutillier, J.C., and Petit, T.L. (1982). Hippocampal mossy fiber pathway development in normal and postnatally lead exposed rats. Experimental Neurology, 75:308-19.

Alfano, D.P., Paniak, C.E., and Finlayson, M.A.J. (1991). Neuropsychological and long-term psychosocial functioning after traumatic brain injury. Journal of Clinical and Experimental Neuropsychology, 13:23.

Alfano, D.P., and Petit, T.L. (1981). Behavioral effects of postnatal lead exposure: Possible relationship to hippocampal dysfunction. Behavioral and Neural Biology, 32:319-33.

Alfano, D.P., and Petit, T.L. (1982). Neonatal lead exposure alters the dendritic development of hippocampal dentate granule cells. Experimental Neurology, 75:275-88.

Alfano, D.P., and Petit, T.L. (1983). Development and plasticity of the hippocampal-cholinergic system in normal and early lead exposed rats. Developmental Brain Research, 10:117-24.

Alfano, D.P., and Petit, T.L. (1985). Postnatal lead exposure and the cholinergic system. Physiology and Behavior, 34:449-55.

Almli, C.R., and Finger, S. (1988). Toward a definition of recovery of function. In: Finger, S., LeVere, T.E., Almli, C.R., and Stein, D.G. (eds). Brain injury and recovery: Theoretical and controversial issues. New York: Plenum Press, 1-14.

Bach-y-Rita, P. (1980). Brain plasticity as a basis for therapeutic procedures. In: Bach-y-Rita, P. (ed). Recovery of function: Theoretical considerations for brain injury rehabilitation. Baltimore: University Park Press, 225-63.

Bach-y-Rita, P. (1988). Brain plasticity. In: Goodgold, J. (ed). Rehabilitation medicine. Toronto: C.V. Mosby, 113-18.

Bach-y-Rita, P., and Bach-y-Rita, E.W. (1990). Biological and psychosocial factors in recovery from brain damage in humans. Canadian Journal of Psychology, 44:148-65.

Bakker, D.J. (1984). The brain as a dependent variable. Journal of Clinical Neuropsychology, 6:1-16.

Bakker, D.J., Moerland, R., and Goekoop-Hoefkens, M. (1981). Effects of hemisphere-specific stimulation on the reading performance of dyslexic boys: A pilot study. Journal of Clinical Neuropsychology, 3:155–59.

Bakker, D.J., and Vinke, J. (1985). Effects of hemisphere-specific stimulation on brain activity and reading in dyslexics. Journal of Clinical and Experimental Neuropsychology, 7:505–25.

Becker, J.B., Curran, E.J., and Freed, W.J. (1990). Adrenal medulla graft induced recovery of function in an animal model of Parkinson's disease: Possible mechanisms of action. Canadian Journal of Psychology, 44:293–310.

Ben-Yishay, Y. (1981). Cognitive remediation after TBI: Toward a definition of its objectives, tasks, and conditions. New York: Institute of Rehabilitation Medicine.

Bond, M.R. (1979). The stages of recovery from severe head injury with special reference to late outcome. International Rehabilitation Medicine, 1:155–59.

Bond, M.R., and Brooks, D.N. (1976). Understanding the process of recovery as a basis for the investigation of rehabilitation for the brain injured. Scandanavian Journal of Rehabilitation Medicine, 8:127–33.

Boyeson, M.G., and Bach-y-Rita, P. (1990). Determinants of brain plasticity. Journal of Neurological Rehabilitation, 3:35–57.

Bracy, O.L. (1983). Computer based cognitive rehabilitation. Cognitive Rehabilitation, 1:7–8.

Brooks, D.N. (1991). The head-injured family. Journal of Clinical and Experimental Neuropsychology, 13:155–88.

Caplan, B. (1982). Neuropsychology in rehabilitation: Its role in evaluation and intervention. Archives of Physical Medicine and Rehabilitation, 63:362–66.

Carlson, N.R. (1986). Physiology of behavior (3rd ed). Boston: Allyn and Bacon.

Chappell, E.T., and LeVere, T.E. (1988). Recovery of function after brain damage: The chronic consequence of large neocortical injuries. Behavioral Neuroscience, 102:778–83.

Chelune, G.J., and Moehle, K.A. (1986). Neuropsychological assessment and everyday functioning. In: Wedding, D., Horton, A.M., and Webster, J. (eds). The neuropsychology handbook: Behavioral and clinical perspectives. New York: Springer, 489–525.

Christensen, A.L., and Uzzell, B. (1988). Neuropsychological rehabilitation. Boston: Kluwer Academic Publishers.

Coleman, P.D., and Flood, D.G. (1988). Is dendritic proliferation of surviving neurons a compensatory response to loss of neighbors in the aging brain? In: Finger, S., LeVere, T.E., Almli, C.R., and Stein, D.G. (eds). Brain injury and recovery: Theoretical and controversial issues. New York: Plenum Press, 235–47.

Cotman, C.W. (1978). Neuronal plasticity. New York: Raven Press.

Cotman, C.W., Matthews, D.A., Taylor, D., and Lynch, G. (1973). Synaptic rearrangement in the dentate gyrus: Histochemical evidence of adjustments after lesions in immature and adult rats. Proceedings of the National Academy of Science, 70:3473–77.

Cotman, C.W., and Nadler, J.V. (1978). Reactive synaptogenesis in the hippocampus. In: Cotman, C.W. (ed). Neuronal plasticity. New York: Raven Press, 227–71.

Cotman, C.W., and Nieto-Sampedro, M. (1985). Progress in facilitating the recovery of function after central nervous system trauma. Annals of the New York Academy of Science, 457:83–104.

Davenport, J.W. (1976). Environmental therapy in hypothyroid and other disadvantaged animal populations. Advances in Behavioral Biology, Vol. 17. New York: Plenum Press.

Davenport, J.W., and Greenough, W.T. (1976). Environments as therapy in the treatment of brain dysfunction. New York: Plenum Press.

Dennenberg, V.H., Woodcock, J.M., and Rosenberg, K.M. (1968). Long-term effects of preweanling and postweanling free-environment experience on rat's problem solving behavior. Journal of Comparative and Physiological Psychology, 66:533–35.

Diamond, M.C., Lindner, B., Johnson, R., Bennett, E.L., and Rosenzweig, M.R. (1975). Differences in occipital cortical synapses from environmentally enriched, impoverished, and standard colony rats. Journal of Neuroscience Research, 1:109–19.

Dikmen, S., Machamer, J., Temkin, N., and McLean, A. (1990). Neuropsychological recovery in patients with moderate to severe head injury: Two-year follow-up. Journal of Clinical and Experimental Neuropsychology, 12:507–19.

Dikmen, S., and Reitan, R.M. (1977). Emotional sequelae of head injury. Annals of Neurology, 2:492–94.

Dikmen, S., Reitan, R.M., and Temkin, N. (1983). Neuropsychological recovery in head injury. Archives of Neurology, 40:333–38.

Diller, L., and Ben-Yishay, Y. (1988). Stroke and traumatic brain injury: Behavioural and psychosocial perspectives. In: Goodgold, J. (ed). Rehabilitation medicine. Toronto: C.V. Mosby, 135–43.

Diller, L., and Gordon, W.A. (1981). Intervention for cognitive deficits in brain injured adults. Journal of Consulting and Clinical Psychology, 49:822–34.

Dunnett, S.B. (1990). Role of prefrontal cortex and striatal output systems in short-term memory deficits associated with ageing, basal forebrain lesions and cholinergic-rich grafts. Canadian Journal of Psychology, 44:210–32.

Feeney, D.M., and Westerberg, V.S. (1990). Norepinephrine and brain damage: Alpha noradrenergic pharmacology alters functional recovery after cortical trauma. Canadian Journal of Psychology, 44:233–52.

Finger, S. (1978). Recovery from brain damage: Research and theory. New York: Plenum Press.

Finger, S. (1989). Reflections on the possible maladaptive consequences of injury-induced reorganization. Neuropsychology, 3:41–47.

Finger, S., LeVere, T.E., Almli, C.R., and Stein, D.G. (1988). Brain injury and recovery: Theoretical and controversial issues. New York: Plenum Press.

Finger, S., and Stein, D.G. (1982). Brain damage and recovery. New York: Academic Press.

Finlayson, M.A.J., Alfano, D.P., and Sullivan, J.F. (1987). A neuropsychological approach to cognitive remediation: Microcomputer applications. Canadian Psychology, 28:180–90.

Fordyce, D.J., Roueche, J.R., and Prigatano, G.P. (1983). Enhanced emotional reactions in chronic head trauma patients. Journal of Neurology, Neurosurgery, and Psychiatry, 46:620–24.

Glick, S.D. (1974). Changes in drug sensitivity and mechanisms of functional recovery following brain damage. In: Stein, D.G., Rosen, J.J., and Butters, N. (eds). Plasticity and recovery of function in the central nervous system. New York: Academic Press, 339–72.

Globus, A., Rosenzweig, M.R., Bennett, E.L., and Diamond, M.C. (1973). Effects of differential experience on dendritic spine counts. Journal of Comparative and Physiological Psychology, 82:175–81.

Goldberger, M.E. (1974). Recovery of movement after CNS lesions in monkeys. In: Stein, D.G., Rosen, J.J., and Butters, N. (eds). Plasticity and recovery of function in the central nervous system. New York: Academic Press, 265–338.

Goodale, M.A., Milner, A.D., Jakobson, L.S., and Carey, D.P. (1990). Kinematic analysis of limb movements in neuropsychological research: Subtle deficits and recovery of function. Canadian Journal of Psychology, 44:180–95.

Gouvier, D., Webster, J.S., and Blanton, P.D. (1986). Cognitive retraining with brain-damaged patients. In: Wedding, D., Horton, A.M., and Webster, J. (eds). The neuropsychology handbook: Behavioral and clinical perspectives. New York: Springer, 278–324.

Greenough, W.T., and Volkmar, F.R. (1973). Pattern of dendritic branching in occipital cortex of rats reared in complex environments. Experimental Neurology, 40:491–504.

Grzesiak, R.C. (1979). Psychological services in rehabilitation medicine: Clinical aspects of rehabilitation psychology. Professional Psychology, 10:511-20.

Halstead, W.E. (1947). Brain and intelligence. Chicago: University of Chicago Press.

Hayes, R.L., Lyeth, B.G., and Jenkins, L.W. (1989). Neurochemical mechanisms of mild and moderate head injury: Implications for treatment. In: Levin, H.S., Eisenberg, H.M., and Benton, A.L. (eds). Mild head injury. New York: Oxford University Press, 54-79.

Holloway, R.L. (1966). Dendritic branching: Some preliminary results of training and complexity in rat visual cortex. Brain Research, 2:393-96.

Jacobson, M. (1978). Developmental neurobiology (2nd ed). New York: Plenum Press.

Jenkins, W.M., Merzenich, M.M., Ochs, M.T., Allard, T., Guic-Robles, E. (1990). Functional reorganization of primary somatosensory cortex in adult owl monkeys after behaviorally controlled tactile stimulation. Journal of Neurophysiology, 63:82-104.

Jennett, B., and Teasdale, G. (1981). Management of head injuries. Philadelphia: F.A. Davis.

Kalat, J.W. (1988). Biological psychology (3rd ed). Belmont, CA: Wadsworth.

Kalsbeek, W.D., McLaurin, R.L., Harris, B.S.H., and Miller, J.D. (1980). The national head and spinal cord injury survey: Major findings. Journal of Neurosurgery, 53:19-31.

Kandel, E.R. (1981). Nerve cells and behaviour. In: Kandel, E.R., and Schwartz, J.H. (eds). Principles of neural science. New York: Elsevier/North-Holland, 14-23.

Kaplan, M.S. (1988). Plasticity after brain lesions: Contemporary concepts. Archives of Physical Medicine and Rehabilitation, 69:984-91.

Kiernan, J.A. (1979). Hypotheses concerned with axonal regeneration in the mammalian nervous system. Biological Review, 54:155-97.

Klein, W.L., Sullivan, J., Skorupa, A., Aguilar, J.S. (1989). Plasticity of neuronal receptors. FASEB Journal, 3:2132-40.

Kolb, B. (1989). Brain development, plasticity, and behavior. American Psychologist, 44:1203-12.

Kolb, B., and Whishaw, I.Q. (1988). Mass action and equipotentiality reconsidered. In: Finger, S., LeVere, T.E., Almli, C.R., and Stein, D.G. (eds). Brain injury and recovery: Theoretical and controversial issues. New York: Plenum Press, 103-16.

Kolb, B., and Whishaw, I.Q. (1990). Fundamentals of human neuropsychology (3rd ed). New York: W.H. Freeman.

Krech, D., Rosenzweig, M.R., and Bennett, E.L. (1960). Effects of environmental complexity and training on brain chemistry. Journal of Comparative and Physiological Psychology, 53:509-19.

Lashley, K.S. (1938). Factors limiting recovery after central nervous lesions. Journal of Nervous and Mental Disease, 88:733-55.

Laurence, S., and Stein, D.G. (1978). Recovery after brain damage and the concept of localization of function. In: Finger, S. (ed). Recovery from brain damage: Research and theory. New York: Plenum Press, 369-407.

LeVere, T.E. (1988). Neural system imbalances and the consequence of large brain injuries. In: Finger, S., LeVere, T.E., Almli, C.R., and Stein, D.G. (eds). Brain injury and recovery: Theoretical and controversial issues. New York: Plenum Press, 15-28.

Levin, H.S., Grossman, R.G., Rose, J.E., and Teasdale, G. (1979). Long-term neuropsychological outcome of closed head injury. Journal of Neurosurgery, 50:412-22.

Levin, H.S., Benton, A.L., and Grossman, R.G. (1982). Neurobehavioral consequences of closed head injury. New York: Oxford University Press.

Levin, H.S., Peters, B.H., Kalisky, Z., High, W.M., Von Laufen, A., Eisenberg, H.M., Morrison, D.P., and Gary, H.E. (1986). Effects of oral physostigmine and lecithin on memory and attention in closed head-injured patients. Central Nervous System Trauma, 3:333-42.

Levin, H.S., Grafman, J., and Eisenberg, H.M. (1987). Neurobehavioral recovery from head injury. New York: Oxford University Press.

Levitt-Gilmour, T.A., and Salpeter, M.M. (1986). Gradient of extrajunctional acetylcholine receptors early after denervation of mammalian muscle. Journal of Neuroscience, 6:1606-12.

Lezak, M.D. (1983). Neuropsychological assessment (2nd ed). New York: Oxford University Press.

Lezak, M.D. (1988). Brain damage is a family affair. Journal of Clinical and Experimental Neuropsychology, 10:111-23.

Lund, R.D. (1978). Development and plasticity of the brain: An introduction. New York: Oxford University Press.

Lux, H.D., and Schubert, P. (1975). Some aspects of the electroanatomy of dendrites. In: Kreutzberg, G.W. (ed). Advances in neurology, Vol. 12. New York: Raven Press, 29-44.

Lynch, G., and Cotman, C.W. (1975). The hippocampus as a model for studying anatomical plasticity in the adult brain. In: Isaacson, R.L., and Pribram, K.H. (eds). The Hippocampus, Vol. 1. New York: Plenum Press, 123-54.

Malec, J., and Questad, K. (1983). Rehabilitation of memory after craniocerebral trauma: Case report. Archives of Physical Medicine and Rehabilitation, 64:436-38.

Mandleberg, I.A., and Brooks, D.N. (1975). Cognitive recovery after severe head injury: Serial testing on the Wechsler Adult Intelligence Scale. Journal of Neurology, Neurosurgery, and Psychiatry, 38:1121-26.

Marshall, J.F. (1984). Brain function: Neural adaptations and recovery from injury. Annual Review of Psychology, 35:277-308.

Mateer, C., and Sohlberg, M.M. (1988). A paradigm shift in memory rehabilitation. In: Whitaker, H. (ed). Neuropsychological studies of non-focal brain injury: Dementia and closed head injury. New York: Springer-Verlag, 202-25.

McClelland, R.J. (1988). Psychosocial sequelae of head injury—anatomy of a relationship. British Journal of Psychiatry, 153:141-46.

McSweeney, A.J., Grant, I., Heaton, R.K., Prigatano, G.P., and Adams, K.M. (1985). Relationship of neuropsychological status to everyday functioning in healthy and chronically ill persons. Journal of Clinical and Experimental Neuropsychology, 7:281-91.

Meier, M.J., Benton, A.L., and Diller, L. (1987). Neuropsychological rehabilitation. New York: Churchill Livingstone.

Meier, M.J., Strauman, S., and Thompson, W.G. (1987). Individual differences in neuropsychological recovery: An overview. In: Meier, M.J., Benton, A.L., and Diller, L. (eds). Neuropsychological rehabilitation. New York: Churchill Livingstone, 71-110.

Miller, E. (1980). The training characteristics of severely head injured patients: A preliminary study. Journal of Neurology, Neurosurgery, and Psychiatry, 43:525-28.

Miller, E. (1984). Recovery and management of neuropsychological impairments. New York: Wiley and Sons.

Miller, W.G. (1986). The neuropsychology of head injuries. In: Wedding, D., Horton, A.M., and Webster, J. (eds). The neuropsychology handbook: Behavioral and clinical perspectives. New York: Springer, 347-75.

Mollgaard, K., Diamond, M.C., Bennett, E.L., Rosenzweig, M.R., and Lindner, B. (1971). Quantitative synaptic changes with differential experience in rat brain. International Journal of Neuroscience, 2:113-28.

Neilson, P.M., Alfano, D.P., and Fink, M.P. (1991). Family stress and ways of coping after neurotrauma. Canadian Psychology, 32(2a):215.

Oddy, M., Coughlan, T., Tyerman, A., and Jenkins, D. (1985). Social adjustment after closed head injury: A further follow-up seven years after injury. Journal of Neurology, Neurosurgery, and Psychiatry, 48:564-68.

Oddy, M., and Humphrey, M. (1980). Social recovery during the year following severe head injury. Journal of Neurology, Neurosurgery, and Psychiatry, 43:798-802.

Oddy, M., Humphrey, M., and Uttley, D. (1978). Subjective impairment and social recovery after closed head injury. Journal of Neurology, Neurosurgery, and Psychiatry, 41:611-16.

Ogden, J.A. (1987). The recovery of spatial deficits in a young man with a fronto-parietal infarct of the right hemisphere. New Zealand Journal of Psychology, 16:72-78.

Petit, T.L., and Alfano, D.P. (1979). Differential experience following developmental lead exposure: Effects on brain and behavior. Pharmacology, Biochemistry, and Behavior, 11:165-71.

Petit, T.L., Alfano, D.P., and LeBoutillier, J.C. (1983). Early lead exposure and the hippocampus: A review and recent advances. Neurotoxicology, 4:79-94.

Petit, T.L., and LeBoutillier, J.C. (1979). Effects of lead exposure during development on neocortical dendritic and synaptic structure. Experimental Neurology, 64:482-92.

Povlishock, J.T., and Coburn, T.H. (1989). Morphopathological change associated with mild head injury. In: Levin, H.S., Eisenberg, H.M., and Benton, A.L. (eds). Mild head injury. New York: Oxford University Press, 37-53.

Prigatano, G.P. (1986). Neuropsychological rehabilitation after brain injury. Baltimore: Johns Hopkins University Press.

Rao, S.M., and Bieliauskas, L.A. (1983). Cognitive rehabilitation two and one-half years post right temporal lobectomy. Journal of Clinical Neuropsychology, 5:313-20.

Reitan, R.M. (1966). A research program on the psychological effects of brain lesions in human beings. In: Ellis, R.M. (ed). International review of research in mental retardation. New York: Academic Press, 153-218.

Reitan, R.M. (1988). Integration of neuropsychological theory, assessment, and clinical applications. The Clinical Neuropsychologist, 2:331-49.

Reitan, R.M., and Wolfson, D. (1988). Traumatic brain injury: Recovery and rehabilitation. Tucson: Neuropsychology Press.

Rosenzweig, M.R. (1980). Animal models for effects of brain lesions and for rehabilitation. In: Bach-y-Rita, P. (ed). Recovery of function: Theoretical considerations for brain injury rehabilitation. Baltimore: University Park Press, 127-72.

Rosenzweig, M.R. (1984). Experience, memory, and the brain. American Psychologist, 39:365-76.

Rosenzweig, M.R., Krech, D., Bennett, E.L., and Diamond, M.C. (1962). Effects of environmental complexity and training on brain chemistry and anatomy: A replication and extension. Journal of Comparative and Physiological Psychology, 55:429-37.

Rosner, B.S. (1970). Brain functions. Annual Review of Psychology, 21:555-94.

Rourke, B.P. (1982). Central processing deficiencies in children: Toward a developmental neuropsychological model. Journal of Clinical Neuropsychology, 4:1-18.

Schallert, T., and Lindner, M.D. (1990). Rescuing neurons from trans-synaptic degeneration after brain damage: Helpful, harmful, or neutral in recovery of function. Canadian Journal of Psychology, 44:276-92.

Schwartz, S. (1964). Effects of neonatal cortical lesions and early environmental factors on adult rat behavior. Journal of Comparative and Physiological Psychology, 57:72-77.

Schwartz, R.D., and Kellar, K.J. (1983). Nicotinic cholinergic receptor binding sites in the brain: Regulation in vivo. Science, 220:214-16.

Sena, D.A. (1986). The effectiveness of cognitive rehabilitation for brain-damaged patients. Journal of Clinical and Experimental Neuropsychology, 8:142.

Skilbeck, C.E., Wade, D.T., Hewer, R.L., and Wood, V.A. (1983). Recovery after stroke. Journal of Neurology, Neurosurgery, and Psychiatry, 46:5-8.

Slavin, M.D., Laurence, S., and Stein, D.G. (1988). Another look at vicariation. In: Finger,

S., LeVere, T.E., Almli, C.R., and Stein, D.G. (eds). Brain injury and recovery: Theoretical and controversial issues. New York: Plenum Press, 165–79.

Sohlberg, M.M., and Mateer, C. (1989). Introduction to cognitive rehabilitation: Theory and practice. New York: Guilford Press.

Smith, A. (April 1974). Diaschisis and neuropsychology. Bulletin of the International Neuropsychological Society, 2–3.

Smith, H.V. (1972). Effects of environmental enrichment on open field activity and Hebb Williams problem solving in rats. Journal of Comparative and Physiological Psychology, 80:163–68.

Stambrook, M., Moore, A.D., Peters, L.C., Deviaenes, C., and Hawryluk, G.A. (1990). Effects of mild, moderate, and severe closed head injury on long-term vocational status. Brain Injury, 4:183–90.

Stein, D.G. (1988a). Practical and theoretical issues in the use of fetal brain tissue transplants to promote recovery from brain injury. In: Finger, S., LeVere, T.E., Almli, C.R., and Stein, D.G. (eds). Brain injury and recovery: Theoretical and controversial issues. New York: Plenum Press, 249–72.

Stein, D.G. (1988b). In pursuit of new strategies for understanding recovery from brain damage: Problems and perspectives. In: Boll, T., and Bryant, B. (eds). Clinical neuropsychology and brain function: Research, measurement, and practice. Washington: American Psychological Association, 13–55.

Stein, D.G., Rosen, J.J., and Butters, N. (1974). Plasticity and recovery of function in the central nervous system. New York: Academic Press.

Tabaddor, K., Mattis, S., Zazula, T. (1984). Cognitive sequelae and recovery course after moderate and severe head injury. Neurosurgery, 14:701–08.

Thornburg, J.E., and Moore, K.E. (1975). Supersensitivity to dopamine agonists following unilateral 6-hydroxydopamine-induced striatal lesions in mice. Journal of Pharmacology and Experimental Therapeutics, 192:42–49.

Tolman, E.C. (1938). The determiners of behavior at a choice point. Psychological Review, 45:1–41.

van Zomeren, A.H., and van den Burg, W. (1985). Residual complaints of patients two years after severe head injury. Journal of Neurology, Neurosurgery, and Psychiatry, 48:21–28.

Volkmar, F.R., and Greenough, W.T. (1972). Rearing complexity affects branching of dendrites in the visual cortex of the rat. Science, 176:1445–47.

von Monakow, C.V. (1911). Localization of brain functions. Journal fur Psychologie und Neurologie, 17:185.

Walsh, K.W. (1978). Neuropsychology: A clinical approach. New York: Churchill Livingstone.

Weddell, R., Oddy, M., and Jenkins, D. (1980). Social adjustment after rehabilitation: A two-year follow-up of patients with severe head injury. Psychological Medicine, 10:257–63.

West, R.W., and Greenough, W.T. (1972). Effect of environmental complexity on cortical synapses of rats: Preliminary results. Behavioral Biology, 7:279–84.

Whishaw, I.Q., Zaborowski, J.A., and Kolb, B. (1984). Postsurgical enrichment aids adult hemidecorticate rats on a spatial navigation task. Behavioral and Neural Biology, 42:183–90.

Will, B.E., Rosenzweig, M.R., and Bennett, E.L. (1976). Effects of differential environments on recovery from neonatal brain lesions, measured by problem solving scores and brain dimensions. Physiology and Behavior, 16:603–11.

Will, B.E., Rosenzweig, M.R., Bennett, E.L., Hebert, M., and Morimoto, H. (1977). Relatively brief environmental enrichment aids recovery of learning capacity and alters brain measures after post-weaning brain lesions in rats. Journal of Comparative and Physiological Psychology, 91:33–50.

Wilson, R.C., Levy, W.B., and Steward, O. (1979). Functional effects of lesion-induced plasticity: Long-term potentiation in normal and lesion-induced temporodentate connections. Brain Research, 176:65–78.

Woodruff, M.L., and Baisden, R.H. (1986). Theories of brain functioning: A brief introduction to the study of the brain and behavior. In: Wedding, D., Horton, A.M., and Webster, J. (eds). The neuropsychology handbook: Behavioral and clinical perspectives. New York: Springer, 23–58.

II

CLINICAL MANAGEMENT

4

Factors Affecting Head Injury Rehabilitation Outcome: Premorbid and Clinical Parameters

ELAINE MACNIVEN

As most patients sustaining head injuries will now survive to live out their expected life span, it is imperative that rehabilitation professionals develop means of predicting functional outcome after head injury in order to facilitate the determination of realistic goals for re-entry into society. It has been reported that the influence of original injury severity on functioning diminishes substantially with time after injury (Brooks, Campsie, Symington, Beattie, and McKinleay, 1986). Thus, the identification of other influences on recovery is becoming increasingly important. The aim of this chapter is to examine factors that contribute to outcome after head injury and their influence on natural recovery.

DEFINING OUTCOME

In order to study variables that influence outcome, it is necessary to formulate an operational definition that allows for both measurement and prediction. Outcome after head injury has been described in numerous ways. To formulate a conceptual framework wherein these outcome measures can be organized and contrasted, it is necessary to adopt a broad definition of outcome. The World Health Organization conceptualization allows for the classification of outcomes in terms of impairment, disability, or handicap, thus providing a basis for a critical review of the existing literature on factors affecting outcome after head injury. Within this perspective, it follows that improvement can relate to reductions in severity in all three areas of classification.

At the most basic level, outcome can be described simply in terms of whether or not a head injury victim lives. Assuming survival, outcome can be defined as ". . . the adequacy with which a patient's lifestyle is resumed including the efficiency with which he performs the activities of daily life" (Levin, Benton, and Grossman, 1982). From this point of view, recovery could be defined as a complete, unimpeded resumption of daily activities.

Thus, final outcome could occur at any point between the level of functioning immediately postinjury and full recovery.

FACTORS AFFECTING THE EXTENT OF RECOVERY

Although a certain amount of recovery reliably occurs (Stein, 1974), there is much variance in both the course and level of recovery experienced by different patients, even when the initial severity of injury is comparable. A number of variables have been proposed to account for this variance. Some of these are demographic factors present prior to injury; others are postinjury features.

Premorbid Characteristics

Age

Age has long been considered an important influence on the level of outcome attained after head injury. It is generally accepted that brain injury will have less deleterious effects on some cognitive parameters if acquired early in life rather than later (Alberico, Ward, Chol, Marmarou, and Young, 1987; Johnson and Almi, 1978; Levin, Ewing-Cobles, and Benton, 1984). However, this relationship is not as simple as it appears. For example, the pattern of recovery from aphasia appears better in younger versus older patients, although residual deficits often persist even in children injured at a very young age (Alajouanine and Lhermitte, 1965; Woods and Teuber, 1978). After the age of 2, the type of aphasia, as well as the cause and severity of damage, appears to contribute more to outcome than does the age of onset (van Dongen and Loolen, 1977).

The recovery of other capacities may also be affected by the age at which the injury was sustained. For example, permanent attention and memory deficits are more likely to occur in older victims of head injury than in younger patients (Levin, et al., 1982). Furthermore, recovery, as measured by autonomous community functioning, was found to reach an asymptote later and was more complete in younger individuals (Carlsson, van Essen, and Lofgren, 1968). Conversely, one study showed that children who had acquired a brain injury in the first 12 months of life were later found to have lower IQ scores than children injured at a later age (Woods, 1980). This suggests the immature brain may actually be more vulnerable to neural and behavioral abnormalities (Brazier, 1975).

Results from a number of experiments have supported the idea that there is functional sparing following selective brain injury in young animals that is not seen in older animals (e.g., Kennard, 1936; 1938; 1940; 1942). Similar age-related effects in recovery have been noted for maze performance in rats (Tsang, 1937), delayed response learning in rhesus monkeys (Akert, Orth, Harlow, and Schlitz, 1960), and roughness discrimination in cats (Benjamin and Thompson, 1959).

Conversely, evidence from other animal studies has failed to show any age-related differences in the magnitude of recovery observed in the learning of a variety of responses following various brain lesions (Brooks and Peck, 1940; Kling and Tucker, 1967; Goldman, 1974). Some investigators have failed to replicate Kennard's findings (Passingham, Perry, and Wilkinson, 1983). It is possible that observed outcome may be more related to the time of testing after onset and to the types of tests used rather than to age (Goldman, 1974).

In general, it appears that the effects of age on recovery following neural damage may be largely related to the capabilities and capacity of the nervous system at critical periods. Harlow, Blumquist, Thompson, Schlitz, and Harlow (1968) showed that response learning in monkeys was unaffected by lesions made at 5 months of age, but damage at 12 months had severe effects. Furthermore, these effects were greater than those of injury occurring at 18 or 24 months. Kolb (1987; 1989) has also shown that there are developmental windows during which lesions have less severe effects on behavior than at other times.

Consequently, there has been debate on the relevance of age as an isolated prognostic indicator. Some studies have shown that age is only important in predicting outcome when considered in conjunction with other variables such as injury severity. (Carlsson, et al., 1968). Similarly, Jennett and Teasdale (1981) reported that in coma lasting longer than 6 hours, the probability of death was much greater in patients over 50 years of age. It also appears that there is less distinction between the outcomes of mild and severe injuries in older patients, and that age provides less protection from the effects of severe injuries (Jennett, Teasdale, Galbraith, Pickard, Grant, Braakman, Avezaat, Maas, Minderhoud, Vecht, Heiden, Small, Caton, and Kurze, 1977). Conversely, one study has reported no relationship between severity of injury and age (Thomsen, 1989).

It has also been shown that age can interact with etiology in determining outcome. For example, stroke victims younger than 60 years of age tend to have a better chance of recovery than older stroke patients or head injury patients of comparable age (Levin, et al., 1982).

Sex

Differences in cognitive functioning associated with sex-related hemispheric specialization have been investigated. On average, females exhibit superior performance on verbal tasks and males surpass females on visuospatial tests (McGlone, 1980; Inglis and Lawson, 1981). These differences are consistent from early in development (Witelson and Pallie, 1973;

Witelson, 1987) and may relate to neuroanatomic asymmetries (De Vries, De Bruin, Uylings, and Corner, 1984; Wittig and Peterson, 1979), particularly in the corpus callosum (de Lacoste-Utamsing and Holloway, 1982; Wada, 1976; Witelson, 1989; Witelson and Pallie, 1973). Consequently, it is reasonable to inquire whether gender has an influence on recovery following brain injury. This issue may be especially relevant to the study of recovery following closed head trauma as the corpus callosum is known to be macroscopically damaged by the acceleration-deceleration forces characteristic of this injury (Adams, Mitchell, Graham, and Doyle, 1977; Strich, 1956) and such damage may result in behavior characteristic of hemispheric disconnection (Rubens, Geschwind, Mahowald, and Mastri, 1977).

Evidence from clinical practice suggests that female patients are less likely to become aphasic following damage to the left hemisphere (McGlone, 1980). Furthermore, there is a relationship between the side of lesion and degree of verbal and nonverbal IQ impairment following injury for males only (McGlone, 1978). Some studies have reported sex differences in emotional status as measured by the MMPI in that males demonstrate greater emotional disturbance both shortly postinjury (MacNiven and Finlayson, 1990a) and at long-term follow-up (Burton and Volpe, 1988; MacNiven and Finlayson, 1990b; Neilson and Alfano, 1990). There have been very few studies of the relationship between sex or gender and recovery of functioning, and these have generally not yielded significant differences (Caplan, McPherson and Tobin, 1985; Carlsson, et al., 1968). However, MacNiven and Finlayson (1990a) reported that although males and females exhibited comparable performance on a test of concept formation and problem solving shortly postinjury, female patients exhibited greater recovery than males when tested at a later date.

Studies of animal models of brain injury have also yielded results suggestive of sex differences in recovery; however, there is an interaction with the site of lesion. Frontal (Stein, 1974) and septal (Flaherty, Powell, and Hamilton, 1979) lesions apparently result in greater behavioral impairments in female rats, while males are more affected by damage to the hippocampus (Loy and Milner, 1980) and caudate nucleus (Anger, 1982).

Sex may play a role in recovery through differences in neurocognitive organization, or through the influence of reproductive hormones. Progesterone and estrogen have been correlated with variation in performance on a number of cognitive tasks (Hampson, 1990), as has testosterone (Gouchie and Kimura, 1991). Gonadal steroids have also been found to play a role in neuronal development (Goy and McEwen, 1980), morphology (Gould, Woolley, Frankfurt, and McEwen, 1990), and dendritic proliferation after insult (Morse, Scheff, and DeKosky, 1986). Such steroids may also be involved in determining right-left asymmetries (Stewart and

Kolb, 1988). Gonadal hormones may also influence recovery of function after brain damage (Attella, Nattinville and Stein, 1987; Roof, Duvdevani, and Stein, 1992). These studies support the notion that sex-related differences in neurophysiology may underlie disparities in recovery. However, in humans, sex may interact with other variables such as motivation, social support systems, and demographic variables which may themselves affect the extent and course of recovery.

Handedness

Cerebral dominance is also an important determinant of individual differences in functioning. With some exceptions, right-handers tend to be left-hemisphere dominant for language functions while visuospatial skills are represented in the right hemisphere. Conversely, about 15% of left-handers have bilateral speech representation and another 15% tend to be right-hemisphere dominant for speech (Springer and Deutsch, 1981). Left-handers generally have more bilateral representation of cognitive functions than do right-handers (Bryden, 1982), and this may be associated with neuroanatomic differences (Witelson, 1989). As left-handed individuals are more subject to industrial or automobile accidents than right-handers (Coran, 1989; Porac and Coran, 1981), it is possible that there is a large number of left-handers among head injury victims (MacNiven, 1993).

MacNiven and Finlayson (1990a) reported a significantly greater number of left-handed females in a sample of closed head injury patients than would be predicted from the population at large. Also, these patients were initially more cognitively impaired than right-handed females, but later improved to a greater degree. These results are consistent with those found in stroke patients (Hecaen, 1979; Luria, 1970; Subirana, 1958; Sarno, Sarno, and Levita, 1971). It is possible that these effects are partially determined by brain asymmetry and influenced by callosal damage at injury; however, a number of demographic variables may also exert effects.

Personality Variables

Victims of head injury may not represent a random sample of the population. Most patients with head injuries are male (Levin, et al., 1982); many of them have a premorbid history of antisocial behaviors, or psychosocial adjustment problems (Fahy, Irving, and Millac, 1967; Jamieson and Kelly, 1973). Children experiencing head injuries have been found to have a history of social (Fuld and Fisher, 1977) or academic difficulties (Fuld and Fisher, 1977; Haas, Cope, and Hall, 1987), and to come from homes in which there was marital discord and higher levels of psychosocial distress

(Klonoff, 1971). A proportion of victims of head injury may have premorbid psychiatric disability including neurotic or psychotic disorders (Kerr, Kay, and Lassman, 1971). Indeed, persons diagnosed as having a psychiatric illness may be more likely to experience motor vehicle accidents which in turn may lead to head injuries (Tsuang, Boor, and Fleming, 1985). Denker (1958) found a higher incidence of premorbid neurotic difficulties in head injured monozygotic twins than in dizygotic twins, suggesting a biologic predisposition to behaviors that may result in a head injury.

Levin and co-authors (1978) have proposed that these maladaptive personality characteristics may have a negative impact on the degree of anticipated recovery. Studies have suggested that premorbid emotional instability is associated with a higher incidence of psychiatric disturbance following brain injury (Adler, 1945; Kozol, 1945; Ruesch and Bowman, 1945; Rutter, 1981) and decreased probability of returning to work (Humphrey and Oddy, 1981). Furthermore, it may be possible to predict postinjury psychiatric symptomology from premorbid personality features (Lishman, 1973).

Alcohol and Other Drugs

Alcohol is an important contributing factor in the occurrence of head injuries resultant from motor vehicle accidents (Haddon and Bradess, 1959; Tsuang, et al., 1985), assaults (Brismar and Tuner, 1982), and domestic accidents (Field, 1976; Hossak, 1972; Kerr, et al., 1971). It has been reported that from one-third (Field, 1976) to one-half or more of head injury victims over the age of 15 had used alcohol at the time of injury (Brismar, Engstrom, and Rydberg, 1983; Jennett and Teasdale, 1981; Sparedo and Gill, 1989). Also, chronic alcoholics may account for up to one-half of severe head trauma victims (Field, 1976; Brismar, et al., 1983). Alcohol intoxication may cause physiologic complications (e.g., hypoxia, hypertension, cerebral edema, altered blood clotting) which may increase insult to the brain (Bakay and Glasauer, 1980; Elmer and Lim, 1985; Howard, 1982; McQueen and Posey, 1975). There is also a higher likelihood of the occurrence of hematomas after head injury after alcohol use (Elmer, Goransson, and Zoucas, 1984; Markwalder, 1981). Alcohol intoxication at the time of injury in motor vehicle accidents has been related to an enhanced mortality rate compared to sober patients (Luna, Maier, Sowder, Copass, and Oreskovich, 1984; Ward, Flynn, Miller, and Blaisdell, 1982); however, one study failed to demonstrate this finding (Huth, Maier, Simonowitz, and Herman, 1983).

Patients having detectable levels of alcohol in their blood at the time of injury had longer periods of coma with lower levels of consciousness than those not having used alcohol (Edna, 1982; Galbraith, Murray, Patel, and Knill-Jones, 1976). Alcohol ingestion may also be related to lower Rancho levels at discharge (Sparedo and Gill, 1989) and may contribute to the total length of hospitalization after head trauma (Brismar, et al., 1983; Edna, 1982; Sparedo and Gill, 1989). Alcohol use also appears to be related to more severe deficits in memory and verbal learning functions (Brooks, Symington, Beattie, Campsie, Bryden, and McKinlay, 1989).

Although alcohol apparently has serious effects on outcome after injury, it is difficult to tease apart the effects of alcohol from other factors associated with alcohol use such as personality variables, socioeconomic status, and social situations. Furthermore, given the adverse consequences of long-term alcohol use on memory, abstract reasoning, and spatial ability (Loberg, 1986; Tarter and Edwards, 1985), it is possible that alcoholics suffering a head injury may be at a disadvantage in terms of potential recovery.

The role of drugs other than alcohol in the occurrence and outcome of brain injury has been largely ignored. Some surveys have suggested that prescription drugs, such as tranquilizers, may be a causal factor in traffic accidents (Honkanen, Ertma, Lioila, Alha, Lukkari, Karlsson, Kiviluoto, and Puro, 1980; Skegg, Richards, and Doll, 1979); however, one group of investigators failed to find a relationship for sedatives (Jick, Hunter, Dinan, Madsen, and Stergachis, 1981). Studies of illegal drug use have consistently shown that cannabis use can increase the chances of automobile accidents (Milner, 1977), and that this is the most frequent drug, other than alcohol, used by victims of motor vehicle accidents (Luna, et al., 1984).

Brismar and coworkers (1983) reported that 25% of their sample of neurotrauma patients had a history of experience with narcotics. Given that some drugs can have detrimental effects on cognitive functioning (Leavitt, 1974), and on the brain itself (Pascual-Leone, Dhuna, Altafullah, and Abderson, 1990), it is possible that this drug use may negatively influence recovery after neurologic injury.

Demographic Variables

Several demographic variables appear to be correlated with increased chance of brain injury. There are more than 4 times as many divorced individuals among patients with head injuries than would be predicted from prevalence rates in the general population (Kerr, et al., 1971). However, it is possible that these people become divorced because of other factors which may also predispose them to a head injury, such as excessive alcohol use or psychiatric disturbance. Nevertheless, it may be important to consider marital status as a prognostic indicator as family functioning may have effects on adjustment and recovery (see Chapter 15).

Socioeconomic status (SES) may also play a role in recovery. A high number of victims have lower SES backgrounds (Field, 1976; Kerr, et al.,

1971; Klonoff, 1971). In general, patients with higher SES tend to have better outcomes than those with a lower socioeconomic level (Najenson, Mendelson, Schecter, David, Mintz, and Groswasser, 1974; Rusk, Block, and Lowman, 1969). Effects of socioeconomic status on recovery are probably confounded by intelligence and education. Hook (1969) reported that patients of higher intelligence were more likely to have better outcomes and coping skills after injury. Similarly, higher premorbid intelligence, as measured by the Armed Forces Qualification Test, predicted better employment prospects for Korean War veterans with head injuries (Dresser, Meirowsky, Weiss, McNeel, Simon, and Caveness, 1973). Benton (1981) also suggested that higher SES and education level were related to better cognitive functioning in elderly subjects; however, one study has failed to find any differences in recovery based on demographic factors (Smith, 1981).

Head injury may predispose an individual to future brain trauma. Annegers and coworkers (1980) found the incidence of a second head injury to be 3 times higher than for the population at large. Furthermore, the incidence of patients experiencing a third head injury was 8 times higher than the expected incidence rate. Similar results were found in children, and boys were more likely to sustain multiple injuries than girls (Klonoff, 1971).

Repeated head injury may have a cumulative effect on functioning. Carlsson, Svardsudd, and Welin (1987), reported that as the number of head injuries experienced by a patient increased, performance on a number of cognitive tasks declined.

POSTINJURY INFLUENCES

Ostensibly, the principal determinant of outcome after closed head injury is the extent of brain damage incurred. This includes both the primary damage sustained at the time of injury, and secondary damage caused by posttraumatic complications such as raised intracranial pressure (ICP), hydrocephalus, or hematomas (Jennett and Teasdale, 1981). In order to document how the severity of damage contributes to outcome, it is necessary to identify methods of measuring and classifying severity.

Coma Depth and Duration

The degree and duration of alterations in level of consciousness can serve as indirect but reliable indices of the extent of brain damage. Deeper levels of unconsciousness of longer durations have been related to poorer overall outcomes (Carlsson, et al., 1968; Gilchrist and Wilkinson, 1979; Klove and Cleeland, 1972; Overgaard, Hvid-Hansen, Land, Pedersen,

Christensen, Haase, Hein, and Tweed, 1973; Ruesch, 1944). However, early investigators measured and defined "coma" in varying ways, and the lack of a standardized description prevented comparisons across studies. The Glasgow Coma Scale (GCS), developed by Teasdale and Jennett (1974), provides a system for rating the level of consciousness based on the best eye opening, verbal, and motor responses observed during the acute postinjury period. The practical reliability of this scale has been well established (Teasdale, Knill-Jones, and Van Der Sande, 1978), and it has been shown to be superior to similar scales, such as the Acute Physiology Score, in its ease of administration and accuracy of prediction (Rocca, Martin, Viviand, Bidet, Saint-Gilles, and Chevalier, 1989).

Extensive studies designed to predict outcome based on the GCS indicated that it could reliably predict the probability of mortality and functional outcome at 6 months after injury across centers, despite differences in treatment strategies (Jennett, et al., 1977; Jennett, Teasdale, Braakman, Minderhoud, Heiden, and Kurze, 1979). Similar findings have been reported in subsequent studies (Bowers and Marshall, 1980; Jennett, Teasdale, Braakman, Minderhound, and Knill-Jones, 1976; Langfitt, 1978; Teasdale and Jennett, 1976; Vogenthaler, Smith and Goldfader, 1989a; 1989b). The GCS has also been found to predict cognitive outcome after head injury (Levin, Grossman, Rose, and Teasdale, 1979) and to relate to general functional recovery (Volpe and McDowell, 1990).

These results are encouraging, but the GCS is not without limitations. A number of physical constraints resulting from trauma and medical interventions limit its applicability in the acute recovery period. Modifications have been undertaken to increase the sensitivity of this measure and have shown some success. For example, one group of researchers added assessment of brainstem reflexes to the standard Glasgow Coma Scale (GCS) (Born, Albert, Hans, and Bonnal, 1985). The resulting Glasgow-Leige Scale (GLS) was found to have greater accuracy in predicting outcome according to Glasgow Outcome Scale (GOS) criteria than the GCS alone (Born, et al., 1985).

The Comprehensive Level of Consciousness Scale (CLOCS) was developed to assess a broader range of spontaneous and elicited responses (Stanczak, White, Gouview, Moehle, Daniel, Novack, and Long, 1984). The CLOCS addresses posture, resting eye position, and general responsiveness in addition to pupillary reflexes and GCS items. Consequently, the CLOCS is thought to be more reliable than the GCS and is more sensitive to subtle changes in a patient's condition. The CLOCS was also shown to be useful in predicting patient outcome on a modified version of the GOS completed at discharge (Stanczak, et al., 1984).

However, some question remains as to the utility of the duration of coma for clinical projection, particularly in that coma length may not be predictive of cognitive outcome on a number of neuropsychologic tests. However, the duration of posttraumatic amnesia has been found to be useful in that regard (Brooks, Aughton, Bond, Jones, and Rizvi, 1980; Shores, 1989).

Posttraumatic Amnesia

The measurement of posttraumatic amnesia (PTA) was first described by Russell (Russell, 1932; Russell, 1934; Russell and Nathan, 1946), who noted that this period could be as long as 18 months in duration, and was related to age and outcome (Symonds and Russell, 1943). By 1961, Russell had refined the concept of PTA to refer to the period following coma during which the patient is unable to store current events in memory (Russell and Smith, 1961). A number of subsequent studies demonstrated that the duration of PTA is negatively correlated with optimal outcome (Bond, 1976; Levin, et al., 1982). However, many of these studies employed a retrospective interview technique which may be open to a number of biases, particularly in brain damaged patients. Indeed, Gronwell and Wrightson (1980) reported that there is some inconsistency between retrospective estimates of PTA duration and prospective evaluation during recovery. There has also been some doubt as to the interrater reliability of PTA assessments (Schacter and Crovitz, 1977; Sisler and Penner, 1975). Consequently, more reliable measurement tools have been devised.

The Galveston Orientation and Amnesia Test (GOAT) is a standardized questionnaire which is administered serially during the acute postcoma phase of recovery (Levin, O'Donnell, and Grossman, 1979). This scale assesses orientation to person, place, and time, as well as memory of current events, and for circumstances preceding the injury. Scores on the test are related to severity of injury indicated by CT scans and GCS scores, and have been found to be predictive of long-term outcome using the GOS (Levin, et al., 1979).

The Oxford Scale (Artiola, Fortuny, Briggs, Newcombe, Ratcliff, and Thomas, 1980) also addresses personal details, orientation, and memories immediately antecedent and following the injury, but it also includes a short recognition memory test. The Oxford PTA Scale has shown good interobserver reliability and has clinical validity (Artiola, et al., 1980).

The Westmead PTA Scale (Shores, Marosszeky, Sandanam, and Batchelor, 1986) is an extension and enhancement of the Oxford Scale that is very brief, and employs a more stringent definition of PTA. There is also evidence that duration of PTA as measured by the Westmead can predict cognitive functioning 2 years after injury (Shores, 1989).

Although the duration of coma and the length of PTA have been invaluable to the determination of prognosis after brain injury, some limitations remain. For example, severe head injury is defined by GCS score of

3–8, and loss of consciousness and/or PTA of longer than 24 hours (Prigatano and Fordyce, 1986). However, PTA can range up to 18 months (Russell, 1934). Consequently, it is possible that other cognitive and functional differences exist among patients suffering long-term PTA. It is unlikely that a PTA duration of 1 week is equivalent in severity and consequences to a PTA lasting over a year. Furthermore, the definition of PTA needs to permit an ultimate end to this condition and allow for the distinction of PTA from permanent memory devastation.

Technological Determination of Severity of Injury

In recent years, the advent of modern technology has made it possible to gain more direct measurement of the severity of brain damage as an alternative to estimates of coma and PTA duration which may be biased, limited, inaccurate, and difficult to assess in some patients. Comprehensive reviews of post head injury neural abnormalities, indicated by neuroimaging, and their relationship to cognitive functioning can be found elsewhere (Ruff, Cullum, and Luerssen, 1989; Wilson, 1990). Consequently, this section will deal selectively with the use of biotechnology in aiding outcome prediction.

Some investigators have used Computerized Tomographic (CT) scanning to detect traumatic lesions in the central nervous system (Gandy, Snow, Zimmerman, and Deck, 1984; Han, Kaufman, Alfidi, Yeung, Benson, Haaga, El Yousef, Clampitt, Bonstelle, and Huss, 1984; Lanksch, Grumme, and Kazner, 1979). This technique has proven to be useful in the detection of cerebral swelling (Kobrine, Timmins, Rajjoub, Rizzoli, and Davis, 1977), focal lesions such as hematomas (Levin, et al., 1986), and contusions (Uzzell, Zimmerman, Dolinskas, and Obrist, 1979; Zimmerman, Bilaniuk, Dolinskas, Gennerralli, Bruce, and Uzzell, 1977). There have been comparatively fewer studies relating CT findings to patient outcome but there may be discrete groups or patterns of CT findings that relate to outcome (Timming, Orrison, and Mikula, 1982). Furthermore, the presence of hematomas detected by CT is related to a higher score on the Halstead Impairment Index (Klove and Cleeland, 1972) and greater memory impairments (Cullum and Bigler, 1986). In general, the use of serial CT scans in combination with other prognostic indicators such as the GCS has been useful in predicting short-term outcome in the acute stages of recovery (Clifton, Ziegler, and Crossman, 1980).

There are some limitations to the usefulness of this technique with closed head injury patients. It is known that the resolution of CT scans is not adequate for the examination of brainstem injury (Gentry, Godersky, and Thompson, 1989). The CT scan may not detect deeper lesions. For example, Snoek and coworkers (Snoek, Jennett, Adams, Graham, and

Doyle, 1979) reported that almost 40% of severe head injury patients had normal CT scans. Consequently, one study has suggested that Magnetic Resonance Imaging (MRI) is more suitable for detecting and characterizing the consequences of closed head trauma (Jordan and Zimmerman, 1990).

It is well known that the anatomic mechanisms of closed head injury involve the mechanical stretching and shearing of nerve fibers which leads to extensive microscopic axonal damage (Adams, Graham, Murray, and Scott, 1982; Strich, 1956). Consequently, CT and MRI scans, which provide primarily structural information, are more limited in assessing the severity of closed head injury and in predicting recovery and ultimate handicap than indices of brain functioning.

Consequently, some investigators have turned to the evaluation of regional Cerebral Blood Flow (CBF) to gain further clinical information. Alterations in CBF can result in ischemic hypoxia which causes necrosis (Levin, et al., 1986). Measurement of regional CBF can determine whether the patient is at risk. Furthermore, CBF is related to level of consciousness and can be used to predict outcome in terms of the GOS (Jaggi, Obrist, Gennarelli, and Langfitt, 1990; Obrist, Gennarelli, Segawa, Dolinskas, and Langfitt, 1979).

Alternatively, Sensory Evoked Potentials (SEPs) represent a noninvasive neurophysiologically based measure of brain function. There are a number of types of SEPs, which give unique information about brain functioning. Somatosensory evoked responses (SSERs) provide information concerning the brainstem, diencephalon, and somatosensory cortex (Allison, Goff, Williamson, and VanGilder, 1980; Cracco and Cracco, 1986). Auditory evoked potentials (AERs) provide further information concerning brainstem functioning, as well as the auditory cortex (Karnaze, Marshall, McCarthy, Klauber, and Bickford, 1982; Seales, Rossiter, Weinstein, and Spencer, 1982). Visual evoked responses (VERs) transverse a number of neuroanatomic regions providing information regarding the optic tracts, as well as the primary and secondary visual cortices (Greenberg, Mayer, and Becker, 1977).

Using evoked potential techniques, it is possible to obtain indices of clinical neurologic status in neuropathologic conditions such as Huntington's Chorea (Ehle, Stewart, Lellelid, and Levinthal, 1984), cerebrovascular disease (Rappaport, Hall, Hopkins, Bellaza, Berrol, and Reynolds, 1977; Rappaport, Hopkins, Hall, Bellaza, Berrol, and Reynolds, 1978), brain tumors (Williamson, Goff, and Allison, 1970), and spinal chord disease (Perot, 1973). Detailed analyses of SEPs in those cases have indicated that particular clinical syndromes may be associated with specific abnormal SEP patterns (see Calloway, Tueting, and Kaslo, 1978, for a review).

SEPs can also contribute greatly to the early assessment of severity and extent of brain injury in comatose patients where few other reliable neurologic indices of damage can be easily obtained (Greenberg and Becker, 1975; Greenberg, Mayer, Becker, and Miller, 1977, Greenberg, Becker, Miller, and Mayer, 1977; Karnaze, Marshall, McCarthy, and Klauber, 1982; Newlon and Greenberg, 1983; Seales, et al., 1979).

In addition to diagnostic capabilities, SEP abnormalities may have predictive power with regard to prognosis. In a high percentage of patients with severe head injuries, the length of time to recovery of consciousness and the presence of residual neurologic difficulty is positively correlated with abnormal SEP responses recorded early in the posttraumatic period (de la Torre, Trimble, Beard, Hanlon, and Surgeon, 1978; Greenberg and Becker, 1975). Furthermore, abnormalities in SEPs recorded shortly after injury allowed a high degree of accuracy in predicting patient outcome in terms of mortality (Bricolo, 1976) and the GOS (Anderson, Bundlie, and Rocksworld, 1984; Greenberg, Newlon, Hyatt, Narayan, and Becker, 1981; Narayan, Greenberg, Miller, Enas, Choi, Kishore, Selhorst, Lutz, and Becker, 1981; Newlon and Greenberg, 1984; Newlon, Greenberg, Hyatt, Enas, and Becker, 1982). Indeed, a comprehensive study of the comparative utility of a number of clinical indicators suggested that SEP abnormalities detected shortly postinjury were more accurate in predicting patient outcome than the GCS, pupillary reflexes, or CT scans (Narayan, et al., 1981). Thus, examination of SEP data early in the posttraumatic period may provide a reliable and valuable basis on which to predict patient outcome.

Etiology

Although the severity of injury is important in the determination of level of functioning both immediately postinjury and during long-term recovery, the type of brain injury can also play a role. It is known that focal injuries tend to have more specific effects on performance, and it is possible that an isolated area of impairment may result, leaving other skills unaffected. This is apparently true for both stroke and trauma, although the recovery of stroke victims may be complicated by their older mean age (Levin, et al., 1986; Meier, et al., 1987).

Closed head injuries tend to cause widespread deficits across a number of areas of functioning. There is also a greater range of individual differences in ability among the population of closed head trauma patients as compared to those with focal injuries (Levin, et al., 1986; Meier, et al., 1990). Furthermore, patients experiencing diffuse injury in addition to focal lesions tended to have poorer outcomes compared to patients with diffuse injury only (Filley, Cranberg, Alecander, and Hart, 1987).

A subset of nonpenetrating brain injuries is composed of patients with anoxic damage in which neurons have been oxygen deprived for some period of time. In general, these patients tend to have significantly poorer outcomes compared to closed head trauma counterparts and any protective effects of young age are minimized in this group (Groswasser, Cohen, and Costeff, 1989; Levati, Farina, Vecchi, Rossanda, and Marrubini, 1982). Finally, regardless of etiology, the presence of secondary insults in the form of multiple trauma (Moore, Stambrook, Peters, Cardoso, and Kassum, 1990), hypoxia, edema, or raised intracranial pressure are also associated with poorer outcomes in the affected patients (Andrews, Piper, Dearden, and Miller, 1990; Miller, Sweet, Narayan, and Becker, 1978).

Emotional Variables

A number of researchers have examined the psychiatric consequences of both diffuse (Jennett, Snoek, Bond, and Brooks, 1981; Kwentus, Hart, Peck, and Kornstein, 1985) and localized head injury (Aita and Ritan, 1948; Dikmen and Reitan, 1978; Fahy, et al., 1967; Fordyce, Roueche, and Prigatano, 1983; Lishman, 1973; Ruesch and Bowman, 1945), as well as stroke (Black, 1975; Folstein, Maiberger, and McHugh, 1977; Robinson and Szetela, 1980). It is also known that brain trauma may provoke the onset of psychiatric disturbance (Haig, 1990). However, there are substantially fewer studies regarding the influence of emotional variables on recovery. Although there has been little direct analysis of this association (Diamond, Barth, and Zillmer, 1988), it is apparent that increased emotional dysfunction is associated with poor cognitive functioning during recovery.

In one study, the authors reported a relationship between neuropsychologic and psychiatric deficits after severe closed head injury in that patients exhibiting good recovery experienced only mild anxiety and depression, while those who were moderately or severely cognitively disabled had more serious psychiatric disorders (Levin, Grossman, Rose, and Teasdale, 1979). Similarly, Nockleby and Deaton (1987) reported that higher levels of distress, as measured by the MMPI, are associated with greater awareness of intellectual impairments.

Barth and colleagues (Barth, Macciocci, Giordani, Rimel, Jane, and Boll, 1983) tested patients at 3 months postinjury and found that 32% had at least one elevated MMPI scale, and that scale 2 was moderately correlated with Impairment Index score. Also, Diamond, et al. (1988), reported elevations of all clinical scales as a result of mild closed head injury, with only 34% of the population being rated as "Normal Nondepressed." A full 50% of these patients were rated as "abnormal" according to the depression classification system of Gilberstadt and Farkas (1961).

Ratings on the Halstead Impairment Index were considered in conjunction with MMPI scores in relation to difficulty in returning to work. This analysis showed that less than 10% of those patients who had problems in returning to work or school had normal MMPI scores or an Impairment Index score of less than 0.6.

Bornstein and his colleagues showed small but significant correlations between Impairment Index scores and scales 1, 2, 3, 7, and 8 for patients recovering from at least minor closed head injury. This result suggests that more extensive neuropsychologic deficits are associated with more serious personality disturbance (Bornstein, et al., 1989a); however, no such relationship was found in another study by the same authors (Bornstein, et al., 1989b).

Studies of focal brain lesions have also reported a relationship between outcome and psychologic functioning. Dikmen and Reitan (1978) demonstrated that patients having emotional difficulties in terms of MMPI profiles also exhibited greater losses of function on a number of neuropsychologic tests. Psychologically disturbed patients were also found to have more impaired functional abilities (Dikmen and Reitan, 1977) and a higher degree of generalized impairment based on the Halstead Impairment Index (Calsyn, Louks, and Johnson, 1982). Similarly, it is possible that there is a negative effect of posttraumatic emotional disturbance on community functioning (Bruckner and Randle, 1972), but one study failed to show such an association (Marsh, Knight, and Godfrey, 1990).

It is difficult to ascertain whether the emotional sequelae of head trauma are manifestations of reactions to deficits and life changes, or are the result of neurochemical or neuroanatomic disruptions. Some studies have shown that the site of lesion is related to the nature of the psychopathology (Gainotti, 1972; Lishman, 1973; Papez, 1937; Robinson and Szetela, 1981; Shaffer, Chadwick, and Rutter, 1975). Furthermore, the extent of personality disruption following injury may be related to the severity of injury (Levin and Grossman, 1978; Prigatano and Fordyce, 1986); however, other investigators found no association between emotional dysfunction and severity of brain damage, as estimated by PTA (Barth, et al., 1983; Brooks and McKinley, 1983), or duration of coma (Rutter, 1981; Shaffer, et al., 1975).

Other reports suggest that there may be alterations in neurochemistry following brain injury characteristic of psychiatric disorders such as depression (Clifton, Ziegler, and Crossman, 1981; Van Woerkom, Teelken, and Minderhound, 1977; Ward, 1966) which may also interact with the site of injury (Kwentus, et al., 1985). Thus, it is possible that emotional disturbance following brain trauma may be associated with the pathophysiology of the injury; however, these reactions may be potentiated by inadequate coping mechanisms.

SUMMARY

It is important to note that there are probably many interactions and correlations between the predictors of recovery after brain damage. On one hand, this can be advantageous. Some studies have shown better predictive power can be obtained when using a number of variables which individually are known to indicate prognosis. However, there appears to be a limit beyond which adding singularly useful variables does not contribute to prognostic success. For example, Braakman, Gelpke, Habbema, Maas, and Minderhound (1980), analyzed the relative contribution of a number of prognostic features to optimal outcome prediction using the GOS. They discovered that only 3–5 were necessary, including age, dimensions of coma, and pupillary reflexes.

Conversely, it has also been suggested that combining factors confounds their interrelatedness. It is difficult to distinguish which features are truly relevant and reliable, and it is virtually impossible to isolate any single causative factors (Brooks, 1989). For example, patients using alcohol at the time of injury are more likely to have accompanying negative personality traits and tend to acquire their injury through violence or falls than in another manner (Brismar, et al., 1983). All of these elements may contribute to outcome, or they may themselves be dependent on another unidentified factor capable of exerting a greater influence on recovery potential.

References

Adams, J.H., Graham, D.I., Murray, L.S., and Scott, G. (1982). Diffuse axonal injury due to nonmissile head trauma in humans: An analysis of 45 cases. Annals of Neurology, 12:557-653.

Adams, J.H., Mitchell, D.E., Graham, D.I., and Doyle, D.E. (1977). Diffuse brain damage of immediate impact type. Brain, 100:489-502.

Adler, A. (1945). Mental symptoms following head injury. A statistical analysis of two hundred cases. Archives of Neurology and Psychiatry, 53:34-43.

Aita, J.A. and Reitan, R.M. (1948). Psychotic reactions in the late recovery period following brain injury. American Journal of Psychiatry, 105:161-69.

Akert, K., Orth, O.S., Harlow, H.F., and Schlitz, F. (1960). Learned behavior of rhesus monkeys following neonatal bilateral prefrontal lobotomy. Science, 132:1944-45.

Alajouinine, T. and Lhermitte, F. (1965). Acquired aphasia in children. Brain, 88:653-62.

Alberico, A.M., Ward, J.D., Choi, S.C., Marmarou, A., and Young, H.F. (1987). Outcome after severe head injury. Journal of Neurosurgery, 67:648-56.

Allison, T., Goff, W.R., Williamson, P.D., and VanGilder, J.C. (1980). On the neural origin of early components of the human somatosensory evoked potential. In: Desmedt, J.E. (ed). Progress in Clinical Neurophysiology, Vol. 7: Clinical Uses of Cerebral, Brain Stem and Spinal Somatosensory Evoked Potentials. Basel: S. Karger, 51-68.

Anderson, D.C., Bundlie, S., and Rocksworld, G.L. (1984). Multimodality evoked potentials in closed head injury. Archives of Neurology, 41:369-74.

Andrews, P.J.D., Piper, I.R., Dearden, N.M., and Miller, J.D. (1990). Secondary insults during intrahospital transport of head injured patients. Lancet, 1:327-30.

Anger, K. (1982). Sex differences in recovery from brain damage after lesions of the caudate nucleus. Worcester, MA: B.A. Thesis, Clark University.

Annegers, J.F., Grabow, J.D., Groover, R.V., Laws, E.R., and Kurland, L.T. (1980). Seizures after head trauma: A population study. Neurology, 30:683–89.

Artiola, I., Fortuny, L., Briggs, M., Newcombe, F., Ratcliff, G., and Thomas, C. (1980). Measuring the duration of posttraumatic amnesia. Journal of Neurology, Neurosurgery, and Psychiatry, 43:377–79.

Attella, M.J., Nattinville, A., and Stein, D.G. (1987). Hormonal state affects recovery from frontal cortex lesions in adult female rats. Behavioral and Neural Biology, 48: 352–67.

Bakay, L. and Glauser, F.E. (1980). Head Injury. Boston: Little, Brown and Company.

Barth, J.F., Macciocchi, S.N., Giordani, B., Rimel, R., Jane, J.A., and Boll, T.J. (1983). Neuropsychological sequelae of minor head injury. Neurosurgery, 13:529–33.

Benjamin, R.M. and Thompson, R.F. (1959). Differential effects of cortical lesions in infant and adult cats on roughness discrimination. Experimental Neurology, 1:305–21.

Benton, A.L. (1981). Aspects of the neuropsychology of aging. Invited Address, Division 40, American Psychology Association, Los Angeles.

Black, F.W. (1975). Unilateral brain lesions and MMPI performance: A preliminary study. Perceptual and Motor Skills, 40:87–93.

Bond, M.R. (1976). Assessment of the psychosocial outcome of severe head injury. Acta Neurochirurgica, 34:57–70.

Born, J.D., Albert, A., Hans, P.P., and Bonnal, J. (1985). Relative prognostic value of best motor response and brain stem reflexes in patients with severe head injury. Neurosurgery, 16:595–601.

Bornstein, R.A., Miller, H.B., and van Schoor, J.T. (1988). Emotional adjustment in compensated head injury patients. Neurosurgery, 23:622–27.

Bornstein, R.A., Miller, H.B., and van Schoor, J.T. (1989). Neuropsychological deficit and emotional disturbance in head injury patients. Journal of Neurosurgery, 70: 509–13.

Bowers, S.A. and Marshall, L.F. (1980). Outcome in 200 consecutive cases of severe head injury treated in San Diego County: A prospective analysis. Neurosurgery, 6:237–42.

Braakman, R., Gelpke, G.J., Habbema, J.D.F., Maas, A.I.R., and Minderhoud, J.M. (1980). Systematic selection of prognostic features in patients with severe head injury. Neurosurgery, 6:362–70.

Brazier, M.A.B. (ed). (1975). Growth and development of the brain. Nutritional, genetic and environmental factors. Vol. 1. International Brain Research Organization Monograph Series. New York: Raven Press.

Bricolo, A. (1976). Electroencephalography in neurotraumatology. Clinical Electroencephalography, 7:184–97.

Brismar, B. and Tuner, K. (1982). Battered women. A surgical problem. Acta Chirurgica Scandinavica, 148:103–05.

Brismar, B., Engstrom, A., and Rydberg, U. (1983). Head injury and intoxication: A therapeutic dilemma. Acta Chirurgica Scandinavica, 149:11–14.

Brooks, D.N. and McKinley, W. (1983). Personality and behavioral change after severe blunt head injury—A relative's view. Journal of Neurology, Neurosurgery, and Psychiatry, 46:336–44.

Brooks, C.M. and Peck, M.E. (1940). Effects of various cortical lesions on development of placing and hopping reactions in rats. Journal of Neurophysiology, 3:66–73.

Brooks, N. (1989). Defining Outcome. (Editorial). Brain Injury, 3:325–29.

Brooks, N., Aughton, M.E., Bond, M.R., Jones, P., and Rizvi, S. (1980). Cognitive sequelae in relationship to early indices of severity of brain damage after severe blunt injury. Journal of Neurology, Neurosurgery, and Psychiatry, 43:529–34.

Brooks, N., Campsie, L., Symington, C., Beattie, A., and McKinlay, W. (1986). The five year outcome of severe blunt head injury: A relative's view. Journal of Neurology, Neurosurgery, and Psychiatry, 49:764-70.

Brooks, N., Symington, C., Beattie, A., Campsie, L., Bryden, J., and McKinlay, W. (1989). Alcohol and other predictors of cognitive recovery after severe head injury. Brain Injury, 3:235-46.

Bruckner, F.E. and Randle, P.H. (1972). Return to work after severe head injuries. Rheumatology and Physical Medicine, 11:344-48. Bryden, M.P. (1982). Laterality. New York: Academic Press.

Burton, L.A. and Volpe, B.T. (1988). Sex differences in emotional status of traumatically brain-injured patients. Journal of Neurological Rehabilitation, 2:151-57.

Calsyn, D.A., Louks, J.L., and Johnson, J.S. (1982). MMPI correlates of the degree of generalized impairment based on the Halstead-Reitan Battery. Perceptual and Motor Skills, 55:1099-102.

Calloway, E., Tueting, T., and Kaslo, S.H. (eds). (1978). Event Related Potentials in Man. New York: Plenum Press.

Caplan, P.J., McPherson, G.M., and Tobin, P. (1985). Do sex-related differences in spatial abilities exist? A multilevel critique with new data. American Psychologist, 40:786-99.

Carlsson, C.A., van Essen, C., and Lofgren, J. (1968). Factors affecting the clinical course of patients with severe head injury. Journal of Neurosurgery, 29:242-51.

Carlsson, G.S., Svardsudd, K., and Welin, L. (1987). Long-term effects of head injuries sustained during life in three male populations. Journal of Neurosurgery, 67:197-205.

Clifton, G.L., Ziegler, M.G., and Crossman, R.G. (1981). Circulating catecholamines and sympathetic activity after head injury. Neurosurgery, 8:10-14.

Coran, S. (1989). Left-handedness and accident-related injury risk. American Journal of Public Health, 79:1040-41.

Cracco, R.Q. and Cracco, J.B. (1976). Somatosensory evoked potentials in man: Farfield potentials. Electroencephalography and Clinical Neurophysiology, 41:460-66.

de Lacoste-Utamsing, C., and Holloway, R.L. (1982). Sexual dimorphism in the human corpus callosum. Science, 216:1431-32.

De La Torre, J.C., Trimble, J.L., Beard, R.T., Hanlon, K., and Surgeon, J.W. (1978). Somatosensory evoked potentials for the prognosis of coma in humans. Experimental Neurology, 60:304-17.

Denker, S.J. (1958). A follow-up study of 120 closed head injuries in twins using co-twins as controls. Acta Psychiatrica Scandinavica, Supplement, 123:1-125.

De Vries, G.J., De Bruin, J.P.C., Uylings, H.B.M., and Corner, M.A. (eds). (1984). Sex differences in the brain: The relation between structure and function. Progress in Brain Research. Vol. 61. Amsterdam: Elsevier Science Publishers.

Diamond, R., Barth, J.T., and Zillmer, E.A. (1988). Emotional correlates of mild closed head trauma: The role of the MMPI. The International Journal of Clinical Neuropsychology, 10:35-40.

Dikmen, S. and Reitan, R.M. (1977). MMPI correlates of adaptive ability deficits in patients with brain lesions. The Journal of Nervous and Mental Disease, 165:247-54.

Dikmen, S. and Reitan, R.M. (1978). Emotional sequelae of head injury. Annals of Neurology, 2:492-94.

Dresser, A.C., Meirowsky, A.M., Weiss, G.H., McNeel, M.L., Simon, G.A., and Caveness, W.F. (1973). Gainful employment following head injury. Archives of Neurology, 29:111-16.

Edna, T.H. (1982). Alcohol influence and head injury. Acta Chirurgica Scandinavica, 148:209-12.

Ehle, A.L., Stewart, R.M., Lellelid, N.A., and Levinthal, N.A. (1984). Evoked potentials in Huntington's Disease: A comparative and longitudinal study. Archives of Neurology, 41:379–82.

Elmer, O. and Lim, R. (1985). Influence of acute alcohol intoxication on the outcome of severe nonneurologic trauma. Acta Chirurgica Scandinavica, 151:305–08.

Elmer, O., Goransson, G., and Zoucas, E. (1984). Impairment of primary haemostasis and platelet function after alcohol ingestion in man. Haemostasis, 14:223–28.

Fahy, T.J., Irving, M.H., and Millac, P. (1967). Severe head injuries. Lancet, 1:475–79.

Field, J.H. (1976). Epidemiology of head injury in England and Wales: With particular application to rehabilitation. Leicester: Printed for H.M. Stationary Office by Wilsons.

Filley, C.M., Cranberg, L.D., Alexander, M.P., and Hart, E.J. (1987). Neurobehavioral outcome after closed head injury in childhood and adolescence. Archives of Neurology, 44:194–98.

Flaherty, C.F., Powell, G., and Hamilton, L.W. (1979). Septal lesions, sex and incentive shift effects on open field behavior. Physiology and Behavior, 22:903–09.

Folstein, M.F., Maiberger, R., and McHugh, P.R. (1977). Mood disorder as a specific complication of stroke. Journal of Neurology, Neurosurgery, and Psychiatry, 40:1018–20.

Fordyce, D.J., Roueche, J.R., and Prigatano, G.P. (1983). Enhanced emotional reactions in chronic head trauma patients. Journal of Neurology, Neurosurgery, and Psychiatry, 46:620–24.

Fuld, P.A. and Fisher, P. (1977). Recovery of intellectual ability after head injury. Developmental Medicine and Child Neurology, 19:495–502.

Gainotti, G. Emotional behavior and hemispheric side of the brain. Cortex, 8:41–55.

Galbraith, S., Murray, W.R., Patel, A.R., and Knill-Jones, R. (1976). The relationship between alcohol and head injury and its effect on conscious level. British Journal of Surgery, 63:128–30.

Gandy, S.E., Snow, R.B., Zimmerman, R.D., and Deck, M.D.F. (1984). Cranial nuclear imaging in head trauma. Annals of Neurology, 16:254–57.

Gentry, L.R., Godersky, J.C., and Thompson, B.H. (1989). Traumatic brain stem injury: MR imaging. Radiology, 171:177–87.

Gilberstadt, H. and Farkas, E. (1961). Another look at MMPI profile types in multiple sclerosis. Journal of Consulting Psychology, 25:440–44.

Gilchrist, E. and Wilkinson, M. (1979). Some factors determining prognosis in young people with severe head injuries. Archives of Neurology, 36:355–59.

Goldman, P.S. (1974). An alternative to developmental plasticity: Heterology of CNS structures in infants and adults. In: Stein, D.G., Rosen, J.J., and Butters, N. (eds). Plasticity and Recovery from Brain Damage. New York: Academic Press, 149–74.

Gouchie, C. and Kimura, D. (1991). The relationship between testosterone levels and cognitive ability patterns. Psychoneuroendocrinology, 16:323–34.

Gould, E., Woolley, C.S., Frankfurt, M., and McEwen, B.S. (1990). Gonadal steroids regulate dendritic spine density in hippocampal pyramidal cells in adulthood. Journal of Neuroscience, 10:1286–91.

Goy, R.W. and McEwen, B.S. (1980). Sexual Differentiation of the Brain. Cambridge, MA: M.I.T. Press.

Greenberg, R.P. and Becker, D.P. (1975). Clinical applications and results of evoked potential data in patients with severe head injury. Surgical Forum, 26:484–86.

Greenberg, R.P., Mayer, D.J., Becker, D.P., and Miller, J.D. (1977). Evaluation of brain function in severe human head trauma with multimodality evoked potentials. 1. Evoked brain injury potentials method and analysis. 2. Localization of brain dysfunction. Journal of Neurosurgery, 47:150–62.

Greenberg, R.P., Becker, D.P., Miller, J.D., and Mayer, D.J. (1977). Evaluation of brain function in severe human head trauma with multimodality evoked potentials. Part 2: Localization of brain dysfunction and correlation with posttraumatic neurological conditions. Journal of Neurosurgery, 47:163-77.

Greenberg, R.P., Newlon, P.G., Hyatt, M.S., Narayan, R.K., and Becker, D.P. (1981). Prognostic implications of early multimodality evoked potentials in severe head injury patients: A prospective study. Journal of Neurosurgery, 55:227-36.

Gronwell, D. and Wrightson, P. (1980). Duration of posttraumatic amnesia after mild head injury. Journal of Clinical Neuropsychology, 2:51-60.

Groswasser, Z., Cohen, M., and Costeff, H. (1989). Rehabilitation outcome after anoxic brain damage. Archives of Physical and Medical Rehabilitation, 70:186-88.

Haas, J.F., Cope, D.N., and Hall, K. (1987). Premorbid prevalence of poor academic performance in severe head injury. Journal of Neurology, Neurosurgery, and Psychiatry, 50:52-56.

Hadden, W. and Bradess, V.A. (1959). Alcohol in the single vehicle fatal accident. Journal of the American Medical Association, 169:1587-93.

Hampson, E. (1990). Estrogen-related variations in human spatial and articulatory-motor skills. Psychoneuroendocrinology, 15:97-111.

Han, J.S., Kaufman, B., Alfidi, R.J., Yeung, H.N., Benson, J.E., Haaga, J.R., El Yousef, S.J., Clampitt, M.M., Bonstelle, C.T., and Huss, R. (1984). Head trauma evaluated by magnetic resonance and computerized tomography: A comparison. Radiology, 150:71-77.

Harlow, H.F., Blumquist, A.J., Thompson, C.I., Schlitz, K.A., and Harlow, M.K. (1968). Behavioral and anatomical sequelae of damage to the infant limbic system. In: Isaacson, R.L. (ed). The Neuropsychology of Development: A Symposium. New York: John Wiley and Sons.

Hecaen, H. (1979). Cortical areas involved in spatial function. Behavioral and Brain Sciences, 2:503-04.

Honkanen, R., Eratma, L., Linnoila, M., Alha, A., Lukkari, I., Karlsson, M., Kiviluoto, O., and Puro, M. (1980). Role of drugs in traffic accidents. British Medical Journal, 281:1309-12.

Hook, O. (1976). Rehabilitation. In: Vinken, P.J. and Bruyn, G.W. (eds). Handbook of Clinical Neurology. Amsterdam: North-Holland Publishing Company, 683-97.

Hossack, D.W. (1972). Investigation of 400 people killed in road accidents with special reference to blood alcohol levels. Medical Journal of Australia, 2:255-58.

Howard, J. (1952). Transactions of the First Conference on Shock and Circulatory Homeostasis. New York: Colies, Macy.

Humphrey, M. and Oddy, M. (1981). Return to work after head injury: A review of postwar studies. Injury, 12:107-14.

Huth, J.F., Maier, R.V., Simonowitz, D.A., and Herman, C.M. (1983). Effect of acute ethanolism on the hospital course and outcome of injured automobile drivers. Journal of Trauma, 23:494-98.

Inglis, J. and Lawson, J.S. (1981). Sex differences in the effects of unilateral brain damage on intelligence. Science, 212:113-16.

Jaggi, J.L., Obrist, W.D., Gennarelli, T.A., and Langfitt, T.W. (1990). Relationship of early cerebral blood flow and metabolism to outcome in acute head injury. Journal of Neurosurgery, 72:176-82.

Jamieson, K.G. and Kelly, D. (1973). Crash helmets reduce head injuries. The Medical Journal of Australia, 2:806-09.

Jennett, B. and Teasdale, G. (1981). Management of head injuries. Philadelphia: F.A. Davis Company.

Jennett, B., Snoek, J., Bond, M.R., and Brooks, N. (1981). Disability after severe head injury: Observations on the use of the Glasgow Outcome Scale. Journal of Neurology, Neurosurgery, and Psychiatry, 44:285-93.

Jennett, B., Teasdale, G., Braakman, R., Minderhoud, J., and Knill-Jones, R. (1976). Predicting outcome in individual patients after severe head injury. Lancet, 1:878-81.

Jennett, B., Teasdale, G., Braakman, R., Minderhoud, J., Heiden, J., and Kurze, T. (1979). Prognosis of patients with severe head injury. Neurosurgery, 4:283-89.

Jennett, B., Teasdale, G., Galbraith, S., Pickard, J., Grant, H., Braakman, R., Avezaat, C., Maas, A., Minderhoud, J., Vecht, C.J., Heiden, J., Small, R., Caton, W., and Kurze, T. (1977). Severe head injuries in three countries. Journal of Neurology, Neurosurgery, and Psychiatry, 40:291-98.

Jick, H., Hunter, J.R., Dinan, B.J., Madsen, S., and Stergachis, A. (1981). Sedating drugs and automobile accidents leading to hospitalization. American Journal of Public Health, 71:1399-1400.

Johnson, D. and Almli, C.R. (1978). Age, brain damage, and performance. In: Finger, S. (ed). Recovery From Brain Damage. New York: Plenum Press.

Jordan, B.D. and Zimmerman, R.D. (1990). Computed tomography and magnetic resonance imaging comparisons in boxers. Journal of the American Medical Association, 12:1670-74.

Karnaze, D.S., Marshall, L.F., McCarthy, C.S., Klauber, M.R., and Bickford, R.G. (1980). Localizing and prognostic value of auditory evoked responses in coma after closed head injury. Neurology, 32:299-302.

Kennard, M.A. (1936). Age and other factors in motor recovery from precentral lesions in monkeys. American Journal of Physiology, 115:138-46.

Kennard, M.A. (1938). Reorganization of motor function in the cerebral cortex of monkeys deprived of motor and premotor areas in infancy. Journal of Neurophysiology, 1:477-97.

Kennard, M.A. (1940). Relation of age to motor impairment in man and in subhuman primates. Archives of Neurology and Psychiatry, 44:377-97.

Kennard, M.A. (1942). Cortical reorganization of motor functions. Studies on series of monkeys of various ages from infancy to maturity. Archives of Neurology and Psychiatry, 48:227-40.

Kerr, T.A., Kay, D.W.K., and Lassman, L.P. (1971). Characteristics of patients, type of accident, and mortality in a consecutive series of head injuries admitted to a neurosurgical unit. British Journal of Preventative and Social Medicine, 25:179-85.

Klonoff, H. (1971). Head injuries in children: Predisposing factors, accident conditions, accident proneness and sequelae. American Journal of Public Health, 61:2405-17.

Klove, H. and Cleeland, C.S. (1972). The relationship of neuropsychological impairment to other indices of severity of head injury. Scandinavian Journal of Rehabilitation Medicine, 4:55-60.

Kobrine, A.I., Timmins, E., Rajjoub, R.K., Rizzoli, H.V., and Davis, D.O. (1977). Demonstration of massive traumatic brain swelling within 20 minutes after injury. Case Report. Journal of Neurosurgery, 46:256-58.

Kolb, B. (1987). Recovery from early cortical damage in rats. 1. Differential behavior and anatomical effects of frontal lesions at different ages of maturation. Behavioral Brain Research, 25:205-20.

Kolb, B. (1989). Brain development, plasticity and behavior. American Psychologist, 9:1203-12.

Kozol, H.L. (1945). Pretraumatic personality and psychiatric sequelae of head injury. Archives of Neurology and Psychiatry, 53:358-64.

Kwentus, J.A., Hart, R.P., Peck, E.T., and Kornstein, S. (1985). Psychiatric complications of closed head trauma. Psychosomatics, 26:8-17.

Langfitt, T.W. (1978). Measuring outcome from head injuries. Journal of Neurosurgery, 48:673-78.

Lanksch, W., Grumme, T., and Kazner, E. (1979). Computed Tomography in Head Injuries. New York: Springer-Verlag.

Leavitt, F. (1974). Drugs and behavior. Philadelphia: W.B. Saunders Company.

Levati, A., Farina, M.L., Vecchi, G., Rossanda, M., and Marrubini, M.B. (1982). Prognosis of severe head injuries. Journal of Neurosurgery, 57:779-83.

Levin, H.S. and Grossman, R.G. (1978). Behavioral sequelae of closed head injury: A quantitative study. Archives of Neurology, 35:720-27.

Levin, H.S., Benton, A.L., and Grossman, R.G. (1982). Neurobehavioral Consequences of Closed Head Injury. New York: Oxford University Press.

Levin, H.S., Ewing-Cobles, L., and Benton, A.L. (1984). Age and recovery from brain damage: A review of clinical studies. In: Scheff, S.W. (ed). Aging and recovery of function in the central nervous system. New York: Plenum Press.

Levin, H.S., Grossman, R.G., Rose, J.E., and Teasdale, G. (1979). Long-term neuropsychological outcome of closed head injury. Journal of Neurosurgery, 50:412-22.

Levin, H.S., O'Donnell, V.M., and Grossman, R.O. (1979). The Galveston Orientation and Amnesia Test. A practical scale to assess cognition after head injury. Journal of Nervous and Mental Disease, 167:675-84.

Lishman, W.A. (1973). The psychiatric sequelae of head injury: A review. Psychological Medicine, 3:304-18.

Loberg, T. (1986). Neuropsychological findings in the early and middle phases of alcoholism. In: Grant, I. and Adam, K. (eds). Neuropsychological Assessment of Neuropsychiatric Disorders. New York: Oxford University Press, 415-40.

Loy, R. and Milner, T.A. (1980). Sexual dimorphism in extent of axonal sprouting in the rat hippocampus. Science, 208:1282-84.

Luna, G.K., Maier, R.V., Sowder, L., Copass, M.K., and Oreskovich, M.R. (1984). The influence of ethanol intoxication on outcome of injured motorcyclists. Journal of Trauma, 24:695-700.

Luria, A.R. (1970). Traumatic aphasia. The Hague: Mouton.

MacNiven, E. and Finlayson, M.A.J. (1990a). Sex differences in emotional status and cognitive recovery after closed head injury. The Clinical Neuropsychologist, 4:305.

MacNiven, E. and Finlayson, M.A.J. (1992). The interplay between emotional and cognitive recovery after closed head injury. Brain Injury, 6 (in press).

MacNiven, E., and Finlayson, M.A.J. (1990c). Sex differences in emotional status and cognitive recovery after closed head injury. The Clinical Neuropsychologist, 4:305.

Markwalder, T. (1981). Chronic subdural hematomas: A review. Journal of Neurosurgery, 54:637-45.

Marsh, N.V., Knight, R.G., and Godfrey, H.P.D. (1990). Long-term psychosocial adjustment following very severe closed head injury. Neuropsychology, 4:13-27.

McGlone, J. (1978). Sex differences in functional brain asymmetry. Cortex, 14:122-28.

McGlone, J. (1980). Sex differences in human brain organization: A critical survey. Behavioural and Brain Sciences, 3:215-27.

McQueen, J. and Posey, J. (1975). Changes in intracranial pressure and brain hydration during acute ethanolism. Surgical Neurology, 4:375-79.

Meier, M.J., Strauman, S., and Thompson, W.G. (1987). Individual differences in neuropsychological recovery: An overview. In: Meier, M.J., Benton, A., and Diller, L. (eds). Neuropsychological Rehabilitation. New York: The Guilford Press, 70-110.

Miller, J.D., Sweet, R.G., Narayan, R., and Becker, D.P. (1978). Early insults in the injured brain. Journal of the American Medical Association, 240:439-42.

Milner, G. (1977). Marijuana and driving hazards. Medical Journal of Australia, 1:208-11.

Moore, A.D., Stambrooke, M., Peters, L.C., Cardoso, E.R., and Kassum, D.A. (1990). Long-term multi-dimensional outcome following isolated traumatic brain injuries and traumatic brain injuries associated with multiple trauma. Brain Injury, 4:379-89.

Morse, J.K., Scheff, S.W., and DeKosky, S.T. (1986). Gonadal steroids influence axon sprouting in the hippocampal dentate gyrus: A sexually dimorphic response. Experimental Neurology, 96:649-58.

Najenson, T., Mendelson, L., Schecter, I., Daviv, C., Mintz, N., and Groswasser, Z. (1974). Rehabilitation after severe head injury. Scandinavian Journal of Rehabilitation Medicine, 6:5-14.

Narayan, R.J., Greenberg, R.P., Miller, J.D., Enas, G.G., Choi, S.C., Kishore, P.R.S., Selhorst, J.B., Lutz, H.A., and Becker, D.P. (1981). Improved confidence of outcome prediction in severe head injury. Journal of Neurosurgery, 54:751-62.

Neilson, P.M. and Alfano, D.P. (1990). Sex-related differences in emotionality after brain injury. Journal of Clinical and Experimental Neuropsychology, 12:52.

Newlon, P.G. and Greenberg, R.P. (1984). Assessment of brain function with multimodality evoked potentials. In: Rosenthal, M., Griffith, E.R., Bond, M.R., and Miller, J.D. (eds). Rehabilitation of the head injured adult. Philadelphia: F.A. Davis, 75-96.

Newlon, P.G., Greenberg, R.P., Hyatt, M.S., Enas, G.C., and Becker, D.P. (1982). The dynamics of neuronal dysfunction and recovery following severe head injury assessed with serial multimodality evoked potentials. Journal of Neurosurgery, 57:168-77.

Nockleby, D.M., and Deaton, A.V. (1987). Denial versus distress: Coping patterns in post head trauma patients. The International Journal of Clinical Neuropsychology, 9:145-48.

Obrist, W.D. Gennarelli, T.A., Segawa, H. Dolinskas, C.A., and Langfitt, T.W. (1979). Relation of cerebral blood flow to neurological status and outcome in head-injured patients. Journal of Neurosurgery, 51:292-300.

Overgaard, J., Hvid-Hansen, O., Land, A.M., Pedersen, K.K., Christensen, S., Haase, J., Hein, O., and Tweed, W.A. (1973). Prognosis after head injury based on early clinical examination. Lancet, 2:631-35.

Papez, J.W. (1937). A proposed mechanism for emotion. Archives of Neurology and Psychiatry, 38:725-43.

Pascuale-Leone, A., Dhuna, A., Altfullah, I., and Anderson, D.C. (1990). Cocaine-induced seizures. Neurology, 40:404-07.

Passingham, R.E., Perry, V.H., and Wilkinson, F. (1983). The long-term effects of removal of sensorimotor cortex in infant and adult rhesus monkeys. Brain, 106:675-705.

Perot, P.L. (1973). The clinical use of somatosensory evoked potentials in spinal cord injury. Clinical Neurosurgery, 20:367-81.

Porac, C. and Coran, S. (1981). Lateral Preferences and Human Behavior. New York: Springer-Verlag.

Prigatano, G. and Fordyce, D. (1986). Cognitive dysfunction and psychosocial adjustment after brain injury, In: Prigatano, G.P. (ed). Neuropsychological rehabilitation after brain injury. Baltimore: Johns Hopkins University Press, 1-17.

Rappaport, M., Hall, K., Hopkins, K., Bellaza, T., Berrol, S., and Reynolds, G. (1977). Evoked brain potentials and disability in brain damaged patients. Archives of Physical and Medical Rehabilitation, 58:333-38.

Rappaport, M., Hopkins, K., Hall, K., Bellaza, T., Berrol, S., and Reynolds, G. (1978). Brain evoked potential use in a physical, medical and rehabilitation setting. Scandinavian Journal of Rehabilitation Medicine, 10:27-32.

Rocca, B., Martin, C., Viviand, X., Bidet, P.F., Saint-Gilles, H.L., and Chevalier, A. (1989). Comparison of four severity scores in patients with head trauma. The Journal of Trauma, 29:299-305.

Robinson, R.G. and Szetela, B. (1981). Mood change following left hemispheric brain injury. Annals of Neurology, 9:447-53.

Roof, R.L., Duvdevani, R., and Stein, D.C. (1992). Gender influences outcome of brain injury: Progesterone plays a protective role. Presented at the 22nd Annual Meeting of the Society for Neuroscience. Anaheim, CA, October, 1992.

Rosenzweig, M.R. (1984). Experience, memory and the brain. American Psychologist, 39:365-76.

Rubens, A.B., Geschwind, N., Mahowald, M.W., and Mastri, A. (1977). Posttraumatic hemispheric disconnection syndrome. Archives of Neurology, 34:750-55.

Ruesch, J. (1944). Intellectual impairment in head injuries. American Journal of Psychiatry, 100:480-96.

Ruesch, J. and Bowman, K. (1945). Prolonged posttraumatic syndromes following head injury. American Journal of Psychiatry, 102:145-63.

Ruff, R.M., Cullum, C.M., and Luerssen, T.G. (1989). Brain imaging and neuropsychological outcome in traumatic brain injury. In: Bigler, E.D., Yeo, R.A., and Turkheimer, E. (eds). Neuropsychological function and brain imaging. New York: Plenum Press, 161-83.

Rusk, H.A., Block, J.M., and Lowman, E.W. (1969). Rehabilitation of the brain-injured patient: A report of 157 cases with long-term follow-up of 118. In: Walker, A.E., Caveness, W.F., and Critchley, M. (eds). The late effects of head injury. Springfield: Charles C. Thomas, 327-32.

Russell, W.R. (1932). Cerebral involvement in head injury. Brain, 55:549-603.

Russell, W.R. (1934). The after-effects of head injury. Edinburgh Medical Journal, 41:129-41.

Russell, W.R. (1935). Amnesia following head injuries. Lancet, 2:762-63.

Russell, W.R. and Nathan, P.W. (1946). Traumatic Amnesia. Brain, 69:183-87.

Russell, W.R. and Smith, A. (1961). Posttraumatic amnesia in closed head injury. Archives of Neurology, 5:4-17.

Rutter, M. (1981). Psychological sequelae of brain damage in children. American Journal of Psychiatry, 183:1533-49.

Sarno, J.E., Sarno, M.T., and Levita, E. (1971). Evaluating language improvement after completed stroke. Archives of Physical Medicine and Rehabilitation, 52:73-78.

Schacter, D.L. and Crovitz, H.F. (1977). Memory function after closed head injury: A review of the quantitative research. Cortex, 13:150-76.

Seales, W., Rossiter, V.S., Weinstein, M.E., and Spencer, J.D. (1979). Brainstem auditory evoked responses in patients comatose as a result of blunt head injury. Journal of Trauma, 19:347-53.

Shaffer, D., Chadwick, O., and Rutter, M. (1975). Psychiatric outcome of localized head injury in children. In: Porter, R. and Fitzsimons, D.W. (eds). Outcome of severe damage to the central nervous system. Ciba Foundation Symposium 34. Amsterdam: Elsevier/Excerptica Medica/North Holland.

Shores, E.A. (1989). Comparison of the Westmead PTA Scale and Glasgow Coma Scale as predictors of neuropsychological outcome following extremely severe blunt head injury. Journal of Neurology, Neurosurgery, and Psychiatry, 52:126-38.

Shores, E.A., Marosszeky, J.E., Sandanam, J., and Batchelor, J. (1986). Preliminary validation of a clinical scale for measuring the duration of posttraumatic amnesia. The Medical Journal of Australia, 144:569-72.

Sisler, G. and Penner, H. (1975). Amnesia following severe head injury. Canadian Psychiatry Association Journal, 20:333-36.

Skegg, D.C.G., Richards, S.M., and Doll, R. (1979). Minor tranquilisers and road accidents. British Medical Journal, 1:917-19.

Smith, A. (1981). Principles underlying human brain functions in neuropsychological sequelae of different neuropathological processes. In: Filskov, S.B. and Boll, T.J. (eds). Handbook of clinical neuropsychology. New York: John Wiley and Sons, 175-226.

Snoek, J., Jennett, B., Adams, Graham, D.I., and Doyle, D. (1979). Computerised tomography after recent severe head injury in patients without acute intracranial haematoma. Journal of Neurology, Neurosurgery, and Psychiatry, 42:215-115.

Sparedo, F.R. and Gill, D. (1989). Effects of prior alcohol use on head injury recovery. Journal of Head Trauma Rehabilitation, 4:75–82.

Springer, S. and Deutsch, G. (1981). Left brain, right brain. San Francisco: W.H. Freeman.

Stanczak, D.E., White, J.G., Gouview, W.D., Moehle, K.A., Daniel, M., Novack, T., and Long, C.J. (1984). Assessment of level of consciousness following severe neurological insult. Journal of Neurosurgery, 60:955–60.

Stein, D.G. (1974). Some variables influencing recovery of function after central nervous system lesions in the rat. In: Stein, D.G., Rosen, J.J., and Butters, N. (eds). Plasticity and recovery of function in the central nervous system. New York: Academic Press.

Stewart, J. and Kolb, B. (1988). The effects of neonatal gonadectomy and prenatal stress on cortical thickness and asymmetry in rats. Behavioral and Neural Biology, 49:244–60.

Stritch, S. (1961). Shearing of nerve fibers as a cause of brain damage due to head injury: A pathological study of twenty cases. Lancet, 2:443–48.

Subirana, A. (1958). The prognosis in aphasia in relation to cerebral dominance and handedness. Brain, 81:415–25.

Symonds, C.P. and Russell, W.R. (1943). Accidental head injuries. Lancet, 1:7–12.

Tarter, R. and Edwards, K. (1985). Neuropsychology of alcoholism. In: Tarter, R. and Van Thiel, D. (eds). Alcohol and the brain: Chronic effects. New York: The Guilford Press, 76–102.

Teasdale, G. and Jennett, B. (1974). Assessment of coma and impaired consciousness: A practical scale. Lancet, 2:81–83.

Teasdale, G. and Jennett, B. (1976). Assessment and prognosis of coma after head injury. Acta Neurochirurgica, 34:45–55.

Teasdale, G., Knill-Jones, R., and Van Der Sande, J. (1978). Observer reliability in assessing impaired consciousness and coma. Archives of Neurology, Neurosurgery, and Psychiatry, 41:603–10.

Thomsen, I.V. (1989). Do young patients have worse outcomes after severe blunt head injury? Brain Injury, 3:157–62.

Timming, R., Orrison, W.W., and Mikula, J.A. (1982). Computerized tomography and rehabilitation outcome after severe head trauma. Archives of Physical Medicine and Rehabilitation, 63:154–59.

Tsuang, M.T., Boor, M., and Fleming, J.A. (1985). Psychiatric aspects of traffic accidents. American Journal of Psychiatry, 142:538–46.

Uzzell, B.P., Zimmerman, R.A., Dolinskas, C.A., and Obrist, W.D. (1979). Lateralized psychological impairment associated with CT lesions in head injury patients. Cortex, 15:391–401.

van Dongen, H.R. and Loolen, M.C.B. (1977). Factors related to prognosis of acquired aphasia in children. Cortex, 13:131–36.

Van Woerkom, T.C.A.M., Teelken, A.W., and Minderhound, J.M. (1977). Difference in neurotransmitter metabolism in frontotemporal-lobe contusion and diffuse cerebral contusion. Lancet, 1:812–13.

Vogenthaler, D.R., Smith, K.R. Jr., and Goldfader, P. (1989). Head injury, an empirical study: Describing long-term productivity and independent living outcome. Brain Injury, 3:355–68.

Vogenthaler, D.R., Smith, K.R. Jr., and Goldfader, P. (1989). Head injury, multivariate study: Predicting long-term productivity and independent living outcome. Brain Injury, 3:369–85.

Volpe, B.T. and McDowell, F.H. (1990). The efficacy of cognitive rehabilitation in patients with traumatic brain injury. Archives of Neurology, 47:220–22.

Wada, J. (1976). Cerebral anatomical asymmetry in infant brains. Symposium on sex differences in brain asymmetry. Presented at meeting of the International Neuropsychological Society, Toronto, Ontario.

Ward, A.A. (1966). The physiology of concussion. In: Caveness, W.F. and Walker, A.E. (eds). Head injury, conference proceedings. Philadelphia: Lippincott, 203-08.

Ward, R.E., Flynn, T.C., Miller, P.W., and Blaisddell, W.F. (1982). Effects of ethanol ingestion on the severity and outcome of trauma. The American Journal of Surgery, 144: 153-57.

Wilson, J.T.L. (1990). The relationship between neuropsychological function and brain damage detected by neuroimaging after closed head injury. Brain Injury, 4:349-63.

Williamson, P.D., Goff, W.R., and Allison, T. (1970). Somatosensory evoked responses in patients with unilateral cerebral lesion. Electroencephalography and Clinical Neurophysiology, 28:566-75.

Witelson, S.F. (1987). Neurobiological aspects of language in children. Child Development, 58:653-88.

Witelson, S.F. (1989). Hand and sex differences in the isthmus and genu of the human corpus callosum. Brain, 112:799-835.

Witelson, S.F. and Pallie, W. (1973). Left hemisphere specialization for language in the newborn. Brain, 96:641-46.

Wittig, M.A. and Petersen, A.C. (eds.) (1979). Sex-related differences in cognitive functioning. New York: Academic Press.

Woods, B.T. (1980). The restricted effects of right-hemisphere lesions after age one: Weschler test data. Neuropsychologia, 18:65-70.

Woods, B.T. and Teuber, H.L. (1978). Changing patterns of childhood aphasia. Annals of Neurology, 3:273-80.

World Health Organization. (1980). International Classification of Impairments, Disabilities, and Handicaps. Geneva: World Health Organization.

Zimmerman, R.A., Bilaniuk, L.T., Dolinskas, C., Gennerralli, T., Bruce, D., and Uzzell, B. (1977). Computed tomography of acute intracerebral hemorrhagic contusion. Computed Axial Tomography, 1:271-80.

5

Medical Management and Principles of Head Injury Rehabilitation

SCOTT H. GARNER
ALEX B. VALADKA

Clinical management of patients with an acquired brain injury requires an understanding of the mechanisms of brain injury, the mechanisms of recovery, and the nature of the learning process. The usual sequence of clinical care includes the stages of acute medical management, early rehabilitation (usually in a specialized rehabilitation setting), and progressive community reintegration. The ultimate goal of rehabilitation is to enable the patient to resume normal living. As Willer points out (Chapter 16), the main goal of rehabilitation should be to reduce "handicap" and to enable the person to resume community living with as much freedom and independence as possible.

Provision of care after head injury has to resolve two antithetical tendencies. Medical management addresses biologic issues and utilizes an approach which seeks to understand and then "fix" the problem. Interventions are done "to" the patient and the approach tends to encourage an attitude of passivity on the part of the patient. Effective rehabilitation demands a different approach. Rehabilitation clinicians seek to improve responsiveness to environmental stimuli, and then elicit active participation in programs which are often demanding, and (contrary to usual institutional medical environments) require effort. Passivity is the "enemy" in the rehabilitation process. Early medical care is oriented to addressing "impairment" issues; rehabilitation must address impairment, disability, and handicap issues. The ultimate concern is to reduce handicap and, although this may be indirectly addressed by treating impairments and disabilities, directly addressing the issues which prevent successful community reintegration should be the most effective. This latter stage is often neglected in traditional rehabilitation. Early treatment focuses on saving life and minimizing the extent of brain injury. This care is delivered by medical staff in an acute care setting in a hospital environment. Rehabilitation, on the other hand, requires a broad range of approaches, particularly at later stages of recovery. A wide array of impairments and disabilities may be present, and appropriate management requires a flexible approach oriented both to the individual's needs and to the demands of the ultimate discharge environment. This may require delivery of service in a variety of institutional or community settings.

MEDICAL MANAGEMENT AFTER SEVERE INJURY

Early medical intervention attempts to attenuate the pathobiologic sequelae of trauma. It does this by keeping in mind two principles: 1) the immediate correction of conditions causing ongoing neuronal damage (see Chapter 2), and 2) prevention of physiologic extremes that may result in secondary insults to a nervous system that is rendered less resistant to such hypotic or hypotensive insults because of the initial trauma.

Early Management

Severity of traumatic brain injury (TBI) is based on the patient's initial score on the Glasgow Coma Scale (GCS) (Teasdale and Jennett, 1974). Mild TBI is generally defined as a GCS score of 13–15; moderate TBI as a GCS of 9–12; and severe TBI as a GCS of 8 or less. Most patients in the latter group are frequently described as comatose, i.e., displaying no signs of arousal or awareness.

Care of victims of TBI begins with the ABC's, i.e., Airway, Breathing, and Circulation. Comatose patients require immediate creation of a secure airway, either with endotracheal intubation or via cricothyroidotomy, to assure adequate ventilation and to protect against aspiration. If the patient is coherent enough to speak and to obey commands, intubation is often withheld if the respiratory and cardiovascular systems are functioning adequately. At the minimum, however, supplemental oxygen is usually used in these cases (Stewart, 1990).

Ventilation

Patients whose respirations appear suboptimal require artificial ventilation at a normal rate in order to assure adequate oxygenation with normocapnia or only minimal hypocapnia. Since the cerebral vascular bed is exquisitely sensitive to the amount of carbon dioxide (CO_2) dissolved in the blood, aggressive hyperventilation can cause a marked reduction in arterial pCO_2, which results in cerebral vasoconstriction. In the short-term, this may cause a decrease in intracranial blood volume, which can lower intracranial pressure (ICP). Such hyperventilation is merely a temporary measure, implemented only until other methods to lower ICP are put into play. When maintained for a prolonged continuous period, excessive hyperventilation may prove harmful and has been associated with a worsened neurological outcome (Ward, et al., 1989).

Cardiovascular

Maintenance of an adequate intravascular volume via infusion of crystalloid or colloid solutions through several large-bore peripheral lines and/or central venous catheter is essential to prevent secondary cerebral insult.

Early Emergency Room Care

Early care often requires steps to rule out significant concurrent injury. These steps ususally include: 1) Chest, pelvis, and cervical spine x-rays; 2) Blood tests with arterial blood gas ascertainment; 3) Insertion of Foley catheter; and, 4) Diagnostic peritoneal lavage (Narayan, 1989). If the patient is suspected of harboring a mass lesion, a bolus of 1 mg/kg of 20% mannitol is administered. An emergency CT scan is done as soon as possible, but if a patient is hemodynamically unstable, then emergent measures to identify and treat serious intrathoracic or abdominal injury (e.g., aortic transection) are given priority. Modern CT scanners can image the entire brain in only a few seconds. If a significant hematoma is identified, then the patient is immediately taken to the operating room for surgical evacuation. In most cases, however, no mass lesion is evident, and the patient is transported directly to the intensive care unit for further monitoring.

Intensive Care Unit

In the intensive care unit, the main thrust of treatment becomes the prevention of secondary insults. Adequate monitoring of blood pressure and oxygenation is essential. Other basic principles of critical care include the prevention of lower extremity venous stasis, documentation of fluid intake and output, and protection of skin integrity through frequent turning or through the utilization of specialized beds that minimize local skin pressure. Adequate nutiritional support is begun as early as possible, since adequate nutrition helps with wound healing and maintains immunologic effectiveness against infection (Bucknall, 1984; Hunt, 1990). Enteral feedings are started with placement of a nasogastric or other tube, or if these are contraindicated, or feedings are not tolerated, then total parenteral nutrition is instituted via a central venous line. High serum glucose levels should be prevented as it has been suggested that high levels may result in further brain injury through the development of cerebral lactic acidosis (Siesjo, et al., 1985; Pulsinelli, et al., 1982; Becker and Gardner, 1985). Victims of severe traumatic brain injury may require intubation or mechanical ventilation for at least several days. If extubation is not possible after approximately 2 weeks, then tracheostomy is usually performed. Minimal hyperventilation is maintained to keep the pCO_2 at approximately 35 mm Hg during the period that ICP control remains a problem. Intracranial pressure monitoring is unique to neurologic critical care. Intracranial pressure is kept below 20 mm Hg, and several interventions may be required to accomplish this goal, such as sedation with a narcotic and/or administration of skeletal muscle relaxants (Miller, et al., 1977).

Intracranial Pressure Elevations

Intracranial pressure elevations require more aggressive treatment. This may include drainage of CSF, administration of mannitol, and administration of furosemide. If intracranial pressure is uncontrollable despite these measures, a follow-up CT scan is required to rule out delayed intracerebral hematomas. If no mass lesion is found, then more drastic steps as barbiturate coma or other surgical procedures (i.e., craniectomy) are done in some settings. Mild hypothermia is also occasionally used to provide cerebral protection and to lower intracranial pressure, but it is not recommended for routine use and is considered an investigational therapy at this time (Clifton, et al., 1992).

Seizures

Most neurosurgeons believe in aggressive pharmacologic prophylaxis against seizures. Diphenylhydantoin sodium (Dilantin) is commonly administered intravenously. After the patient can tolerate enteral medications, a switch to carbamazepine (Tegretol) is often preferred, since Tegretol is felt to cause less sedation and less interference with cognitive functioning (Smith, et al., 1987). However, this continues to be an area of controversy (Meador, et al., 1991). Prolonged treatment with Dilantin in situations where seizure risk is low is not recommended, and a recent controlled trial (Temkin, et al., 1990) suggests the benefit of phenytoin prophylaxis is limited to the first week.

Complications

As early complications are many, constant vigilance to potential problems is required. Adequate treatment of fevers, pulmonary aspiration, and posttraumatic seizures may help to prevent further insult to the central nervous system. To date, there are no pharmacologic interventions that have been shown to protect damaged neurons from further injury. Agents which act as CSF buffers (e.g., tromethamine), or other agents thought to act as free-radical scavengers, have not yet been shown to be of clinical benefit (Ward, et al., 1989). In summary, the acute management focuses on medical/surgical treatment to reverse impairments based on pathophysiologic disturbances caused by trauma. Early identification and removal of mass lesions and maintenance of homeostasis are primary goals of treatment. Aggressive interventions are usually required in patients with severe injuries, while the management of moderate and mild head injury is generally supportive.

Common Medical Issues During Rehabilitation

Medical problems are treated in the context of a comprehensive rehabilitation program. Vigilance to homeostasis provides the backdrop upon which other therapies are based. Ongoing homeostasis is achieved through adequate care of skin and adequate nutritional intake (with the use of enteral tube or TPN systems if needed). Avoidance of lung aspiration and protection of airway through use of tracheostomy tube may be required. Maintenance of joint range of motion, early removal of Foley catheters, and resumption of bowel function through bowel programs are general measures that need to be considered in most cases. Medical problems can occur in most organ systems and vigilance to the possibility of medical complications is required, particularly when progress fails to occur. Late deterioration requires consideration of current intracranial collections of fluid, development of cerebral infection with abscess development, and development of a dynamic hydrocephalus reflecting impaired or obstructive fluid flow. (Cope, et al., 1988; Kalisky, et al., 1985). In this section common medical problems briefly addressed include frequently seen neurologic, orthopaedic, and endocrine problems. Recent detailed medical reviews are also available (Rosenthal, et al., 1990).

Cranial Nerve Injury

Cranial nerve injury is common. Anosmia as a result of cranial nerve I injury may be present in up to 20% of patients (Berrol, 1989). Injury to cranial nerve III, IV, and VI can result in diplopia, and involvement of optic nerve and central visual tracts can result in field defects. Injury to cranial nerve VIII is common even in mild injuries, and hearing impairment, tinnitus, and vertigo are often disabling and a frequent source of frustration to patients. (Berrol, 1989).

Epilepsy

Epilepsy is an area of concern to patients, their families, and their physicians because of the potential impact on driving and vocation. Late posttraumatic epilepsy is noted more often in situations where there have been early seizures (first week after injury), focal cerebral injury in the setting of depressed skull fractures with dural penetration, focal neurologic signs, or posttraumatic amnesia lasting longer than 24 hours

(Jennett, 1990). As in early treatment, anticonvulsants other than phenytoin have been recommended for long-term treatment and current practice favors selection of carbamazepine and valproic acid over phenytoin or phenobarbital (Gualtieri, 1991). If prophylactic anticonvulsants have been continued inappropriately, then difficulty may arise if discontinuation is considered at later stages of recovery as patients are often reluctant to make changes which theoretically might increase their risk of seizures. This argues for medication withdrawal early in the recovery period if risk factors for seizures are low (see also Chapter 12).

Motor Disturbances

Motor disturbance and orthopaedic problems prevent mobilization and limit bed movement. It is not uncommon for appropriate orthopaedic intervention to be delayed because it is felt that the patient will not survive or fail to improve significantly to benefit from the intervention in question. This often results in inadequately treated fractures with resultant deformities and contractures which prevent resumption of mobility at later stages of recovery and then becomes a significant cause of disability (Yarkony, et al., 1987). Current treatment is characterized by aggressive orthopaedic operative interventions which minimizes the need for bed rest and allows activity as early as possible (Kernohan, 1984). Motor impairments are much more common than sensory impairment and caused by a variety of injuries to upper motor neuron, cerebellar, and basal ganglia structures. This can result in a variety of patterns of functional loss as well as excessive motor activity characterized by spasticity (Griffith, E.R., et al., 1990). (See Chapter 6.)

Spasticity

A comprehensive treatment approach to spasticity is as important in brain injury as it is in other disorders causing spasticity (Glenn and Whyte, 1990). This includes appropriate skin care, normalization of bladder and bowel function, and adequate nonforceful passive range of motion. Temperature modalities (heat and cold), vibration, and functional electrical stimulation may have a role in specific cases. Static or dynamic splints (splints or casts) are often helpful particularly when one joint or one extremity is problematic. More aggressive orthopaedic or neurosurgical interventions may be required at later stages of recovery if functional motor deficits are limiting independence. Management of spasticity with medication is problematic as the side effects of the front-line antispasticity medications available (i.e., diazepam, baclofen, and dantrolene) can affect cognition and thus prevent appropriate participation in the rehabilitation process. However, if generalized spasticity is present and causing progressive loss of range and interfering with functional motor activity, then dantrolene may be the most appropriate medication to try. Its mechanism of action is at the level of the muscle fiber and not as likely to affect cognitive function (Young, et al., 1981).

Heterotopic Ossification

Heterotopic ossification is a common musculoskeletal problem noted in the traumatic brain injury population with an incidence of 11%-20% (Garland, et al., 1983). Early treatment recommendations include nontraumatic range of motion and pharmacologic intervention with etidronate disodium or anti-inflammatory medication (such as Indomethacin or Ibuprofen). Prophylaxis with agents like etidronate disodium may have a role after severe injury (Spielman, et al., 1983). Surgical approaches are helpful but a delay of 12-18 months is usually recommended to allow adequate bone maturity to minimize the possibility of recurrence after resection (Garland, 1985). Postsurgical coverage with an anti-inflammatory medication is often recommended to prevent recurrence. Earlier resection would be helpful if recurrence could be prevented through other means, as delayed resection prevents patients from fully participating in rehabilitation and there may be shortening of the muscle and other periarticular tissue which often prevent satisfactory outcome. The role of low dose radiotherapy, which has been used successfully in preventing recurrence after surgical hip procedures, has not been addressed in this population but merits further investigation (Anthony, et al., 1989).

Endocrine

Endocrinologic complications are uncommon and when seen are a result of injury to hypothalamic and pituitary structures (Crompton, 1971). Pituitary and hypothalamic lesions have been noted in up to 50% of all cases of fatal head injury (Korblum, et al., 1969). An anterior pituitary workup is recommended in cases where endocrinologic symptoms are present, when recovery is poor, or when injury makes this lesion suspect (e.g., basal skull fracture) (Horn, et al., 1990). Posterior pituitary disorders are more common and widely recognized. Inappropriate ADH secretion may be a cause of hyponatremia and is usually an early problem (Ishakawa, et al., 1987) and one easily confounded by iatrogenic interventions like fluid loading or drug side effects. Diabetes insipidus is caused by a reduction in ADH secretion and results in hypernatremia and hyperosmolarity. Treatment of diabetes insipidus may be required with a synthetic ADH analog such as desmo-vasopressin acetate (DDAVP) via nasal insufflation.

POSTACUTE CARE

Principles of Rehabilitation

Prognostic outcome determinations are becoming more precise (see Chapter 4) but it is usually impossible to make absolute predictions about a given individual. Rehabilitation workers are usually reluctant to impose unproven limitations on a patient and prefer to allow him/her to define their own limitations by working to achieve all that can be accomplished. A network of clinical services are required to meet these goals because of the variety of problems encountered and the variety of social environments into which patients must be reintegrated (Woods and Eames, 1989). Service delivery varies, depending on the nature and availability of health care and community services. There are usually barriers to the provision of adequate service which usually boil down to a lack of resources. Service delivery is an area of ongoing change and controversy. Uncontrolled studies support the following assumptions: 1) Rehabilitation care is cost effective when compared to no treatment (Aronow, 1987); 2) Early rehabilitation results in more rapid recovery and is cost effective when compared to rehabilitation care at a later stage of recovery (Cope and Hall, 1982); and 3) High intensity rehabilitation results in reduced length of stays and is ultimately cost effective (Blakerby, 1990). The comprehensive treatment team in rehabilitation is an accepted norm, but care delivery by rehabilitation teams has come under recent scrutiny and it is clear that the traditional interdisciplinary service delivery model has not been subjected to experimental study. It is a traditional time honored model that requires evaluation (Keith, 1991). Traditional rehabilitation programs have been criticized for ignoring the "handicap dimension" and failing to impact on community reintegration (see Chapters 16 and 17). Rehabilitation treatment requires the skills of many different professionals and in most cases this is provided through the agency of a multi- or interdisciplinary team. The difficulties with these models of service delivery include fragmented care, division of responsibility, and "isolated therapy," where therapy is provided outside of the settings where the skills will be used (Orelove, et al., 1985).

Transdisciplinary Model

A transdisciplinary model (Leland, et al., 1988) has been put forward as a more appropriate team model for treatment of head injury patients. This approach targets the learning of functional skills relevant to the individual, in relation to their designated environment. Generalization of skills is planned for and a significant portion of retraining may occur in "real world" situations. This model of care is provided by a small number of "primary therapists" with consultation provided by other disciplines as needed. Interventions include procedures to ensure transfer of treatment to the natural setting. The use of smaller numbers of therapists in each patient's care leads to a better therapeutic relationship. Behavioral change in this system relies as much as possible on social processes and a positive relationship with the patient. This model has particular value in situations where environmental control is necessary (in cases of posttraumatic amnesia or disordered executive control; see below). The transdisciplinary approach deals with important goals which have significant social value in the patient's long-term living environment. Social utility as a goal is a philosophy consistent with the approach proposed by behavioral analysts (Baer, 1968), and there has been a gradual introduction of behavioral technology interventions in the management of head injury patients (Matarazzo, et al., 1982; Goldstein, et al., 1983). The increasing use of behavioral technology has been called for by Wood (1990), who notes the unarguable success of behavioral methods in brain injury rehabilitation has failed to influence the general design of rehabilitation programs. He argues that behavioral methods should not be restricted to "controlling deviant behavior" but encourages a broader application to patients with functional handicap in the process of adapting to disability. A "learning/behavioral" foundation for brain injury rehabilitation will likely receive more emphasis in the future.

Coma Stimulation Program

A common problem in head injury, regardless of other impairments, is the management of coma and rehabilitation during coma emergence. The early utilization of the Glasgow Coma Scale (Teasdale and Jennett, 1974) and its widespread adoption in acute treatment centers is related to the correlation between coma and the patterns of injury caused by head trauma (see Chapter 2). In general, severe injury is correlated with deep coma. The emergence from coma is tracked by most clinical scales and reflects the recovery process as arousal and cognitive functioning improves. Outcome scales, such as the Glasgow Outcome Scale (Jennett, and Bond, 1975) and the Disability Rating Scale (Rappaport, et al., 1977), reflect recovery of independent functional ability and assume normalization of cognitive function. The Levels of Cognitive Function Scale (Hagen, et al., 1979), commonly known as the "Rancho Scale," lacks the reliability of other scales but has been widely adopted because it addresses the issue of "cognitive" recovery and directly identifies difficulties with arousal, restlessness, aggression, participation, memory, and executive ability. Comprehensive rehabilitation must be able to provide interventions for patients in various stages of "cognitive/behavioral recovery" as reflected in the "Rancho Scale."

Rancho Los Amigos Scale (Adapted from Hagen and Malkmus, 1979)

Level I	Unresponsive to all stimuli.
Level II	Inconsistent, nonpurposeful, nonspecific reactions to stimuli; responds to pain, but response may be delayed.
Level III	Inconsistent reaction directly related to type of stimulus presented; responds to some commands; may respond to discomfort.
Level IV	Disoriented and unaware of present events with frequent bizarre and inappropriate behavior; attention span is short and ability to process information is impaired.
Level V	Nonpurposeful random or fragmented responses when task complexity exceeds abilities; patient appears alert and responds to simple commands; performs previously learned tasks but is unable to learn new ones.
Level VI	Behavior is goal-directed; responses are appropriate to the situation with incorrect responses because of memory difficulties.
Level VII	Correct routine responses that are robot-like; appears oriented to setting, but insight, judgment, and problem solving are poor.
Level VIII	Correct responding carryover of new learning; no required supervision, poor tolerance for stress, and some abstract reasoning difficulties.

The general goals of treatment of the emerging coma patient can be roughly classified as: 1) To obtain consistent, discrete responses to environmental stimuli; 2) To engage in participatory activity; and 3) To encourage progressive independence in the activities required to successfully reintegrate into the community.

During the medical management of coma there should be a concurrent attempt to manage the environment around the coma patient. If it is not planned it will be done in a haphazard way, with poor understanding of the environmental impact of potentially depriving or overstimulating conditions (e.g., turning, hygiene, tracheal stimulation, and feeding). The goal of this rehabilitation stage is to improve arousal and responsiveness.

Coma stimulation programs continue to be a source of controversy. Recent reviews of these programs (Ellis, et al., 1990; Wood, 1991) note the lack of consistent definition. The two common terms used are coma and vegetative state. Coma exists in the early period after injury and usually lasts no longer than 3–4 weeks. It is characterized by state of unconsciousness in which there is neither arousal nor awareness. Eyes remain closed and there are no sleep/wake cycles present.

The vegetative state describes a condition when the patient demonstrates no signs of cognition but may return to wakefulness with the eyes open in response to verbal stimuli. Sleep/wake cycles, normal blood pressure, and normal respiration are present. However, patients in this state show no organized, discrete motor responses and are unable to engage in verbal interaction. "Persistent" is applied when this latter condition does not change and does not appear to be improving. Berrol (1990) suggests that the term "persistent vegetative state" be used only after 1 year has elapsed.

It is important to rule out pertinent conditions such as the "locked-in" syndrome, where damage has occurred to the ventral pons (usually due to a vascular insult) with resultant anarthria and paralysis. Such patients have conscious awareness of their environment and stimulation programs are not appropriate (Zasler, et al., 1990). The natural recovery history of patients in the vegetative state is not well studied but, in general, most patients "wake up" within the first 3 months, a smaller number between 3–6 months, and a very small number between 6–12 months. Recovery after 1 year is extremely rare and generally not to be expected (Zasler, et al., 1991).

The rationale for coma stimulation programs revolves around the need to avoid the well known negative effects of sensory deprivation, and to systematically attempt to change the environment to engage the patient in a response which is more specific and less reflexive and generalized. Attempts to standardize assessment have occurred through the use of newer measurement tools such as the *Sensory Stimulation Assessment Measure* (Ellis, et al., 1990), and the *Western Neurosensory Stimulation Profile* (Ansell, et al., 1989). These assessment instruments allow clinicians to be more sensitive to minor clinical improvements or to deterioration.

Appropriate care should certainly ensure management that minimizes morbidity and identifies conditions which could prevent recovery (e.g., posttraumatic epilepsy, posttraumatic hydrocephalus, subdural hematomas). Good nursing care to prevent problems with skin, respiratory, bowel/bladder, is appropriate and seating and appropriate orthotics are required. Family involvement, education, and counselling are also important elements of this phase of treatment.

Wood (1991) also argues that habituation to environmental stimulation occurs when environments fail to control certain sensory input such as overexposure to radio or television in the background. Thus, he recommends limiting the use of television or radio and reducing ambient noise to a low level with discrete therapeutic presentations of stimuli.

Coma stimulation programs are quite variable in approach and to date there is little evidence to support the efficacy of coma stimulation programs. Cerebral glucose metabolism studies in patients in the vegetative state do not show dynamic physiologic cerebral function change consistent with cognitive processing, and this raises the question of whether stimulation can have any effect on an unresponsive brain (Zasler, et al., 1991).

In summary, then, the early phase of recovery from a rehabilitation perspective is to monitor patients in an appropriate manner, to facilitate arousal and vigilance, and to encourage engagement so that participation in a more formal rehabilitation program can occur.

Rehabilitation in Settings of Prolonged (or Persistent) Amnesia or Severe Executive Control Dysfunction

During the period of posttraumatic amnesia, there is severe anterograde memory disorder in association with other problems such as disorientation and restlessness. There may be poor participation in rehabilitation programs because of confusion, agitation, or inappropriate behavior. In addition, patients with behavioral deficits, or excesses, as a result of frontal lobe injury may have severe problems with initiation, poor compliance, or impulsivity. These behavioral problems may effectively prevent participation in a traditional multidisciplinary program. This stage is often a transitory one after severe injury and so designated programs are usually not instituted in most cases. However, when these clinical situations persist, systematic assessment and programming is required, and intervention with behavioral methodologies may be most helpful. Often, the other alternative is to immobilize by physical or chemical restraint, which may result in a vicious cycle with further escalation countered by further restraint.

Wood (1990a) points out that brain injury rehabilitation programs are being polarized into two main schools of thought; one which emphasizes a model of procedural learning in which a behavioral approach predominates; the other which emphasizes a declarative model of learning dominated by a cognitive rehabilitation perspective.

Procedural Learning

Procedural learning focuses on conditioning procedures which allow future participation in the designated environment of choice. Procedural learning assimilates information in a form closely related to the way it is intended to be used with the awareness of the environmental conditions.

The procedural approach can be used to establish a collection of habits which can be applied automatically without having to think about alternative response strategies, and new skills can be learned even with some patients who are deemed amnesic and unable to learn (Verfaellie, et al., 1991; Goldstein, and Oakley, 1985).

Declarative Learning

In declarative learning, one attempts to improve the person's understanding or awareness (actually self-control) of relationships between events in their world. The goal is to allow the person to be able to select a particular response from a number of alternatives and attempts to preserve the notion of freedom of choice for the individual. A declarative learning approach demonstrates that a person "knows about things" as opposed to "knowing how to do things" (Reese, 1989). "Knowing how" means behaving with regularity while "knowing about things" means being able to state or know what should happen but not necessarily behaving consistently (not behaving with regularity). The commonly observed gap between words and actions in "frontal lobe" disorders underlines the need to pay more attention to actions, particularly in patients with self-control difficulties. There is a need to investigate how both approaches can be used to maximize functioning, and this area of conflict remains as a collaborative challenge to professionals in the next decade.

Medication

Behavioral underpinnings are not limited to environmental interventions but can also be applied to other interventions such as medication. Large scale randomized controlled trials of pharmacologic agents often cannot be carried out because of a lack of appropriate patients and appropriateness for a given individual cannot be assessed. The use of single subject experimental designs has not been widely utilized in medical practice, but may be useful in identifying useful pharmacologic agents for individuals with persistent problems. Use of medication to reduce confusion and improve participation (see Chapter 12; Cassidy, 1990) can be individually assessed using behavioral methodology, such as "N of 1" study designs (Guyatt, et al., 1988).

The Milieu

Environmental control is helpful for patients who have prolonged or persistent amnesia or difficulty with executive abilities. The best environment is structured to provide clear and immediate feedback on performance of skills which are ecologically relevant to the designated community setting. The social milieu should focus on interpersonal interactions which allow for the development of skills in preparation for less sheltered settings (Wood, 1990).

Prioritization of program needs is based on the requirements of the ultimate designated environment. Treatment of impairment and disability are not precluded in this model. A treatment curriculum (e.g., physical training, speech therapy) can be integrated into a comprehensive treatment program which incorporates behavioral management strategies in the context of functional skill building.

BEYOND PTA

As patients become more aware, more participatory, and are able to utilize executive abilities, the need for environment control lessens, but a behavioral framework may still be useful as there is always a need to ensure skill building with attention to the concept of generalization (see Chapter 7). Even the teaching of cognitive skills (e.g., problem solving strategies) can be cast into a behavioral framework with appropriate testing for generalization which can ensure the relevance of the problem solving strategy in the chosen environment (Foxx, et al., 1989; see Chapter 13). Most patients recovering from severe injury require treatment at this stage of recovery and most rehabilitation efforts for moderate and mild injuries falls into this category.

The ideal site for this stage of rehabilitation needs to be flexible and is often best defined considering both the patient's clinical needs and the availability, location, and quality of the ultimate living environment (see Chapter 18). Some patients are able to benefit from living at home and accessing necessary outpatient day services, while others benefit from a more controlled environment. Ideally, all communities should develop a network of services which range from structured settings to less controlled environments.

Rehabilitation goals should be *"prioritized"* and should focus on the problems which are most relevant for the *individual,* ("I want to drive", etc.). Ongoing rehabilitation in the community may sometimes be impeded by the limitation of having to access a multidisciplinary model care, as institutional care is sometimes required when there is a need to access more than one discipline "skill set" at a time. Yet, patients can continue to make functional gains for years after injury (Bach-y-Rita, et al., 1980) when living in the community, particularly with access to a therapist who ensures appropriateness of program and motivation (Bach-y-Rita et al., 1988). The failure of rehabilitation workers to reach into the community may be overcome if alternative models of service delivery are considered (like the transdisciplinary model). Rehabilitation can then occur in a variety of community settings and may more directly ensure community reintegration and relevance of treatment goals.

A comprehensive continuum of care (see Chapter 18) is needed for the wide variety of problems experienced in this group (Wood, 1989). Persons suffering from the sequelae of head injury may continue to require treatment or support for extended periods of time (sometimes a lifetime).

MILD HEAD INJURY

Patients who have had a mild head injury sometimes require attention as they are often not flagged by the medical system as having problems, yet the ongoing difficulty with pain and cognitive symptoms can often create severe functional limitations (Binder, 1986). There is an increasing recognition of pathophysiologic changes (see Chapter 2) after mild injury, and these neuropathologic alterations may underlie many of the symptoms experienced by this group of patients. However, overlap with other syndromes such as *posttraumatic stress disorder* make it difficult to rule out psychogenic factors contributing to the functional difficulties (Grant, and Alves, 1987). Most patients recover after 3 months, and management interventions, such as education, counselling, cognitive interventions, and gradual reactivation, may be helpful (Wrightson, 1989).

SUMMARY

Medical management attempts to limit the injurious neurobiologic processes induced by trauma. At the present time, these are limited to approaches which attempt to reduce intracranial pressure and prevent secondary physiologic extremes which can exacerbate the initiating damage.

As recovery from severe (and in most cases of mild or moderate) injury occurs, medical management is supportive and attempts to be vigilant to the possible complications produced by injury to the brain and to other organ systems.

Rehabilitation programs attempt to engage the patient in participatory therapeutic activity. This may require structured treatment settings initially and less restrictive options as improvement occurs. The goal of successful community reintegration should guide all rehabilitation interventions.

References

Ansell, B.J., and Keenan, J.E. (1989) The western neurosensory stimulation profile: The tool for assessing slow to recover head injury patient. Archives of Physical Medicine and Rehabilitation, 70:104–08.

Anthony, P., Keys, H., Evarts, C., Rubin, P., and Lush, C. (1987). Prevention of heterotopic bone formation with early postoperative irradiation in high risk patients undergoing total hip arthroplasty: Comparison of 10.00 Gy vs. 20.00 Gy schedules. Int. J. Radiation Oncology Biol. Phy., 11:365–69.

Aronow, H. (1987). Rehabilitation effectiveness with severe brain injury: Translating research into policy. Journal of Head Trauma and Rehabilitation, 2(3):24–36.

Bach-y-Rita, P. (ed). (1980). Recovery of function: Theoretical consideration for brain injury rehabilitation. Baltimore: University Park Press.

Bach-y-Rita, P., Lazarus, J., Boyeson, M.C., Balliet, R., and Dyers, J. (1988). Normal aspects of motor function as a basis of early and post acute rehabilitation. In: Delisa, J.A. (ed). Rehabilitation medicine principles and practice. Philadelphia: J.B. Lippincott Co.

Baer, D.M., Wolfe, M., and Risley, T.R. (1968). Some current dimensions of applied behavioural analysis. Journal of Applied Behavioural Analysis, 1:91–97.

Berrol, S. (February 1989). Cranial nerve dysfunction in traumatic brain injury. In: Horn, L.J., and Cope, D.N. (eds). Physical medicine and rehabilitation—State of the art reviews. Philadelphia: Hanley and Belfus, Inc., 85–93.

Berrol, S. (October 1990). Persistent vegetative state. In Physical Medicine and rehabilitation—State of the art reviews. Philadelphia: Hanley and Belfus Inc. 4(3).

Binder, L.M. (1986). Persisting symptoms after mild head injury: A review of the postconcussive syndrome. Journal of Clinical and Experimental Neuropsychology, 8:323–46.

Blackerby, W.F. (1990). Intensity of rehabilitation and length of stay. Brain Injury, 4:167–73.

Bucknall, J.E. (1984). Factors affecting healing. In: Bucknall, T.E., and Ellis, H. (eds). Wound healing for surgeons. London: Bailliere Tindall, 62–63.

Cassidy, J.W. (1990). Pharmacological treatment of posttraumatic behavioral disorders: Aggression and disorders of mood. In: Wood, R.L. (ed). Neurobehavioral sequelae of traumatic brain injury.

Clifton, G.L., Allen, S., Berry, J., and Koch, S.M. (1992). Systemic hypothermia in treatment of brain injury. J. Neurotrauma, 9: Supp. 2.

Cope, D.N., and Hall, K. (1982). Head injury rehabilitation: Benefit of early intervention. Archives of Physical Medicine and Rehabilitation, 63:433–37.

Cope, D.N., Date, E.S., and Mar, E.Y. (1988). Serial computerized tomographic evaluations in traumatic brain injury. Archives of Physical Medicine and Rehabilitation, 69(7):483–86.

Crompton, M.R. (1971). Hypothalamic lesions following closed head injury. Brain, 94-172.

Ellis, D.W., and Rader, M. (October 1990). Structured sensory stimulation. In: Sandal, M.W., and Ellis, D.W. (eds). Physical medicine and rehabilitation—State of the art reviews: The coma emerging patient, 4(3).

Foxx, R.M., Marella, R.C., and Marchand-Martella, N.E. (1989). The acquisition, maintenance, and generalization of problem solving skills by closed head injured adults. Behavior Therapy, 20:61–76.

Garland, D.E., Blum, C.G., and Waters, R. L. (1980). Periarticular heterotopic ossification in head injured adult: Incidence and location. Journal of Bone and Joint Surgery (American), 62A:1143–46.

Garland, D.G., Hanscon, D.A., Keenan, M.A., Smith, C., and Moore, T. (1985). Resection of heterotopic ossification in the adult with head trauma. Journal of Bone Joint Surgery (American), 67A:1261–69.

Glenn, M.B., and Whyte, J. (1990). The practical management of spasticity in children and adults, Philadelphia: Lea and Febiger.

Goldstein, G., and Ruthven, L. (1983). Rehabilitation of the brain-damaged adult. New York: Plenum Press.

Goldstein, L.H., and Oakley, D.A. (1985). Expected and actual behavioral capacity after diffuse reduction in cerebral cortex: A review and suggestion for rehab techniques with the mentally handicapped and head injured. British Journal of Clinical Psychology, 24:13–24.

Grant, I., and Alves, W. (1987). Psychiatric and psychosocial disturbances in head injury. In: Levin, H.S., Grafman, J., and Eisenberg, H.M. (eds). Neurobehavioral recovery from head injury. Oxford Press, Chapter 17.

Griffith, E.R., and Mayer, N.H. (1990). Hypertonicity and movement disorders. In: Rosenthal, M., Griffith, E.R., Bond, M.R., and Miller, J.D. (eds). Rehabilitation of the adult and child with traumatic brain injury. Philadelphia: F.A. Davis Co., Chapter 10.

Gualtieri, T., and Cox, D. (1991). The delayed neurobehavioural sequelae of traumatic brain injury. Brain Injury, 5(3):219–32.

Guyatt, G., Sackett, D., Adachi, J., Roberts, R., Chong, J., Rosenbloom, D., and Keller, J. (1988). A clinician's guide for conducting randomized trials in individual patients. Canadian Medical Assoc. Journal, 139:497–503.

Hagen, C., Malkmus, D., and Durham, P. (1979). Levels of cognitive function. In: Rehabilitation of head injured adults: Comprehensive physical management. Downy, California Profess. Staff Assoc. of Rancho Los Amigos Hosp, Inc.

Hagen, C., and Malkmus, D. (1979). Intervention strategies for language disorders secondary to head trauma. Atlanta: American Speech-Language-Hearing Association.

Hunt, J.K. (1990). Soft tissue healing. In: Border, J.R., Allgower, M., Hausen, S.T. Jr., and Ruedi, T.P. (eds). Blunt multiple trauma: Comprehensive pathophysiology and care. New York: Marcel Dekker, 100, 102.

Ishikawa, A., Toshikozu, S., Kaneko, K., et al. (1987). Hyponatremia responsive to fluid cortisone acetate in elderly patients after head injury. Annals of Internal Medicine, 106:187–91.

Jennett, B., and Bond, M.R. (1975). Assessment of outcome in severe brain damage and a practical scale. Lancet, 1:482–84.

Jennett, B. (1990). Posttraumatic epilepsy. In: Rehabilitation of the adult and child with traumatic brain injury. Rosenthal, M., Griffith, E.R., Bond, M.R., and Miller, J.D. (eds). Philadelphia: F.A. Davis Co.

Kalisky, S., et al. (1985). Medical problems encountered during rehabilitation of patients with head injury. Archives of Physical Medicine and Rehabilitation, 66:25–28.

Keith, R.A. (1991). Comprehensive treatment team and rehabilitation. Archives of Physical Medicine and Rehabilitation, 72:269–74.

Kernohan, J., Dakin, P.K., Beacon, J.P., and Bayley, J.I.L. (1984). Treatment of major skeletal injuries in patients with a severe head injury. British Medical Journal, 288:1822–23.

Klingbeil, G., and Cane, P. (1985). Anterior hypopituitarism: A consequence of head injury. Archives of Physical Medicine and Rehabilitation, 66:44–46.

Kornblum, R., and Fisher, R. (1969). Pituitary lesions in craniocerebral injuries. Archives Path., 88:242–48.

Leland, M., Leurs, F.D., Henman, S., and Corilla, R. (June 1988). Rehab Counselling Bulletin, 31:89–97.

Matarazzo, R., and Greif, E. (1982). Behavioral approaches to rehabilitation. New York: Springer Publishing Company.

Meador, K.J., Loring, D.W., Allen, M.E., Zamrini, E.Y., Moore, E.E., Abney, O.L., and King, D.W. (1991). Comparative cognitive effects of carbamazepine and phenytoin in healthy adults. Neurology, 41:1537–40.

Miller, J.D., Becker, D.P., Ward, J.D., Sullivan, H.G., Adams, W.E., and Riegner, M.J. (1977). Significance of intracranial hypertension in severe head injury. J. Neurosurg., 47:503–16.

Narayan, R.K. (1989). Emergency room management of the head-injured patient. In: Becker, D.P., and Gudeman, S.K. (eds). Textbook of head injury. Philadelphia: W.B. Saunders, 23–66.

Orelove, F.P., and Sobsey, D. (1987). Designing transdisciplinary programs. In: Orelove, F.P., and Sobsey, D. (eds). Educating children with multiple disabilities: A transdisciplinary approach. Baltimore: Brookes Pub. Co., Chapter 1.

Pulsinelli, W.A., Waldman, S., Rawlinson, E., and Plum, F. (1982). Moderate hyperglycemia augments ischemic brain damage: A neuropathologic study in the rat. Neurology, 32:1239–46.

Rappaport, M., Hall, K.M., Hopkins, K., Belleza, T., and Cope, D.N. (1982). Disability Rating Scale for severe head trauma: Coma to community. Archives of Physical Medicine and Rehabilitation, 63:118–23.

Reese, H.W. (1989). Rules and rule governance: Cognitive and behavioristic views. In: Hayes, S.C. (ed). Rule governed behavior—Cognition, contingencies and instructional control. New York: Plenum Press, 3–84.

Siesjo, B.K., and Wieloch, T. (1985). Brain injury: Neurochemical aspects. In: Becker, D.P., and Povlishock, J.T. (eds). NIH central nervous system trauma status report. Richmond: William Byrd Press, 518.

Smith, D.B., Mattsen, R.H., Cramer, J.A., Collins, J.F., Novelly, R.A., Croft, B., and the Veterans Admin. Epilepsy Cooperative Study Grp. (1987). Results of a nationwide Veterans Administration cooperative study comparing the efficacy and toxicity of carbamazepine phenobarbital, phenytoin, and primidone. Epilepsia 28 (suppl):550–58.

Spielman, G., Generallia, T.A., and Rogers, C.R. (1983). Disodium etidronate: Its role in preventing heterotopic ossification in severe head injury. Archives of Physical Medicine and Rehabilitation, 64:539–42.

Stewart, R.D. (1990). Airway management in trauma resuscitation. In: McMurtry, R.Y., and McLellan, B.A. (eds). Management of blunt trauma. Baltimore: Williams and Wilkins, 46.

Teasdale, G., and Jennett, B. (1974). Assessment of coma and impaired consciousness: A practical scale. Lancet (2):81–83.

Tomkin, N.R., Dikmen, S.S., Urilensky, A.J., Keihm, J., Chabal, S., and Winn, H.R. (1990). A randomized double-blind study of phenytoin for the prevention of posttraumatic seizures. New England Journal of Medicine, 323:497–502.

Verfaellie, M., Bauer, R.M., and Bowers, D. (1991). Autonomic and behavioral evidence of "implicit" memory in amnesia. Brain and Cognition, 15:10–25.

Ward, J.D., Chai, S., Marmaeau, A., Moulton, R., Muizllaar, J.P., DeSalles, A., Becker, D.P., Kantas, H.A., and Young, H.F. (1989). Effect of prophylactic hyperventilation on outcome in patients with severe head injury. In: Hoff, J.T., and Betz, A.L. (eds). Intracranial pressure VII. Balin: Springer-Verlag.

Wood, R.L., and Eames, P. (1989). Models of brain injury rehabilitation. Baltimore: Johns Hopkins University Press.

Wood, R.L. (1990a). Neurobehavioural paradigm for brain injury rehabilitation. In: Wood, R.L. (ed). Neurobehavioural sequelae of traumatic brain injury. London: Taylor and Francis.

Wood, R.L. (1990). Conditioning procedures in brain injury rehabilitation. In: Wood, R.L. (ed). Neurobehavioural sequelae of traumatic brain injury. London: Taylor and Francis.

Wood, R.L. (1991). Critical analysis of the concept of sensory stimulation for patients in vegetative states. Brain Injury, 5:401–09.

Wood, R.L. (ed). (1990). The neurobehavioural sequelae of traumatic brain injury. London: Taylor and Francis.

Wrightson, P. (1989). Management of disability and rehabilitation services after mild head injury. In: Levin, H., Eisenberg, H.M., and Berton. A.L. (eds). Mild head injury. Oxford University Press.

Yarkony, G., and Sahgal, V. (1987). Contractures: A major complication of craniocerebral trauma. Clinical Orthopaedics, 219:93–96.

Young, R.R., and Delwaide, P.J. (1981). Drug therapy: Spasticity Part I. New England Journal of Medicine, 304:28–33.

Young, R.R., and Delwaide, P.J. (1981). Drug therapy: Spasticity Part II. New England Journal of Medicine, 304:96–99.

Zasler, N.D., Kreutzer, J., and Taylor, D. (in press). Coma stimulation and coma recovery, A critical review. Neuro. Rehab., 1(4):34–55.

6

Assessment and Treatment of Physical Impairments Leading to Disability After Brain Injury

CAROLYN GOWLAND
CYNTHIA A. GAMBAROTTO

"In the context of a health experience an impairment is any loss or abnormality of psychological, physiological or anatomical structure or function" (World Health Organization (WHO), 1980). Physical impairments resulting from brain injury, whether they be mechanical or motor, cause functional losses affecting both disability and handicap. The individual who as a result of brain trauma is saddled with such impairments as paresis, spasticity, rigidity, abnormal movement, lack of coordination, loss of fine motor dexterity, or tremor will find the business of carrying out normal daily functions compromised. Ultimately, such impairments lead to significant losses in independence, control over the environment and productivity (WHO, 1980; Weintraub and Opat, 1989).

Figure 6.1 shows the linking of impairments with the underlying disease or disorder, and the resulting disability and handicap. Impairment, disability, and handicap are not simply linear in relationship. "Handicap may result from impairment without the mediation of a state of disability, for example, abnormal movements or a deformed limb even in the absence of disability may constitute a very real disadvantage to the individual" (WHO, 1980). Also, the degree of the resultant handicap can be mediated by the attitude, motivation, and social support of the individual. Impairments can mean different things to different people depending on how they interfere with lifestyle (Wood, 1989, p. 83).

Physical impairments also can be mediated by other impairments. For example, a client's perception, communication, cognition, and behavior can influence the rehabilitation of impairments. The purpose of this chapter is to discuss the clinical management of physical impairments in the brain injured. Major impairments are identified and their management process described. This is followed by a discussion of brain injury rehabilitation when the specific goal of treatment is the prevention or remedia-

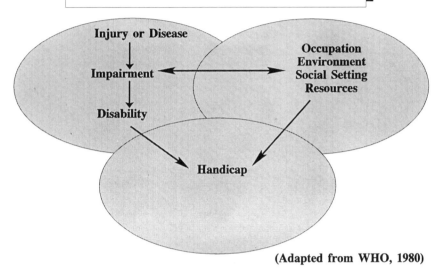

(Adapted from WHO, 1980)

Figure 6.1. Adapted from the World Health Organization's International Classification of Impairment, Disability and Handicap (ICIDH) (WHO, 1980). Handicap is dependent on how the ICIDH components interact with environmental factors.

tion of physical impairment. Commonly used standardized measures and the relevant literature on effectiveness are referenced.

CLINICAL MANAGEMENT PROCESS

The clinical process is made up of the delivery of client care from first referral to last follow-up. The application of scientific principles to the clinical process is essential for effective management. The clinical process can be depicted in 10 steps (Fig. 6.2).

Step 1: Initial Assessment—Gather Data

The major physical impairments are sensorimotor in nature and include disorders of postural control, voluntary movement, sensation, muscle tone, range of motion, strength, coordination, involuntary movements, and fitness. These impairments lead to physical disabilities and handicaps (Fig. 6.3).

In order to manage the client's physical problems information on various factors that mediate the impairments are needed as part of a clinical database. Cost effective practice dictates that the time spent on gathering

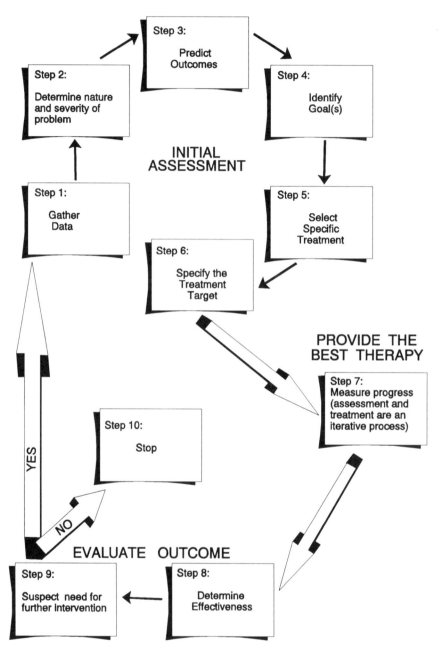

Figure 6.2. Ten steps to the systematic management of brain-injured clients in the clinical setting.

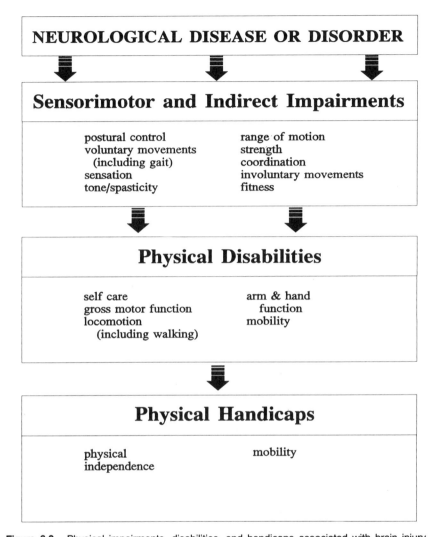

Figure 6.3. Physical impairments, disabilities, and handicaps associated with brain injury.

findings is unjustified unless the information is needed for goal setting, selection of treatment, or the evaluation of outcome (Umphred, 1985).

Step 2: Determine Nature and Severity of Problems

From the data gathered, the nature and severity of a client's physical impairment problems are identified. The importance of these impairments and their interactions with cognition, communication, and behavior are then considered along with the client's disabilities, handicaps, and potential for change.

Step 3: Predict Outcomes

In many individuals, sensorimotor impairments resulting from brain injury have a good prognosis. Some degree of physical sequelae persists in approximately 50% of those who regain consciousness, while 25% have no neurophysic sequelae (Smith, 1985, p. 254).

Although outcome prediction in the brain injured is imprecise, knowledge of the prognostically significant signs, symptoms, characteristics, and behaviors of the individual can help in predicting probable outcome.

Prognosis must be considered when selecting treatment goals, planning preventative strategies, and advising the family (Jennett, Teasdale, and Knill-Jones, 1975, p. 309).

Step 4: Identify Goal(s)

Sackett, Haynes, and Tugwell (1985), remind us that the successful accomplishment of three tasks leads to the rational treatment of any patient (Fig. 6.4). These tasks are to identify the goals of treatment, select the specific treatment, and specify the treatment target. Within the impairment, disability, and handicap framework, the perspective of goal setting is shifted from the medical model, which emphasizes curing the underlying disorder, to a multifaceted rehabilitation model that considers prevention, remediation, restoration, adaptation, and adjustment.

Step 5: Select Specific Treatment(s)

The best available information on effectiveness of treatments should be used to determine the choice of treatment (Sackett, et al., 1985). This information comes from three sources: valid theory, evidence in the research literature, and demonstration in the clinical setting.

The scheme for critically appraising the effectiveness literature that was originally developed by Sackett (1986), and modified by physiotherapists for consensus statements in the neurodevelopmental field, is quite useful for this purpose. The levels of evidence are defined as follows (Campbell, 1990):

Level A: The effectiveness of the therapy is supported by one or more well controlled studies with high statistical power.

Level B: The effectiveness of the therapy is supported by at least one study employing randomly assigned control groups.

Level C: The effectiveness of the therapy is supported by one or more studies lacking randomly assigned control groups, such as single subject research designs.

THE EIGHT ULTIMATE GOALS OF TREATMENT

REMEDIATE

1. Cure the underlying disorder or impairment
2. Relieve the current symptom
3. Restore function

PREVENT

4. Prevent direct and indirect impairment
5. Prevent deterioration in function

COMPENSATE

6. Optimize function
7. Minimize handicap
8. Optimize admustment to permanent impairment
   and disabiltiy

(Adapted from Sackett et al., 1985)

Figure 6.4. Eight ultimate goals for managing the physical impairments, disabilities, and handicaps of the brain-injured.

Step 6: Specify the Treatment Target

Having selected the best treatment, consider what is to be expected as a reasonable outcome, the treatment target. This guides the therapist to know when to stop treatment, change its intensity, or switch to some other treatment (Sackett, et al., 1985). When an individual achieves a target, review the goals, reconsider the treatment being given, and either discontinue treatment or specify a new treatment target (Rinehart, 1990, p. 333).

Step 7: Provide the Best Therapy and Measure Progress

While treatment is being provided with as much technical skill as possible, assessment and treatment interact in a constant iterative way and progress should be objectively assessed on an ongoing basis. The complexity of the relationships among various impairments (e.g., physical, cognitive, communicative, and behavioral) requires that physical rehabilitation of the brain-injured individual not occur in isolation. Members of the health care team must work together in a cooperative effort to optimize the client's rehabilitation potential.

Single case experimental design methodology, where the effect of treatment on the individual is systematically evaluated, is suitable for measuring clinical progress. If client problems are not responding to care as predicted, treatment goals and the treatment plan should be re-examined.

Step 8: Evaluate Outcome in Order to Determine Effectiveness

When treatment is completed, client outcomes relating to the specified targets, and responses to treatment are measured.

Step 9: Assess Need for Further Intervention

Clients with chronic impairment or disability leading to persistent handicap require systematic, long-term management and follow-up.

Step 10: Stop

Only when the individual reaches the status of the healthy disabled, i.e., free from handicap, can vigilance stop.

ASSESSMENT AND TREATMENT OF THE SPECIFIC IMPAIRMENTS

As is shown in the description of the clinical process, client management starts with careful measurement. The information gained from standardized, validated measures lays the groundwork for the development of systematic, scientific practice which will enhance clinicians' judgments about the problems that will respond to intervention, the prediction of outcomes, and the effectiveness of therapies. Measurements selected should be valid for the purpose for which they are intended.

Although the use of nonstandardized measures is being gradually abandoned as valid ones become available, insufficient standardized clinical measures of impairment exist and we still must often rely on descriptive assessments and clinical impressions. Laboratory tests and equipment, such as the pendulum drop test (Bajd and Bowman, 1982) or expensive isokinetic equipment, often do not readily lend themselves to the clinical setting. Although a comprehensive listing of suitable measures is not attempted here, examples of popular standardized clinical measures are cited in the sections describing the impairments they measure.

Although it is generally accepted that recovery from brain injury is influenced by the quality, intensity and duration of rehabilitation, it is often not clear which elements of rehabilitation are essential to recovery. Little hard data are available to help clinicians decide how much, when, or what kind of treatment to provide.

There is Level C evidence (see Step 5 above) supporting the use of early intensive rehabilitation (within 5-weeks posttrauma), including physical and occupational therapy, psychology, and nursing. Length of hospitalization, as well as bowel, bladder, and psychologic impairment were found to be altered significantly as a result of the early introduction of a coordinated, intensive, multidisciplinary treatment approach (Cope and Hall, 1982). There is also a positive effect on client's self-esteem which may facilitate future cognitive remediation. Early stimulation, including upright sitting or standing, has been shown to increase alertness and normalize sleep patterns (Manzi and Weaver, 1987). Because physical recovery generally precedes and may facilitate cognitive reintegration, it would seem appropriate to introduce therapy to enhance physical performance as early as possible (Berrol, 1989; Wood, 1989). Early treatment can prevent or minimize such complications as loss of range of movement and respiratory problems. It can also result in an earlier return of postural control and movement. Manzi and Weaver (1987), in their book on the acute care phase, provide a detailed description of this early rehabilitation.

POSTURAL CONTROL AND VOLUNTARY MOVEMENT

Impairment in postural control and voluntary movement is by far the most common and disabling of all physical impairments in this population. Addressing these impairments is the largest responsibility of those working on physical rehabilitation following brain trauma.

The current theories underlying normal motor control and motor learning (described in the 23 contributions to the Movement Science Series in the December, 1990, and the January, February and March, 1991, editions of Physical Therapy) are challenging traditional approaches to the retraining of posture and movement in clients with neurologic disorders. Academicians and clinicians are examining these theories and efforts are being made to incorporate this thinking into treatment regimens and, where necessary, to modify current approaches.

The traditional neurodevelopmental model of motor control was hierarchical. According to this view, "the behavioral repertoire of the newborn infants is dominated by simple reflexes. These reflexes represent the functioning of subcortical, phylogenetically primitive centers in the brain. In the normally maturing infant, early reflexes diminish, disappear, or are integrated into more mature motor patterns. These changes reflect the maturation of a hierarchically organized nervous system as the cortex increasingly assumes control of motor functions, the reflexes are inhibited or form the basis of more functional movements. . . . The almost exclusive dependence on neural maturation, however, suggests that experience, including therapist intervention, can have only limited effects on motor recovery. . . . It is widely recognized that theories that rely heavily, if not exclusively, on neural explanations of behavior are incomplete" (Kamm, Thelen and Jensen, 1990). Motor control and motor learning are now viewed as dependent on a dynamic system (Newton, 1990). The dynamic systems model for motor control does not assume that one subsystem has privilege over other subsystems, but rather "behavior is an emergent property of the interaction of multiple subsystems" (Kamm, et al., 1990). Several motor control models representing the neural regulation of posture and movement have been proposed to depict the brain's regulation of motor behavior. Although "all models have limitations and are constantly changing as researchers gain new information" (Newton, 1990), these provide a useful basis for understanding the complex interactions of the musculoskeletal and neurologic networks with the environment that result in motor behavior (Newton, 1990, p. 44; Durant, Lord, and Domholdt, 1989). Motor control problems result with brain injury and can be due to disorders in the planning, programming, or executing of movement (Brooks, 1986).

Motor learning theory comes largely from the study of motor skill acquisition in normal individuals. Essential aspects of learning include practice, attention to the task, feedforward, and feedback of both performance (knowledge of performance—KP) and results (knowledge of results—KR) (Schmidt, 1988). Considerations that have been shown to increase learning include relevance and importance of the task to the learner, motivation, and variety. Feedback comes in two forms, intrinsic and extrinsic. Intrinsic feedback is provided internally from the senses and includes kinaesthetic, visual, cutaneous, vestibular, and auditory signals, while extrinsic feedback comes from outside and is usually augmentative in nature. The verbal or gestural feedback on performance that is usually provided by a therapist can be referred to as augmentative or extrinsic. Although verbal feedback can guide the learning of a skill and be highly motivating, immediate and constant extrinsic feedback tends to decrease learning. This would probably be particularly so with brain-injured individuals who are already slow in processing information. Verbal instructions should be directed at changing only one or two things at a time and should not interfere with the learner developing motor problem solving strategies. Also, some margin of error should be allowed (in the language of motor learning theorists, an acceptable bandwidth), before any shortcomings on the performance are mentioned. Too frequent and too detailed correction are to be avoided (Schmidt, 1988, p. 452; Winstein, 1991; Mulder, 1991). Highly skilled and experienced therapists appear to use techniques to enhance motor learning intuitively. These techniques may be "analogous to the faded, intermittent bandwidth, and delayed KR conditions (found in learning theory), although their rationale from the perspective of motor learning principles may not be well understood" (Winstein, 1991).

Lee, Swanson, and Hall (1991) point out the learning of motor skills in neurologically healthy subjects is a highly cognitive process. Thus, the ultimate mode of application of the motor learning principles to the cognitively impaired, brain-injured population is still unclear. Attention and memory are key factors in learning since what is learned must have some meaning or degree of importance to the individual doing the learning (Moore, 1980, p. 75). Umphred (1990, p. 65) notes that learning in brain injured individuals is often slower and in some cases may be impossible. As well as attention and memory deficits, impaired judgment and insight also interfere with learning. If the learning is not relevant, compliance with treatment regimens becomes a problem. Compliance tends to improve if the learning is relevant to client goals. Often brain damaged clients will work on functional activities such as walking, but not on strengthening exercises for the weak lower extremity muscles that contribute to poor gait. In these cases, the goal of strengthening is best accomplished concurrently with the functional task.

Working on altering impairments through the practice of functional tasks not only benefits the client because it provides a meaningful context in which to learn, it also directly results in earlier attainment of functional independence. Additionally, while observing how the client is performing the task, the therapist can easily observe how and which of the impairments are limiting the function and thus require primary attention. For example, weakness of hip extensors commonly limits bed mobility, and practicing this functional task accomplishes the dual goals of increased hip strength and improved bed mobility. Functional tasks, such as sitting and standing, are very useful for training righting, protective, balance, and equilibrium reactions, the major postural control impairments. Transfers, walking, and recreational games can be used to promote coordinated voluntary movement and strength.

Although currently no evidence of the effectiveness of strategies using motor learning theory in the brain injured is available, undoubtedly motor control and motor learning theory will be instrumental in guiding the future development of treatment principles and techniques. This new knowledge should also result in updating the theoretical rationale underlying more traditional treatment approaches.

Theories of motor control and learning alone will not be enough since the rehabilitation of posture and movement in brain-injured individuals does not consist solely of the acquisition of skill. Common problems that result from severe brain injury include paralysis, reflexive movement, and spasticity. In early stages of severe brain injury, many of the subsystems of the brain which are normally involved in the production of movement, particularly the cortical subsystem, become inactive and the primitive, phylogenetically older, components of the CNS motor systems are responsible for what movement does occur. Initially, basic postures and primitive reflexes may be lost. The reestablishment of the "primitive" postural system does not rely as heavily on strategies that require cognition as the phylogenetically newer structures which are highly involved in the production of skilled movement. Moore (1980, p. 67) reminds us that damaged "older CNS systems cannot be reawakened by utilizing the highly cognitive techniques that are applicable for rehabilitating the neo-systems." Rather these older, more automatic, systems need to be reestablished "by having the client use them in the manner in which they once functioned, i.e., as . . . unconscious, bilateral, primitive patterns" (Moore, 1980, p. 67). When first overcoming paresis, the attempt to gain stability may be accompanied by an adaptive mechanism of reducing mobility. If mobility is not soon introduced through facilitation however, paucity of movement and total body rigidity may result. To encourage both stability and mobility superimposed on this stability—terms originated by Rood (Stockmeyer, 1967)—facilitation techniques, moving surfaces and inflatable equipment such as mattresses and large balls can be used. The goal is to reestablish automatic movements and postural reactions, ". . . thus renewing the patient's acquaintance with experiences of movement of which he has been deprived for some time" (Evans, 1981, p. 104).

Moving in synergies, which occur early in the recovery period, would appear to enable the nervous system to begin to reorganize itself subcortically. This subcortical organization precedes cortical integration. External facilitatory and inhibitory stimuli foster the establishment and reintegration of this system. This is done by stimulating proprioceptive, cutaneous, vestibular, and visual receptors. Vibration, stretch, touch, pressure, and resistance are applied with enough external control and guidance to assure that basic postural and movement patterns are possible (Moore, 1980). The basic elements of posture and movement include the spinal reflexes with the limb synergies, the brainstem reflexes, and righting reactions. In the comatose, unresponsive patient, such stimulation may be the only way of augmenting brain function (Cohadon, Richer, Reglade, and Dartigues, 1988). During the early phases of rehabilitation, the performance of gross motor activities in prone, supine, sitting, kneeling, crawling and standing is advocated to achieve spontaneous movement and functional motor performance (Rinehart, 1990). The key principles of treatment are to encourage head and trunk mobility and stability with midline and vertical orientation, followed by limb movement, weight bearing, and weight shifting.

Traditional neurodevelopmentally based treatment approaches concentrated on techniques aimed at reintegrating the older systems in order to bring about normal postural control and movement. The approach was originated by Bobath (1978) and Rood (Stockmeyer, 1967), but over the years has been modified with advancement of new theoretical and clinical knowledge. Good examples of current application for the brain injured client are offered by Rinehart (1990, 1983), Berrol (1989), Charness (1986), and Evans (1981). Throughout her text, Charness, particularly, provides helpful information for moving the client through various functional positions from supine to standing. Although the neurodevelopmental approach will probably continue to find a place in the early treatment of postural and movement impairments in the brain injured, new theoretical models are being advanced, particularly for the study and treatment of balance and equilibrium.

A complex interactive systems model is currently being proposed for the study of postural control in the brain injured. As is the case in motor learning, this model originated from the study of subjects with a normal nervous system. According to this model, during the accomplishment of a task, balance emerges from a complex interaction of biomechanical, motor, and sensory aspects, and is modified by environmental constraints such as the position of the body or body part relative to gravity (Shumway-Cook and Olmscheid, 1990; Horak, 1987). Biomechanical components include available range of motion, alignment of skeletal segments, and muscle strength and endurance. The motor component involves the complex motor programs which control the positioning of the center of body mass within defined limits, while the sensory components include the visual, vestibular, and somatosensory systems which perceive orientation relative to the environment including gravity (Horak, 1987; Shumway-Cook, et al., 1990).

A sensory loss will interfere with the feedback which is needed for learning. In the absence of normal feedback, alternate feedback modes are available to some extent due to the built in redundancies of the nervous system. For example, vision can compensate to some extent for a proprioceptive loss by providing feedback on performance. Charness (1986, pp. 69–76) outlines several possible sensory deficits, the corresponding area of brain damage or dysfunction, clinical manifestations, functional implications, and possible treatment strategies.

The Sensory Organization Test is designed to clinically assess the influence of the senses on postural stability in standing. The reliability of this measure is not reported but one study does report its concurrent validity (DiFabio and Badke, 1990). Other measures suitable for use with a brain damaged population are available to assess aspects of balance. These include the "Get Up and Go" Test (Mathias, Nayak, and Isaacs, 1986), the Postural Stress Test (Wolfson, Whipple, Amerman, and Kleinberg, 1986), and the Berg Scale (Berg, Wood-Dauphinee, Williams, and Gayton, 1989).

It is postulated that once the deficient sensory system(s) are identified, those specific systems can be targeted in treatment. Charness (1986, pp.

69–78) and Herdman (1990) provide suggestions for treatment targeted at specific sensory and vestibular systems respectively. Both authors emphasize careful assessment, augmentation of functioning systems, alternate system compensation, and practice. Herdman in particular relates the treatment of various vestibular disturbances to etiology, i.e., central versus peripheral and unilateral versus bilateral. For unilateral and bilateral vestibular losses, treatment focuses on visuomotor exercises for improving gaze stability. In the case of peripheral vestibular disturbance, habituating or adapting by slowly and repeatedly adopting the vertigo producing position is suggested.

Charness (1986) provides suggestions for augmenting proprioceptive input, listing stretch, resistance, joint compression, weight bearing, and EMG biofeedback as suitable techniques. Therapy can also be focused on treating faulty biomechanical or motor systems (Horak, 1987).

The application of knowledge from the basic sciences also is resulting in a new and innovative approach to gait training. Recent advances in the use of treadmill training with postural support and reduced weight bearing have had some success in improving the quality and efficiency of gait in spinal cord and hemiplegic patients. Visintin and Barbeau suggest that "... progressive weight bearing during treadmill locomotion may be an effective strategy to retrain neurologically impaired gait" (Visintin and Barbeau, 1989). Recently, Level C evidence of the effectiveness of this technique has been published (Danakas, Barbeau, Arsenault, and Riley, 1991).

TONE, SPASTICITY AND RANGE OF MOTION

The development of joint and muscle contractures that reduce range of motion and interfere with function are common impairments in severely brain injured (Lehmkuhl, Thoi, Baize, Kelley, Krawczyk, and Bontke, 1990). The most common sites for contractures are the elbow, wrist, fingers, hip, knee, and ankle (Carr and Shepherd, 1980, p. 202; Evans, 1981). Contractures result primarily from prolonged, severe muscle tone imbalance and prolonged immobilization in any one position. Because of this close relationship between tone, spasticity, and contractures, these three topics are dealt with together.

"Spasticity is a disorder of spinal proprioceptive reflexes, manifested clinically as tendon jerk hyperreflexia and an increase in muscle tone that becomes more apparent the more rapid the stretching movement. It is a common but not inevitable consequence of lesions that damage descending pathways, including the pyramidal tracts, at any level—cortex, internal capsule, brainstem, or spinal cord" (Burke, 1988). Stiffness, during either active or passive movement, and contracture formation are clinical manifestations arising from severe spasticity. Not all of the stiffness and contracture is the result of abnormal firing of motor units. Non-neural factors, including decreased compliance of muscle, are responsible for some of the increased resistance to passive stretch. The rapid loss of sarcomeres when a muscle, particularly one that is contracting, is immobilized in a shortened position, plays a significant role in contracture formation (Burke, 1988).

The pendulum drop test provides an objective measure of spasticity in certain muscle groups (Bajd, et al., 1982). This test measures spasticity by quantifying the passive restraint offered by a stretched muscle during free falling passive movement (the pendulum drop). Perhaps a more clinically applicable means of measuring spasticity because it is simpler and less expensive, is the handheld dynamometer which has been shown to be reliable for use on a similar population (Malouin, Borteau, Bonneau, Pichard, and Bravo, 1989). The Modified Ashworth Scale of muscle spasticity is an even simpler clinical measure that rates spasticity on an ordinal scale. This measure also has demonstrated reliability (Bohannon, 1987). Joint range of motion can be reliably measured using a goniometer (Horger, 1990). Gajdosik and Bohannon (1987) remind us that reliability with a goniometer depends on clinicians adopting standardized methods for goniometric use.

Treatment is first aimed at preventing contractures by minimizing the × adverse effects of abnormal tone and immobilization. To preserve the integrity of muscle, positioning is used to maintain muscle length, while facilitation activates weak antagonists, and inhibition generally induces relaxation. Joint mobility is maintained as much as possible through the use of passive range of motion exercises and accessory joint motions. Prolonged (longer than 20 minutes) positioning with the muscle elongated is by far the most important of these techniques.

When preventative measures fail, prolonged passive lengthening using positioning, orthoses, serial casting, and splinting, as well as neurolytic blocks and surgery, can effectively reduce contractures. Several authors endorse the use of casts to maintain and increase joint range of motion in the traumatic brain injured population (Keenan, 1987; Zablotny, 1987; Leahy, 1988; Conine, Sullivan, Mackie, and Goodman, 1990; Lehmkuhl, et al., 1990; Barnard, Dill, Eldredge, Held, Judd, and Nalette, 1984). There is a substantial body of Level C evidence in the literature examining the effectiveness of casting. To summarize, serial casting has been found to be effective in the acute stage postinjury (Kent, Hershler, Conine, and Hershler, 1990; Conine, et al., 1990), and nonbivalved casts are preferable to bivalved (Imie, Eppinghaus, and Boughton, 1986). In the pediatric literature there is Level A evidence (one or more well controlled studies) showing inhibitive casting is effective in reducing contracture (Bertoti, 1986; Hinderer, et al., 1988).

STRENGTH

Although there is controversy as to whether traditional means of measuring muscle strength should be used in patients with brain lesions (Bohannon, 1989; Rothstein, Riddle, and Finucane, 1989), weakness due to output paresis in this population is unquestionably a problem. Imbalanced and inadequate recruitment of motor units which results in an inability to generate sufficient force is an important reason for poor motor performance whenever the pyramidal tracts are damaged (Sahrmann, 1977; Rosenfalck and Andreassen, 1980; Knutsson and Martensson, 1980; Tang and Rymer, 1981; Whitley, Sahrmann, and Norton, 1982; Colebatch, Gandevia, and Spira, 1986). Abnormal recruitment and rate modulation of motor neurons lead to inefficient muscle activation, early loss of force, increased effort and the clinical perception of weakness (Katz and Rymer, 1989). In the brain injured, disturbances with muscle recruitment and timing that result in muscle weakness may have a more profound effect on motor behavior than abnormal muscle tone (Rinehart, 1983). Additionally, disuse and inactivation lead to atrophy with an accompanying loss of strength.

Although the question of the validity of muscle strength measures with this population remains unanswered, clinicians are promoting some form of assessment of muscle strength (Duncan, 1990, p. 266). The most common test of muscle strength, Manual Muscle Test, grades groups of muscles (Medical Research Council, 1976). Variations of this standard method with numerical or alphabetical grading schemes were recently described by Schneider and Gabriel (1990, p. 406).

Because the recognition of the problem of weakness in this population is recent, little evidence of treatment effectiveness is reported. Indirect evidence might be inferred from the EMG biofeedback literature. Level C evidence of the effectiveness of feedback in improving function has been gathered over the last decade and a half (Korein, Brudny, Grynbaum, Sachs-Frankel, Weisinger, and Levidow, 1976). Presumably, improved recruitment of motor units with secondary improvements in muscle strength would have accompanied these functional gains.

In the individual where movement is dependent on primitive reflexes and synergies, it is generally held that traditional strengthening techniques should be avoided. Similarly, most therapists will refrain from directly strengthening muscles when efforts result in abnormal movements, unwanted increases in tone, and decreased movement.

CEREBELLAR INCOORDINATION

"Ataxia is a general term used to describe the lack of coordination displayed by individuals with cerebellar lesions" (Urbscheit, 1990, p. 597). It includes disturbances of posture and balance of the head, trunk, and extremities; dysmetria; disturbances of gait; movement decomposition; and dysdiadochokinesia.

A few clinical measures are available for assessing impairments in coordination (Fugl-Meyer, Jaasko, Leyman, Olsson, and Steglind, 1975; Kurtzke, 1983; Schmitz, 1988). However, none of these has been evaluated for reliability, validity, or the ability to detect change. Clinicians using these measures should be aware of these limitations and if possible attempt to address them for their own purposes.

Although the availability of an effective treatment is questionable at the present time, the neurodevelopmental approach described earlier is commonly used (Urbscheit, 1990). There is some agreement that joint approximations and other techniques, such as weight bearing, that emphasize stability and augment the proprioceptive information to the cerebellum, help symptomatically (Berrol, 1989; Charness, 1986; Carr, et al., 1980). Several techniques for treating ataxia are commonly echoed in the literature. These include 1) focusing on stable posture in the trunk and limb girdles, 2) augmenting proprioception by the use of joint compression, 3) introducing tasks of increased complexity, starting with the reinforcement of a stable posture and progressing by adding small range movements then large range movements, 4) feedback on performance, and 5) repetition. Some degree of impairment may be compensated for by the use of weighted cuffs, "fixing" of the trunk or limbs, or the use of elasticized therapeutic bands. However, the symptoms are often permanent and an often important goal of treatment is to optimize the client's adjustment to this impairment.

INVOLUNTARY MOVEMENTS

Although dyskinesia is not usually the most common impairment in the brain injured, several types are associated with involvement of the basal ganglia. These include dystonias, choreiform movements, athetosis, and Parkinsonian symptoms including akinesia, bradykinesia, muscular rigidity, and persistent tremor. Drug management can often help. There is little evidence of the long-term effectiveness of physical treatment approaches which are primarily symptomatic. As is the case with coordination impairments, the symptoms are often permanent and an important goal of treatment is to optimize the client's adjustment to the disabling losses.

FITNESS

Components of fitness include muscle strength, aerobic fitness, flexibility, muscle endurance, and anthropometry (Fitness and Amateur Sport

Canada, 1987). Prolonged immobilization, decreased level of physical activity, and altered metabolism all contribute to a generally reduced level of fitness in the brain injured.

The Canadian Standardized Test of Fitness (CSTF) (Fitness and Amateur Sport Canada, 1987) gives instructions for measuring all components of fitness and is suitable for use with the mildly involved. A screening questionnaire, the Physical Activity Readiness Questionnaire—PAR-Q— the purpose of which is to determine suitability to participate in a vigorous fitness program, accompanies the CSTF. However, like Hunter, Tomberlin, Kirkikis and Kuna (1990) found, modifications to a standard fitness protocol may be required for clients with severe ataxia or spasticity of lower limb muscles.

Another method for assessing aerobic fitness is heart rate monitoring during submaximal cycle ergometry. This is widely reported as a safe means of determining fitness in apparently healthy individuals (Astrand and Rodahl, 1986; American College of Sports Medicine, 1986; Golding, 1980) and is suitable for use on the majority of brain injured clients who are capable of undertaking a fitness program. Astrand and Rodahl (1986, p. 376), however, caution of a 10%–15% standard error in prediction of maximal oxygen uptake from submaximal exercise tests.

Once it is established that a client's autonomic and homeostatic functions respond appropriately to increased activity, a fitness program can begin. Offering Level C evidence, Hunter, et al. (1990), found a 3-month fitness training program was effective on a group of 12 brain-injured subjects who were a minimum of 1 year postinjury. They concluded that their results indicate that decreased fitness in this population can be reversed by training (Hunter, et al., 1990).

With impaired balance and coordination, bicycle ergometry provides a useful alternative to a treadmill or stairs during assessment and training. For individuals with severe impairments involving the lower limbs, arm ergometry often suffices. Because a smaller muscle mass is used, clients may fatigue more easily (Hunter, et al., 1990). This might prevent them from attaining an adequate training workload.

Standardized protocols for strengthening and improving flexibility are suitable for use on the majority of the brain injured who are participating in a fitness program. Astrand and Rodahl (Astrand, et al., 1986) provide a description of standard protocols. Since reduced cognition, memory and motivation are often problems with the brain injured, fitness training through the use of therapeutic games is often of benefit.

It is presumed that paying increased attention to the fitness needs of this population could benefit the recipients considerably, however, considerable study of these benefits and suggestions for revising standardized assessment and training protocols are needed.

SUMMARY

Physical impairments in individuals with brain injury are part of the complex interactive problem set of this population. The use of a dynamic systems model can be of value in depicting the various physical impairments and their relationships with other disabilities and handicaps. Because of their relationship with the underlying brain trauma, and the multiple disabilities and handicaps that result, physical impairments can no longer be viewed in isolation. The understanding of these relationships is derived from the WHO framework, the International Classification for Impairments Disabilities and Handicaps (WHO, 1980). Current management of physical impairments in the brain injured is undergoing change resulting from the aspiration of health professionals to be more scientific in their practice. The professions are seeking to provide evidence that therapies have demonstrated effectiveness and are based on valid theories. Batteries of measures for efficiently measuring the physical impairments are generally not available, and those that are, generally are inadequately standardized and evaluated. Clinical measures of impairment resulting from brain trauma with good psychometric properties are needed. The description of the step-by-step process involved in clinical care, the clinical process, can be a useful means of examining the scientific requirements of the process.

New models of practice for dealing with the physical impairments commonly seen in individuals with CNS damage are emerging. For the most part, these models use a dynamic systems approach, are based on current theories, and are backed by research findings which often come from information gained on normal function. As the theoretical knowledge of movement science develops, it is postulated that there are needed changes in the method by which posture and movement (including gait) are trained. However, treatment protocols applicable to the brain injured population are only in the process of being developed, and there is currently little evidence of the effectiveness of these new approaches to therapy. Traditional methods of treatment such as Neurodevelopmental Therapy (NDT) continue to be used but have undergone revision as theoretical and clinical knowledge advances. More and more, clinicians will be required to apply systematic approaches for evaluating the effectiveness of treatments in the clinical setting and will need to select measures which are valid for these purposes. The relationship between the art and science of practice must be a close one if brain injured individuals with physical impairments are to be provided optimal care.

References

American College of Sports Medicine (1986). Guidelines for exercise testing and prescription. Philadelphia: Lea and Febiger.

Astrand, P.O., and Rodahl, K. (1986). Textbook of work physiology: Physiological bases of exercise. New York: McGraw Hill.

Bajd, T., and Bowman, B. (1982). Testing and modelling of spasticity. Journal of Biomedicine of England, 4:90–95.

Barnard, P., Dill, H., Eldredge, P., Held, J.M., Judd, D.L.M., and Nalette, E. (1984). Reduction of hypertonicity by early casting in a comatose head injured individual. Physical Therapy, 64(10):1540–42.

Berg, K., Wood-Dauphinee, S., Williams, J.I., and Gayton, D. (1989). Measuring balance in the elderly: Preliminary development of an instrument. Physiotherapy Canada, 41(6):304–11.

Berrol, S. (1989). The treatment of physical disorders following brain injury. In: Wood, R.L., and Eames, P. (eds). Models of brain injury rehabilitation. Baltimore, MD: Johns Hopkins University Press, 100–16.

Bertoti, D.B. (1986). Effect of short leg casting on ambulation in children with cerebral palsy. Physical Therapy, 66(10):1522–29.

Bobath, B. (1978). Adult hemiplegia: Evaluation and treatment. London: Wm. Heinemann.

Bohannon, R.W. (1989). Is the measurement of muscle strength appropriate in patients with brain lesions? A special communication. Physical Therapy, 69(3):225–36.

Bohannon, R.W. and Smith, M.B. (1987). Interrater reliability of a modified Ashworth scale of muscle spasticity. Physical Therapy, 67:206–07.

Bond, M.R. (1990). Standardized methods of assessing and predicting outcome. In: Rosenthal, M., Griffith, E.R., Bond, M.R., and Miller, J.D. (eds). Rehabilitation of the adult and child with traumatic brain injury. Philadelphia: F. A. Davis, 59–74.

Brooks, V.B. (1986). The neural basis of motor control. New York: Oxford University Press.

Burke, D. (1988). Spasticity as an adaptation to pyramidal tract injury. Advances in Neurology, 47:401–22.

Campbell, S.K. (1990). Proceedings of the consensus conference on the efficacy of physical therapy in the management of cerebral palsy. Pediatric Physical Therapy, 2(3):123–76.

Carr, J.H., and Shepherd, R.B. (1980). Physiotherapy in disorders of the brain. London: Wm. Heinemann.

Charness, A. (1986). Stroke/head injury: A guide to functional outcomes in physical therapy management. Rockville, MD: Aspen.

Cohadon, F., Richer, E., Reglade, C., and Dartigues, J.F. (1988). Recovery of motor function after severe traumatic coma. Scandinavian Journal of Rehabilitation and Medicine, 17:75–85.

Colebatch, J.G., Gandevia, S.C., and Spira, P.J. (1986). Voluntary muscle strength in hemiparesis: Distribution of weakness at the elbow. Journal of Neurology, Neurosurgery and Psychiatry, 49:1019–24.

Conine, T.A., Sullivan, T., Mackie, T., and Goodman, M. (1990). Effect of serial casting for the prevention of equinus in patients with acute head injury. Archives of Physical Medicine and Rehabilitation, 71:310–12.

Cope, D.N., and Hall, K. (1982). Head injury rehabilitation: Benefit of early intervention. Archives of Physical Medicine and Rehabilitation, 63:433–37.

Danakas, M., Barbeau, H., Arsenault, A.B., and Riley, E. (1991). A preliminary study of the effects of a locomotor training program for spastic paraparetic subjects. Physiotherapy Canada, 43:A–17.

DiFabio, R.P., and Badke, M.B. (1990). Relationship of sensory organization to balance function in patients with hemiplegia. Physical Therapy, 70(9):542–48.

Duncan, P.W. (1990). Physical therapy assessment. In: Rosenthal, M., Griffith, E.R.,

Bond, M.R., and Miller, J.D. (eds). Rehabilitation of the adult and child with traumatic brain injury. Philadelphia: F.A. Davis, 264–83.

Durant, T.L., Lord, L.J., and Domholdt, E. (1989). Outpatient views on direct access to physical therapy in Indiana. Physical Therapy, 69(10):850–57.

Evans, C.D. (1981). Physiotherapy: Assessment and treatment of disordered motor function. In: Evans, C.D. (ed). Rehabilitation after severe head injury. Edinburgh: Churchill Livingston, 91–113.

Fitness and Amateur Sport Canada. (1987). Canadian standardized test of fitness (CSTF). Ottawa, ON: Fitness and Amateur Sport Canada.

Fugl-Meyer, A.R., Jaasko, L., Leyman, I., Olsson, S., and Steglind, S. (1975). The post-stroke hemiplegic patient: A method for evaluation of physical performance. Scandinavian Journal of Rehabilitation Medicine, 7:13–31.

Gajdosik, R.L., and Bohannon, R.W. (1987). Clinical measurement of range of motion. Physical Therapy, 67:1867–72.

Golding, L.A. (1980). Exercise physiology. In: Long, C. (ed). Prevention and rehabilitation in ischemic heart disease. Baltimore: Williams and Wilkins.

Hagen, C. (1979). Levels of cognitive functioning. Rehabilitation of the head injured adult: Comprehensive physical management. Downey, CA: Rancho Los Amigos Hospital.

Harris, S.R. (1990). Therapeutic exercises for children with neurodevelopmental disabilities. In: Basmajian, J.V., and Wolf, S.L. (eds). Therapeutic exercise. Baltimore: Williams and Wilkins, 163–76.

Herdman, S.J. (1990). Treatment of vestibular disorders in traumatically brain-injured patients. Journal of Head Trauma Rehabilitation, 5(4):63–76.

Hinderer, K.A., Harris, S.R., Purdy, A.H., Chew, D.E., Staheli, L.T., McLaughlin, J.F., and Jaffe, K.M. (1988). Effects of "tone-reducing" vs. standard plaster casts on gait improvement of children with cerebral palsy. Developmental Medicine and Child Neurology, 30:370–77.

Horak, F.B. (1987). Clinical measurement of postural control in adults. Physical Therapy, 67:1881–85.

Horger, M.M. (1990). The reliability of goniometric measurements of active and passive wrist motions. American Journal of Occupational Therapy, 44(4):342–48.

Hunter, M., Tomberlin, J., Kirkikis, C., and Kuna, S.T. (1990). Progressive exercise testing in closed head-injured subjects: Comparison of exercise apparatus in assessment of physical conditioning program. Physical Therapy, 70(6):363–71.

Imie, P.C., Eppinghaus, C.E., and Boughton, A.C. (1986). Efficacy of nonbivalved and bivalved serial casting on head injured patients in intensive care. Physical Therapy, 66:748–48.

Jennett, B., Teasdale, G., and Knill-Jones, R. (1975). Prognosis after severe head injury. In: Ciba Foundation Symposium 34, Outcome of severe damage to the central nervous system. Amsterdam: Elsevier, 309–24.

Kamm, K., Thelen, E., and Jensen, J.L. (1990). A dynamical systems approach to motor development. Physical Therapy, 70(12):763–55.

Katz, R.T., and Rymer, W.Z. (1989). Spastic hypertonia: Mechanisms and measurement. Archives of Physical Medicine and Rehabilitation, 70(2):144–54.

Keenan, M.A. (1987). The orthopedic management of spasticity. Journal of Head Trauma Rehabilitation, 2(2):62–71.

Kent, H., Hershler, C., Conine, T.A., and Hershler, R. (1990). Case-control study of lower extremity serial casting in adult patients with head injury. Physiotherapy Canada, 42(4):189–91.

Knutsson, E., and Martensson, C. (1980). Dynamic motor capacity in spastic paresis and its relationship to prime mover dysfunction, spastic reflexes and antagonistic co-ordination. Scandinavian Journal of Rehabilitation Medicine, 12:93–106.

Korein, J., Brudny, J., Grynbaum, B., Sachs-Frankel, G., Weisinger, M., and Levidow, L.

(1976). Sensory feedback therapy of spasmodic torticollis and dystonia: Results in treatment of 55 patients. Advances in Neurology, 114:375–403.

Kurtzke, J.F. (1983). Rating neurological impairment in multiple sclerosis: An expanded disability status scale. Neurology, 33:1444–52.

Leahy, P. (1988). Pre-casting worksheet—an assessment tool: A clinical report. Physical Therapy, 68:72–74.

Lee, T.D., Swanson, L.R., and Hall, A.L. (1991). What is repeated in a repetition? Effects of practice conditions on motor skill acquisition. Physical Therapy, 71(2):150–56.

Lehmkuhl, I.D., Thoi, L.L., Baize, C., Kelley, C.J., Krawczyk, L., and Bontke, C.F. (1990). Multimodality treatment of joint contractures in patients with severe brain injury: Cost, effectiveness, and integration of therapies in the application of serial/inhibitive casts. Journal of Head Trauma Rehabilitation, 5(4):23–42.

Malouin, F., Borteau, M., Bonneau, C., Pichard, L., and Bravo, G. (1989). Use of a hand-held dynamometer for the evaluation of spasticity in a clinical setting: A reliability study. Physiotherapy Canada, 41:126–34.

Manzi, D.B., Weaver, P.A. (1987). Head injury: The acute care phase. Thorofare, NY: Slack.

Mathias, S., Nayak, U.S.L., and Isaacs, B. (1986). Balance in elderly patients: The "get-up and go" test. Archives of Physical Medicine and Rehabilitation, 67:387–89.

Medical Research Council (1976). Aids to the examination of the peripheral nervous system. London: Her Majesty's Stationary Office.

Miller, J.D., Pentland, B. and Berrol, S. (1990). Early evaluation and management. In: Rosenthal, M., Griffith, E.R., Bond, M.R., and Miller, J.D. (eds). Rehabilitation of the adult and child with traumatic brain injury. Philadelphia: F.A. Davis, 21–51.

Moore, J.C. (1980). Neuroanatomical considerations relating to recovery of function following brain lesions. In: Bach-y-Rita, P. (ed). Recovery of function: Theoretical considerations for brain injury rehabilitation. Baltimore: University Park Press, 9–90.

Mulder, T. (1991). A process-oriented model of human motor behavior: Toward a theory-based rehabilitation approach. Physical Therapy, 71(2):157–63.

Newton, R.A. (1990). Motor control. In: Umphred, D.A. (ed). Neurological rehabilitation. St. Louis, MO: C.V. Mosby, 43–52.

Rinehart, M. (1990). Strategies for improving motor performance. In: Rosenthal, M., Griffith, E.R., Bond, M.R., and Miller, J.D. (eds). Rehabilitation of the adult and child with traumatic brain injury. Philadelphia: F.A. Davis, 331–48.

Rinehart, M. (1983). Considerations for functional training in adults after head injury. Physical Therapy, 63:1975–82.

Rosenfalck, A., and Andreassen, S. (1980). Impaired regulation of force and firing pattern of single motor units in patients with spasticity. Journal of Neurology, Neurosurgery and Psychiatry, 43:907–16.

Rothstein, J.M., Riddle, D.L., and Finucane, S.D. (1989). Is the measurement of muscle strength appropriate in patients with brain lesions? A special communication. Physical Therapy, 69(3):230–35.

Sahrmann, S.A. (1977). The relationship of voluntary movement to spasticity in the upper motor neuron syndrome. Annals of Neurology, 2:460–65.

Sackett, D.L. (1986). Rules of evidence and clinical recommendations on the use of anti-thrombotic agents. Chest, 89(Suppl.):2–3.

Sackett, D.L., Haynes, R.B., and Tugwell, P. (1985). Clinical epidemiology. A basic science for clinical medicine. Toronto: Little, Brown and Co.

Schmidt, R.A. (1988). Motor control and learning: a behavioral emphasis. Champaign, IL: Human Kinetics.

Schmitz, T.J. (1988). Coordination assessment. In: O'Sullivan, S.B., and Schmitz, T.J.

(eds). Coordination testing. Physical rehabilitation: Assessment and treatment procedures (2nd ed). Philadelphia: F.A. Davis, 121–34.

Schneider, J.W. and Gabriel, K.L. (1990). Congenital spinal cord injury. In: Umphred, D.A. (ed). Neurological rehabilitation. St. Louis, MO: C.V. Mosby, 397–422.

Shumway-Cook, A., and Olmscheid, R. (1990). A systems analysis of postural dyscontrol in traumatically brain injured patients. Journal of Head Trauma Rehabilitation, 5(4):51–62.

Smith, S.S.(1985). Traumatic head injuries. In: Umphred, D.A. (ed). Neurological rehabilitation. St. Louis: C.V. Mosby, 249–88.

Stockmeyer, S.A. (1967). An interpretation of the approach of Rood to the treatment of neuromuscular dysfunction. American Journal of Physical Medicine, 46(1):900–56.

Tang, A., and Rymer, W.Z. (1981). Abnormal force—EMG relations in paretic limbs of hemiparetic human subjects. Journal of Neurology, Neurosurgery and Psychiatry, 44:690–98.

Teasdale, G., and Jennett, B. (1974). Assessment of coma and impaired consciousness. Lancet, 81–84.

Umphred, D.A. (1990). Neurological Rehabilitation (2nd ed). St. Louis, MO: C.V. Mosby.

Umphred, D.A. (1985). Neurological Rehabilitation. St. Louis, MO: C.V. Mosby.

Umphred, D.A. (1983). Conceptual model of an approach to the sensorimotor treatment of the head injured client. Physical Therapy, 63(12):1983–87.

Urbscheit, N.L. (1990). Cerebellar dysfunction. In: Umphred, D.A. (ed). Neurological rehabilitation. St. Louis, MO: C.V. Mosby, 597–618.

Visintin, M., and Barbeau, H. (1989). The effects of body weight support on the locomotor pattern of spastic paretic patients. Canadian Journal of Neurological Sciences, 16(3):315–25.

Weintraub, A.H., and Opat, C.A. (1989). Motor and sensory dysfunction in the brain-injured adult. In: Horn, L.J., and Cope, D.N. (eds). Traumatic brain injury. Philadelphia: Hanley and Belfus, 59–84.

Whitley, D.L., Sahrmann, S.A., and Norton, B.J. (1982). Patterns of muscle activity in the hemiplegic upper extremity. Physical Therapy, 62:641.

Winstein, C.J. (1991). Knowledge of results and motor learning—implications for physical therapy. Physical Therapy, 71(2):140–49.

Wolfson, L.I., Whipple, R., Amerman, P., and Kleinberg, A. (1986). Stressing the postural response: A quantitative method for testing balance. American Geriatrics Society, 34:845–50.

Wood, R.L. (1989). A salient factors approach to brain injury rehabilitation. In: Wood, R.L., and Eames, P. (eds). Models of brain injury rehabilitation. Baltimore: Johns Hopkins University Press, 75–99.

World Health Organization (WHO) (1980). International classification of impairments, disabilities and handicaps. Geneva: World Health Organization.

Zablotny, C. (1987). Using neuromuscular electrical stimulation to facilitate limb control in the head-injured patient. Journal of Head Trauma Rehabilitation, 2(2):28–33.

7

Functional Assessment and Intervention

GORDON MUIR GILES

Rehabilitation effectiveness may be measured by the outcome for the patient and his or her family, but should include a consideration of the cost to society of providing or not providing services. In most cases, the patient and family will be more satisfied with greater independence. It is widely accepted that an independent member of society is less costly to the community than one who requires prolonged care. The focus of rehabilitationists should not be on recovery in and for itself, but on the improvement of real world functional performance. A preoccupation with impairment may not only lead to unrealistic expectations and frustrations for the patient and family, but to an injudicious use of health care monies. Immense resources may be expended to provide services for individuals who are unlikely to develop a significantly higher level of functional independence while individuals who could be considerably more independent with only limited help receive no assistance at all.

The development of an integrated model of service delivery is complicated by the absence of consensus regarding the most effective method of intervention, and its timing or duration. The study of outcome from rehabilitation has been hampered by the inexact nature of the outcome measures used, and by the diversity of populations studied. Although some general programmatic approaches have shown positive findings (Prigatano, et al., 1984; Eames and Wood, 1985) it is difficult to determine what specific aspects of the programs resulted in improvement. Individuals recover from brain injury. The rapidity of this process in the early stages of recovery demonstrates that a neurophysiologic process or processes, other than learning, underlies this improvement. Although the nature of the factors responsible for early rapid recovery are unknown, therapists have attempted to potentiate the process by stimulating the patient during this stage of recovery. There are some animal studies (Black, Markowitz, and Cianci, 1975) and anecdotal reports (Shaw, Brodsky, and McMahon, 1985) which support the usefulness of this type of intervention. There is, however, no robust evidence of a specific therapy effect (e.g., one type of motor skills retraining method over another) nor for a need for specific timing or duration.

A study by Cope and Hall (1982) is frequently used as evidence of the superiority of early over late intervention for brain-injured individuals. In Cope and Hall's study, severely brain-injured patients in an acute rehabilitation setting were divided retrospectively into early and late rehabilitation admission groups (admitted before and after 35 days postinjury). Two groups of 16 and 20 patients were matched for length of coma, age, level of disability, and neurosurgical procedures performed. The groups differed on measures of cognitive functioning and continence. The researchers found that late admission patients required twice as much rehabilitation to reach a standard discharge criteria as did the early admission group. Outcome at 2-year follow-up was comparable. Unfortunately, no reasons are given as to why the late group was not admitted to rehabilitation sooner. It is possible that the reason some patients were admitted to rehabilitation later was because they were more impaired to begin with, leaving the subsequent differences between the two groups uninterpretable.

In the postacute recovery period, therapists have attempted to directly address the cognitive substrata of perception, attention, memory, judgment and reasoning, and other "skills." Recently, a consensus has emerged that attempts to retrain the cognitive substrata of memory are ineffective. No such consensus exists for the other areas mentioned. The advantage of these basic cognitive interventions, were they to be effective, would be the "trickle down" effect improvement in basic cognitive skills would have on all aspects of the patient's functioning. So, for example, an improvement in attention would improve the patient's memory functioning, work performance, etc. The disadvantage of attempting to remediate basic cognitive functioning is that this type of intervention is of unproven efficacy, so that a good deal of the patient's time and effort may be devoted to a pointless task and result in no actual functional improvement. As an alternative to addressing basic cognitive deficits, some therapists have attempted to train brain-injured patients in compensatory approaches to specific deficits (Wilson and Moffat, 1984). Unfortunately, patients are often taught techniques without adequate consideration being given to whether the likely improvement in the patient's quality of life warrants the effort required for them to learn the compensatory technique. Patients must be able to transfer the compensatory strategy to novel situations encountered in the real world. Brain-injured individuals can often learn strategies, but be unable to apply them. Compensatory behaviors which are most successful, are those which the individuals may overlearn to the point of automaticity. Compensatory techniques which, despite overlearning, remain effortful (such as visualization strategies in memory retraining) are usually too demanding to be used outside the training sessions.

As an alternative to the above approaches, specific task approaches train the patient to perform a specific functional behavior. Single case, or small group, studies have demonstrated the efficacy of functional task training with brain-injured adults in the areas of continence (Cohen, 1986), self-feeding (Hooper-Row, 1988), transfers (Goodman-Smith and Turnball, 1983), personal hygiene (Giles and Clark-Wilson, 1988; Giles and Shore, 1989), mobility and community skills (Giles and Clark-Wilson, 1993), social skills (Gajar, et al., 1984; Brotherton. et al., 1988), and behavioral control (Eames and Wood, 1985). In specific task training, the therapist attempts to teach the patient to perform a specific functional task. The intervention may or may not involve task specific compensatory training. (For example, a hemianoptic patient who is being taught to cross the street may be trained to overcompensate by turning their head to the left. Since there are many activities that involve scanning left to compensate for a visual field deficit, it is helpful if the patient is taught to do this in as many situations as possible.) Elsewhere we have advocated what we have called a neurofunctional approach, which involves an attempt to restructure the patient's way of approaching the world by training specific routines across many functional settings. It is hoped that the patient will be able to generalize the skills learned in functional settings to novel settings (a bottom-up approach) (Giles and Clark-Wilson, 1993). Using the terminology of the World Health Organization (WHO, 1980), what is taught is intended to reduce the patient's disability or handicap. The intervention must address a behavior of clinical importance and to an extent which makes a real difference. What is or is not worth learning may vary from patient to patient, and depends on the general severity of the patient's impairments and likely future living environment. In most cases training must be complete enough to be self-perpetuating by the time the patient is discharged from the treatment setting, or it will not be maintained.

Functional retraining may best be conceptualized as part of an intervention strategy with three major components: 1) pharmacological/medical interventions, 2) functional retraining (which includes motor skills retraining), and 3) behavioral/environmental manipulation which provides the patients with the most beneficial learning environment. Functional retraining must consider the learning characteristics of the patient in the design and implementation of programs. Since attention, memory, and problem solving deficits are central to many of our patient's problems, these areas must be considered in the development of retraining programs. A theoretical framework for considering these deficits will be discussed before an outline of a system of functional retraining is described.

ATTENTION DEFICIT
Automatic and Control Processing

Shiffrin and Schneider (1977) describe attention in terms of attention-dependent controlled processing and attention-independent automatic processing. Controlled processing is capacity limited and is required for new learning to occur. During the learning phase of an activity, the unskilled individual relies heavily on feedback about his performance and consciously attends to the activity (controlled processing). This focused attention continues during the practice stage of response acquisition. Once the action is learned, the individual's performance is controlled by a series of "prearranged instruction sequences" which act independently of feedback (automatic processing), leaving the individual free to concentrate on other aspects of the same or different tasks. Automatic processing occurs without conscious control, and places only limited demands on the information processing system. Observations of individuals following severe brain injury, suggest that activities which were previously automatic are disrupted by brain injury. Levin, Goldstein, High, and coworkers (1988), administered free recall and frequency of occurrence tasks to patients with severe brain injury and a control group. In their first experiment, Levin and associates (1988), found that both free recall (an effortful task), and judgment of relative frequency of occurrence (an automatic task), were impaired in 15 brain-injured patients relative to the control group. In a second experiment, the authors corroborated this finding, and showed that estimates of frequency were also impaired in a different group of 16 brain-injured patients. Shiffrin and Schneider (1977) have described two types of attentional system breakdown: divided attentional deficits and focused attentional deficits.

Divided Attentional Deficit

A divided attentional deficit (DAD) (Schneider, Dumais, and Shiffrin, 1984) indicates a failure of the capacity limited attentional system to accommodate all the information necessary for optimum task performance. For example, in gait retraining a patient may be able to ambulate with standby assistance, unless a person walks across their visual field or says "Good morning," whereupon they lose their balance. This failure constitutes a divided attentional deficit, because the patient had insufficient attentional capacity to walk and attend to any other information. A study by Stuss, et al. (1989), using a complex reaction time task, confirmed the existence of DAD among brain-injured patients. Patients are slow in tasks which require consciously controlled information processing, and demonstrate an inability to process multiple pieces of information rapidly. Stuss, et al. (1989), found this to be so even in mildly injured patients.

Focused Attentional Deficit

A focused attentional deficit (FAD) typically occurs when an unfamiliar response is required to a stimulus, which already has an overlearned response linked to it (Schneider, Dumais, and Shiffrin, 1984). Continuous attention from the individual may be required to suppress this automatic behavior. Stuss, et al. (1989), developed a series of computer tasks designed to assess focused attentional deficits; the research design examined the ability to suppress a previously learned complex level of processing when a simpler level of processing was demanded. A complex reaction time computer program task which required multiple discrimination (shape, internal line orientation, color) was followed by a task, the outward appearance of which was identical to this complex task, but which required a far less complex level of discrimination. Although both patients and controls were informed of the change, the patients were less able than the controls to inhibit the processing of redundant information. The concept of FAD depends to some extent on a Hullian notion of habit strength. For example, when attempting to reach a destination, we may deviate from the correct route to another route of greater familiarity which it partially overlaps. Once arriving at the familiar (and in this case unwanted) destination, we may realize that it was reached on "autopilot." Individuals with brain injury may be extremely inattentive in this sense and have a reduced ability to sustain their attention on new tasks. Below we will suggest that individuals with brain injury are also less likely to spontaneously monitor their behavior for errors on an ongoing basis, making them more susceptible to this type of error.

Selectivity

Performance of virtually all tasks is influenced by the presence of competing attentional demands (Kewman, Yanus, and Kirsch, 1988). The ability to selectively attend depends on discriminating task-relevant information from competing background stimuli. For example, following traumatic brain injury, individuals have more difficulty than the nonneurologically impaired in filtering out distracting verbal information from relevant verbal information (Kewman, Yanus, and Kirsch, 1988). Part of the difficulty in maintaining selective attention may be due to an inability to suppress responses to novel or irrelevant stimuli. As a task is practiced, novel and irrelevant stimuli become less distracting as the individual habituates to them (Lorch, Anderson, and Well, 1984). In Solokov's (1963) view, habituation occurs because repeated presentation allows the individual to construct a mental representation of the irrelevant stimuli as irrelevant. There is no evidence, however, to suggest that generalization of the habituation process occurs.

Attention and Memory

Long-term memory storage can be conceptualized under the headings procedural and declarative (Tulving, 1983). Declarative memory has its greatest development in man (Squire, 1986). Information in this store is available to introspection. Declarative memory may be divided into semantic and episodic memory. Episodic memory stores information about temporally dated events, and the temporal-spatial relations between these events (Tulving, 1972). It refers to "historical" information specific to the individual. Semantic memory is organized knowledge about the world, which is normally not tied to context (it includes the majority of information learned in institutional education, e.g., scientific facts and historical dates) (Tulving, 1972). Tulving maintains that the retrieval of information (from the episodic or semantic memory systems) constitutes an episode. One implication of this theory is that the act of remembering is recorded in the episodic memory store thus changing its overall contents. Episodic memory is the most vulnerable to impairment. Though deficits in acquiring new semantic information probably occur in tandem with episodic memory deficits, semantic memory stores may still be accessed, and learning may take place via frequent repetition of to-be-remembered information.

Procedural memory can be thought of as the store of acquired patterns of behavior not necessarily mediated by cognition. Procedural "knowledge" is not available to introspection, information is accessed through performance. Learning may occur without the subject being aware that learning has taken place. Nissen and Bullemer (1987) examined the attentional requirements of procedural learning to determine whether attention is necessary for procedural learning as it is for introspectively available forms of knowledge acquisition. A computerized serial reaction time task was used. A light appeared at one of four locations. Subjects pressed one key out of a set of four located directly below the position of the light. Learning was evaluated by measuring facilitation of performance on a repeating 10-trial stimulus sequence about which the subjects were naive. In nonneurologically impaired subjects there was considerable improvement in performance when this was the only task; however, when given in a dual-task condition (a condition reducing the subjects' ability to attend to the task), learning of the sequence, as assessed by verbal report and performance measures, was minimal. Patients with Korsakoff's syndrome were also able to learn the sequence in the single task condition, despite their lack of awareness of the repeating pattern. Nissen and Bullemer (1987) conclude that improved performance in the task, which is dependent on procedure memory, required the subject to attend to it.

There is increasing interest in the role of procedural memory in the acquisition of complex behaviors. Lewicki and coworkers, in a series of experiments (Lewicki, Hill, and Bizot, 1988; Lewick, Czyzewska, and Hoffman, 1987), have examined the ability of individuals to acquire relatively complex procedural knowledge. Results confirm that nonconsciously acquired knowledge can automatically be utilized to facilitate performance, but of particular note in the reports of Lewicki and colleagues, is the extreme complexity of the tasks employed. Although the skill acquisition is likely to be via procedural learning, the tasks were far more complex than those normally thought to be subserved by this memory system.

Problem Solving and Planning

Freedman, Bleiberg, and Freedland (1987), examined the ability of closed brain-injured patients to forward plan, using a relatively simple conditioning paradigm (a shuttlebox analog avoidance task). When compared to a group of patients after a cerebrovascular accident, the closed brain-injured patients demonstrated greater anticipatory behavior deficits, despite the fact that the two groups did not differ on escape behavior, and that the closed brain-injured group were equivalent or better on performance of individual tests of the Halstead-Reitan Battery and Wechsler scales. Neither clarification of the instruction, additional trials nor enhancement of the warning cue, appeared to ameliorate the anticipatory behavior deficit. The authors suggested that patients with anticipatory behavior deficits would show deficits in situations where current behavior should be regulated on the basis of expected future consequences. Vilkki (1988), using a task similar to the token test but with more ambiguity, found patients with frontal lobe deficits fail to identify the appropriate categories for sorting. Cicerone, Lazar, and Shapiro (1983), found that subjects with frontal lobe lesions failed to systematically explore a hypothesis (general concept formation) and failed to discard an inappropriate hypothesis. The authors suggest that the deficit may be the result of disturbance of an attentional control mechanism which is involved in the ongoing monitoring of feedback from the environment and segregates relevant from irrelevant sources of information. Brain-injured individuals may not engage in the internal behaviors necessary for planning, and subsequently executing, complex dependant sequences of action. Shallice and Evans (1978) attempted to explicate some of these issues using a novel research protocol. They noticed that many of their patients who had frontal lobe impairment, demonstrated a gross inability to produce adequate cognitive estimates. The authors asked the patients questions which tapped areas of knowledge which most people possess, but which require material to be accessed and manipulated in novel ways. Answering such questions adequately involves the selection of an appropriate plan to answer the question and check possible answers mentally for error. Examples of the questions included: "On average how many TV programs are shown on one TV channel between 6:00 pm and 11:00 pm?" and "What is the length of an average man's spine?" In the latter question, one must compare the spontaneous estimate of an average persons height with the percentage of an individual's height accounted for by his spine. The patients with anterior lesions performed considerably worse than either patients with posterior lesions or normal controls. The authors interpret this finding as a deficit in planning and checking answers against multiple types of data for bizarreness and inconsistency.

In order to carry out complex behaviors which require the initiation of novel behaviors through time, it is necessary to develop a plan and then initiate a check act/wait cycle (Reason, 1984). Once the plan is developed the individual compares "plan time" with real time in order to determine whether he needs to initiate a plan component or wait. For example, in order to get to an appointment 45 minutes across town, we intermittently check the time throughout the day so as to leave at an appropriate time. Each time we look at the clock we decide if we need to leave or wait. As the time for leaving approaches, we look at the clock with greater frequency and also begin to adjust our other activities so as to allow us to leave on time. Many of our patients, particularly those with marked frontal lobe impairment appear unable to initiate this type of planning behavior. Developing neither action plans nor the "drive" required for the check act/wait cycles. The author found it particularly instructive to observe some severely injured patients doing their laundry. It rapidly became apparent that the severely brain-injured patients were unable to check to see if their laundry was dry. The absence of checking could not be accounted for by memory impairment (the patients when questioned were aware that their clothes were in the dryer), nor by lack of knowledge about the laundry procedures involved, nor by lack of motivation. The patients, nonetheless, required an external cue to enable them to initiate the behavior. Many therapists attempt to have the patient practice problem solving and reasoning to overcome these deficits. The author believes these types of interventions to be misdirected. What the patient cannot do is spontaneously develop and monitor a novel dependent sequence of actions. Rather than have the patient attempt to improve their responses to novelty we attempt to have patients overlearn needed behavioral sequences. Some types of novelty can be accommodated by training the patient in the use of a diary or other form of external memory aid. The overlearning of frequent checking of the diary must be a component of this retraining.

Functional Assessment

Functional assessment may make use of a range of evaluation techniques. Methods include observation, questionnaires, check list and rating scales, and standardized assessment tools. Of these methods the most important is observation. Functional assessment determines current level of functioning and assists in the determination of optimal forms of retraining. The functional assessment is central to the selection of goals and target behaviors required for the rehabilitation teams integrated treatment plan. Functional assessments should be conducted under conditions as close as possible to those the person will experience following rehabilitation. Functional assessment, therefore, differs from other types of testing which demand highly standardized conditions. The rigorous control of variables necessary for the pursuit of science is sacrificed in favor of ecologic validity. There are many variables which influence performance in real world situations, for example, the presence of setting events, cues, or environmental conditions. The ability to make accurate observations is a skill acquired with training and experience. Most therapists do not emphasize observation. This may be due to lack of appreciation of the importance of establishing a picture of what the client does unconstrained by external cues or demands. Observational assessment methods are described more concretely under the discussion of concrete retraining methods below.

Functional Retraining

Severe brain-injury often results in the loss or disruption of patterns of adaptive behavior. Additionally, the individual's ability to reacquire adaptive patterns of behavior is impaired. The frequency of disruption of basic self-care skills has been estimated at 5%–15% (Jennet and Teasdale, 1981; Jacobs, 1988). The disruption of more complex self-care skills appears to be more common (Jacobs, 1988). The extent and location of brain injury places constraints on human learning, but the ability to acquire new behaviors is retained in all but the most profoundly injured. Having discussed some of the factors which lead to the disruption of functional behaviors, we consider how we might retrain a cognitively impaired brain-injured person on a functional task. Let us take, as a concrete example, how we might train an individual with severe memory impairment to cross the street. Having performed a task analysis, we determine that crossing the street safely consists of stopping at the curbside, looking in both directions, and then walking directly across the street, when there are no motor vehicles within a certain distance (depending on the patients speed of ambulation, street width, and so forth). Having performed the task analysis we can develop a program of verbal prompts, the purpose of which is to elicit from the patient the appropriate behavior and direct the patient's attention to the factors in the task which lead to success or failure. The first time the patient practices street crossing is an "episode." It is processed, and the specific to-be-learned activity is associated with the specific street intersection, the traffic which is passing, and other incidental information. This episode may not be available later for introspection, but a certain priming effect will have occurred. On the second occasion retraining occurs, only certain aspects of the situation will have been held constant, for instance, the specific instructions given. As this street crossing routine is repeated always using the same prompts, the street crossing "episodes" are not retained (or at least are not recallable). The street crossing memory becomes an abstraction of many specific memory traces, all inevitably slightly different, that eventually produces the generalized memory structure of "crossing streets." This experience becomes prototypical, and the patient develops a habit of crossing the street in the way which has been practiced. In optimum cases, the patient no longer chooses to cross the street in a certain manner, the patient just "knows" that this is how to cross the street. Initially during treatment, there is an attempt to reduce the possibility of failure to a minimum by the cues given (see Warrington and Weiskrantz, 1968, 1974, on cued recall in amnesia). As performance improves, cues may be faded. The task practiced must be ultimately performable given the fixed aspects of the patients deficits (if the therapist attempts to teach behaviors which are beyond the patient's cognitive ability the program will fail). Although apparently banal, this is a central issue which is often overlooked in functional skills retraining programs.

The role of the functional skills trainer is to determine the functional skill to be trained, develop methods which allow the patient to perform the task with the minimum amount of new learning, and develop a method which directs the patient's attention to the central components of the task.

Programming may be thought to exist on a behavioral-cognitive behavioral continuum. All treatment centers around modifying the patient's previous responses (Giles and Clark-Wilson, 1988) and replacing them with new and more adaptive ones via practice. More cognitively preserved patients can be assisted to attend to, and interrupt, inappropriate behaviors and replace them with more adaptive behaviors themselves. What can be taught also depends on the patient's cognitive abilities. Functional skills which require the patient to cope with novelty require a more complex set of cognitive abilities. For example, complete functional use of a diary always involves decisions about what information to write down. Practice in how to make entries and what information to enter reduces the difficulty of these tasks, but the patient must, nevertheless, be able to categorize a particular event as one of the classes of events which are recorded and initiate the recording. Training programs which attempt to address a general behavior, such as reduce a social skills deficit or develop use of a memory book in a severely impaired patient, should include the following three stages: 1) A cognitive overlearning element which is an attempt to focus the patient's attention on the behavior or area of skills deficit and then develop a verbal label for the behavior. The therapist discusses the long-term consequences of the behavior or skill deficit with the patient. The therapist emphasizes its inconvenience and the benefits likely to accrue to the patient from changing it. If the patient has severe deficits, this cognitive component may need to be reviewed one or more times per day and may continue throughout or beyond the other program elements. 2) Sessional practice of required behaviors. Here the patient practices the behavior for a short period of time in an environment controlled by the therapist. The patient must be able to produce the behavior with only moderate effort in this controlled environment before progressing to the 24-hour program approach. 3) In stage 3 there is an attempt to target each instance of the behavior throughout the day. This type of intervention requires an interdisciplinary team and a high level of staff training. Each time the patient exhibits the target behavior, a staff member responds in a predetermined manner, usually so as to have the patient attend to the behavior, categorize it as an instance of the target behavior, suppress it, and replace it with an alternative or incompatible behavior. Training of less severely impaired patients may take place in settings which can exert less control over patient behavior. However, the process of skill acquisition may be conceptualized in a similar way: cognitive overlearning, sessional practice generalized response acquisition.

In the author's experience, the degree to which a behavior becomes automatic influences its durability. Behaviors which are possible to develop to a high degree of automaticity, such as washing and dressing (and which are practiced repeatedly), are extremely robust. Behaviors which require to be consciously initiated by the subject, such as use of a memory book, require more specific and ongoing environmental support.

In addition to the above, central to the operation of functional retraining programs, is the development of an appropriate rehabilitation culture or holding environment. For a discussion of the development of rehabilitation culture see Giles and Clark-Wilson (1993).

Reinforcement and Skill Building

A reinforcing event is one which increases the likelihood of the behavior which immediately precedes it being repeated. Reinforcers may be primary or secondary. Primary reinforcers are intrinsically desirable (such as social attention, praise, and candy). Secondary reinforcers are points or tokens which may be traded for primary reinforcers. There is some evidence that reinforcement aids learning (Dolan and Norton, 1977; Lashley and Drabman, 1974). The reason that reinforcement increases learning is unknown but may be related to the ability of reinforcement to direct attention toward the to-be-learned aspects of the practiced behaviors.

Task Analysis

Task analysis involves a process of dividing tasks into component parts, which can be taught as units, and chained together into a functional whole. The analysis provides a method of organizing behaviors so as to make them easier to learn. The components of a task analysis may be converted to verbal or visual prompts, and the learner's attention is directed to each step of the activity sequentially. These can be built into subgroups of contiguous core skills and/or identified as functional clusters of behavior. These clusters can be taught as a single instructional step to learners who are more competent. A functional cluster is defined as a sequence of 2–4 component, contiguous "core skills" that have a meaningful relationship, and constitute an identifiable, and potentially teachable, segment of a whole task. An example of a core skill might be establishing an appropriate sitting posture. An example of a functional cluster might be all the steps that go into preparing for a wheelchair transfer. When using a task analysis to develop a set of verbal cues, the number of cues depends on the patient's ability. For example, in developing a washing and dressing program, some patients require only a few prompts, such as "wash your face," to produce complex behavioral chains. Other patients require several prompts, for example, "pick up the washcloth," "put soap on the washcloth," "wash your face," "rinse the washcloth." O'Reilly and Cuvo (1989) used an interesting variant of this procedure in attempting to train self-treatment of cold symptoms to an anoxic brain-injured adult. Three levels of cuing were used. Generic prompts (nonspecific subject headings), specific prompts (based on a specific step-by-step task analysis), and individualized prompts where specific prompt sequences were provided only when the client failed to provide the appropriate behavior to the generic prompt.

Where clients were able to respond to verbal prompts to carry out procedures, we have found it most effective to use a whole task system in which prompts are provided for each step until the task is completed. An exception to this general rule applies to clients who are so slow that attempting to train the whole task is too demanding. Where this is the case, specific functional clusters may be selected.

Prompts

Events which facilitate the production of a behavior are called prompts (or cues). A prompt assists an individual to produce the target behavior, which may then be reinforced. In many instances, prompts are available in the environment, but they are no longer sufficient to guide behavior or they have lost their meaning entirely (e.g., arriving at a busy road junction no longer cues safe street crossing routines). The therapist adds additional prompts to those already available in the environment. Therapists can facilitate the learning of skills with differing types of prompts; verbal instruction, written lists, physical touch, or guidance. Once the skill is reliably carried out, the prompt can be faded until performance occurs without the additional aid to initiation.

Shaping

Shaping refers to the reinforcement of closer and closer approximations to the desired behavior. Tasks are graded in difficulty so they are achievable. As competency is demonstrated the task requirements are increased. For example, one patient seen by the author would pace the corridors of the treatment facility when not engaged in an activity by staff. The goal of intervention was to have the patient sit with others and engage in appropriate conversation. Initially, he was reinforced (with attention and food) if he remained in the unit day room; later he was only reinforced if he was sitting down; and finally only if engaged in appropriate conversation.

Control of a Behavior by Antecedents

For many clinicians, applied behavioral analysis, when applied to brain-injured persons, has been synonymous with an operant conditioning model. Antecedents may be altered in an attempt to change behavior. This is a method of setting the environmental conditions—the stimulus events—so as to increase the possibility that the patient will emit the desired behavior. Elsewhere we reported the use of posters containing specific information in an attempt to "prime" the individual in certain activities (Giles and Clark-Wilson, 1988). The control of specific antecedents may be particularly useful in working with patients with profound memory impairment. Zencius, Wesolowski, Burke, and McQuade (1989), compared the effect of altering antecedents with the effect of varying consequences in three patients with marked memory disorder following severe brain injury. Zencius and coworkers (1989) found that posting a sign regarding break times at the work station of the first patient they studied drastically reduced the number of unauthorized breaks. In another client, the most effective way to increase cane usage, a goal of the rehabilitation team, was to provide her with a cane to use during her morning ADLs. This technique was found to be more effective than social praise, a contract for money, or someone to escort her to get her cane when she was found without it. In a third patient, the authors found that a map and a written daily schedule was more powerful than a contract for money in increasing therapy attendance. The alteration in the antecedents produced behavioral improvement, whereas attempts to alter behavior by manipulating consequences had proved to be at best only marginally successful (for a fuller discussion see Giles and Clark-Wilson, 1993).

Overlearning

Overlearning refers to the practice of a skill well beyond the point where the patient is able to produce the behavior. Overlearning increases the chances that the skill is consolidated—has become automatic—and reduces the amount of effort required for performance. When a skill becomes automatic, it becomes the easiest behavior to initiate from an array of possible behaviors (i.e., the possibility of an interference error is reduced). The goal of rehabilitation can often best be met by having the individual engage in overlearning. For example, a street crossing program should not be terminated on meeting the functional criteria, but on meeting criteria plus a certain number of practice sessions designed to make the behavior automatic. The number of additional sessions required to develop automaticity is unclear. Automaticity is assessed by ongoing monitoring on the patient's behavior in conjunction with distractions.

Fading

Verbal cues may be faded by forming clusters of prompts from the task analysis after the individual has learned to complete the behavior in response to the original prompts. Another method of fading is to increase the time between completion of the previous behavior and the provision of the subsequent prompt. This delay procedure should only be used, however, when the patient has already developed the skill to the point where they can be 80%–90% correct, as otherwise they are likely to "practice" the propagation of incorrect responses—a situation to be avoided. Questions like "What's next?" or instructions telling the individual to "go ahead" can help the individual initiate the activity and decreases dependence on prompts.

Encore Procedure

When an individual demonstrates an infrequently displayed skill without prompting, he or she can be prompted to produce several more correct responses. For example, CP was learning to attract people's attention appropriately before asking questions or making requests in social skills training sessions. On any occasion when she asked appropriately, such as by saying the persons name, or saying "excuse me" (rather than by screaming or banging objects) and then asking a question, she was given social, and occasionally tangible, reinforcement and asked to repeat the sequence of behaviors again, whereupon she was reinforced again.

Highlighting

Many individuals after brain injury have problems in distinguishing the central aspects of a task. Highlighting refers to a strategy that promotes the discrimination of the crucial elements of an activity by exaggerating the perceptual salience of some stimulus features. Prompts are progressively faded once the patient is consistently making correct discriminations. Highlighting might be achieved by emphasizing phrases, pointing, touching, or by providing specific reinforcement.

More cognitively oriented intervention should involve consideration of the foregoing factors, but, in addition, should maximize use of the patients own retained learning ability. The therapists role becomes to supervise the patient in setting their own goals, and developing their own strategies to perform functional tasks. For example, a patient who has been working on improving their community mobility might set themselves the task of finding the way to a specific novel location. The patient would then have to develop for themselves, with the assistance of the therapist, a knowledge of the parameters involved in the task, e.g., available means of transportation, time requirements, cost, route finding methods, and so forth. Initially, limited time periods should be set aside for the individual to "self-schedule," as they may find the activity stressful, may become inactive without continuous support, become sidetracked, or demonstrate behavioral deterioration. As the patient shows increasing competencies, longer periods of time and more complex tasks can be set for the patient. Eventually, long periods of the treatment day should be devoted to the patient pursuing their own goals, periodically "checking in" with the therapist who can ensure that they remain critically self-aware. The therapist's goal is to set tasks and direct the patients' attention on how their current experience can be incorporated into strategies to improve their future functioning. Tasks might include enrolling in evening classes, college programs, or finding social activities. Interactions with individuals after brain injury should be designed to facilitate learning. Two techniques central to this type of intervention are goal statements and debriefing.

Goal Statements

The incorporation of goal statements in each session has a number of advantages in helping brain-injured individuals learn. It may increase participation, help the patient attend to the to-be-learned aspect of their activities (this discriminatory aspect may need to be repeated throughout the session), and it communicates respect from therapist to patient. For patients with lack of insight, it orients them to their deficits and cues them as to how the to-be-undertaken therapeutic activity will help them achieve their own goals. Therapists may wish to present the session as a scientific endeavor, in which either the therapist or the patient are allowed to have incorrect notions, but in which an empirical question is examined. With some patients, however, active agreement with the therapeutic intervention is not attainable, and the therapist seeking agreement will only sidetrack the patients and derail the therapeutic endeavor. The therapist is not advised to abandon the goal of developing functional skills by waiting until the patient knows that he has deficits. Goal-directing statements, for example, for 5 minutes at the beginning of each session and interspersed statements throughout, orienting patients to these issues is frequently indicated. For example, "As you know as a result of your severe brain injury you have needed some help in washing and dressing yourself. We are working with you every morning so that you can develop a system to be independent. You can now perform all but three of the activities of washing and dressing completely independently."

Debriefing

Regular debriefing about performance (knowledge of results) is indicated in producing positive behavioral change. Telling the patient that they have done well is encouraging, but nonspecific and damaging if untrue. Feedback about results should be concrete and accurate, written materials that the patient can refer to, such as graphs or logs, should be used where possible.

ASSESSMENT AND TRAINING IN SPECIFIC SKILL AREAS
Self-Feeding

Patients may have difficulty in the motor control of eating and drinking or in regulating their consumption. Inadequate eating and drinking may result from oral motor disorders, decreased arousal, akathisia, ataxia dyspraxia, or other motor disorders. Motor control deficits may be complicated by lowered frustration tolerance and behavior disorder. Assessment of oral motor functioning may be performed by the occupational therapist or the speech therapist. Assessment and treatment of oral motor dysfunction is an area of specialized practice, and the interested reader is referred to the materials listed in the references (Lazarus and Logemann, 1987; Logemann, 1983; see Chapter 9). Adaptive equipment may be useful in the acute stages of recovery and make eating considerably less stressful for the patient. Training the patient in appropriate positioning to maximize stability and control to decrease the effects of abnormal tone, may have a significant effect on eating. Hooper-Roe (1988) has described a successful self-feeding program with a profoundly impaired and uncooperative patient who had previously been fed by nasogastric tube for 2½ years.

Patients may attempt to overfeed or hydrate themselves. Damage to the food regulatory centers in the hypothalamus may be implicated. A condition similar to the hyperorality which may follow herpes simplex encephalitis may follow brain trauma. Memory deficits frequently occur in conjunction with the disorder so that the patient has no memory of having eaten. These patients are notoriously difficult to treat. Limiting the patients access to food may be warranted (see Chapter 13).

Transfers

Being able to transfer without assistance is an important component of independent functioning. Failure to transfer independently is usually the result of a combination of motor control and cognitive deficits, so a transfer training program should consider both types of deficits. Both the ease and fluency of motor control and the organization of the activity are disrupted. Assessment involves observing the patient in order to determine why they fail to transfer safely. A transfer training program should be designed so that it can function as a functional cluster and be used in other training programs. Real muscles (unlike mental ones) become stronger and more efficient with exercise; however, we prefer to have this happen by gradually decreasing the assistance provided to the patient while they perform the real functional task, rather than during an exercise program. A tripartite frame of reference should be used during the implementation of a transfer training program. The sessional practice can be used to perfect the patient's positioning, and the verbal cues and the program can be used on a 24-hour basis as soon as the staff can be trained to carry it out safely. The program may also be rehearsed verbally with the patient so as to accelerate the patient's grasp of the organization of the movement. Table 7.1 provides a typical transfer training program.

Washing and Dressing

Washing and dressing deficits may occur as a result of cognitive or motor control dysfunction. Since a large number of factors may contribute to washing and dressing difficulties, a detailed assessment is essential to arrive at an adequate formulation of the patient's problems. We observe the patient's behavior on three mornings to the prompt "Do what you would normally do to get washed and dressed in the morning." The patient is reprompted if they have not engaged in any washing and dressing related activities for 5 minutes. If the patient is not performing adequately, more specific cues can be provided. The therapist looks for

Table 7.1.
Transferring from Wheelchair to Chair

---

1. Position wheelchair by the side of the chair
2. Put brakes on
3. Remove footrests
4. Sit well (previously established core skill involving feet flat on the ground and with a space between them with toes under knees back straight and head in midline)
5. Clasp hands—stretch elbows
6. Lean forward
7. Stand up
8. Pivot
9. Check for chair
10. Reach forward and sit down

---

why performance breaks down, the complexity of behavior a patient can perform to a cue (for example, a patient may only be able to produce adequate washing behavior to the prompt "Wash your face" if the words "Use soap, rinse, and dry" are added), and any relatively fixed functional cluster behaviors the patient displays spontaneously. By embedding retained skills in the program, the amount of new learning required of the patient is reduced. Wherever possible, we use a whole task approach with verbal cues derived from a task analysis. Central to the success of a washing and dressing program is that a method be developed which allows the patient to be independent and which is consistent with the patient's other physical rehabilitation goals. Patient's with motor control impairments often require physical assistance, particularly in positioning or transfers at the beginning of a program of washing and dressing training. Design of the program must, however, consider a realistic estimate of the patient's improvement, so that realistic goals can be determined. Motor components of retraining programs should be consistent with each other. For example, if the patient is being taught to stand, with the aim of having the patient ambulate, the patient can be taught to stand during a dressing program rather than arch on the bed. The new physical routines, such as transferring or standing, may require multiple cues and physical assistance initially, and are usually the most difficult sequences for the patient to learn. In addition, learning to place the separate activities of washing in a fixed, and therefore nonrepetitive, sequence may be difficult. Both the order of washing and physical routines may be rehearsed verbally throughout the patient's day. Initially, in the verbal practice sessions, the patient should be cued sufficiently to ensure that they produce the correct answer, as one does not want the patient to practice producing the wrong answer (reducing false positive errors). The patient can be verbally and/or tangibly reinforced for correct answers and told "No. That was incorrect" when they make an error. My colleague, Jo Clark-Wilson, has reported the successful use of a computer program as an adjunctive training device in this procedure (Clark-Wilson, 1988). As the patient learns, so prompts may be consolidated. The patient continues to perform the same routine but requires progressively fewer prompts. Fading may also be accomplished by pausing for long periods before providing the next cue and encouraging the patient to go on to the next task, or by asking what comes next. Patients who are behaviorally disregulated are often at their most aggressive during personal hygiene activities.

COMMUNITY MOBILITY

Street Crossing

Clinical experience suggests that unsafe street crossing is extremely common following brain injury. Many deficits may underlie the patient's problems in street crossing (hemianopia, neglect, perceptual disorders, attention disorder, impulsivity). Street crossing is a functional skill which was automatic prior to injury, but which requires conscious attention following injury. In order to assess the patient, the therapist should accompany the patient on a short trip in the community. The therapist can establish a route which includes a number of different types of streets to cross, both pedestrian protected and unprotected. On leaving the facility the therapist should explain to the patient the purpose of the session. The therapist should walk a foot or so behind the patient so as to stop him or her, if necessary, from walking into traffic. If the patient crosses the street safely during the early part of the assessment, the therapist should engage the patient in unrelated conversation to see if the patient can maintain safe behavior when distracted. Patients with relatively mild deficits may only require a small number of sessions designed to concentrate their attention on safe street crossing in order to achieve an acceptable standard. More handicapped patients, and those with specific perceptual deficits (e.g., left neglect), require a specific street crossing program. Starting with one or two intersections may assist in the development of an initial schema before introducing more variations (different intersections).

Topographic Orientation

Navigating novel environments may be problematic for many patients. Memory impairment, as well as deficits in topographic orientation, may severely impair the patient's community mobility. Some patients have difficulty in learning to find their way in new environments. Other patients can no longer find their way around what should be familiar environments. Benton (1985) views these deficits as dependent on perceptual and attentional deficits. Although topographic disorientation does occur more frequently in patients with neglect, there do appear to be patients without marked perceptual or attentional deficits who have lost previous geographic schema or have a specific learning deficit for route finding. An unimpaired person should be able to travel an unfamiliar route for 5 minutes with 2–3 turns, and have no difficulty in finding his or her way back. If the patient is able to perform adequately on this test, and the patient is otherwise safe, the therapist may proceed to more complex routes and have the patient navigate to more distant points independently. If the patient fails, the therapist may need to know how many times the patient needs to walk a route to learn it. Where the patient continues to have difficulty even after multiple trials, the therapist should investigate whether the patient can successfully read a map or follow printed directions on a checkoff board. Many patients will only be able to follow overlearned routes, but being able to get to even a limited number of sites may considerably increase quality of life.

Physical Deficits

Many patients have physical deficits which impair their community mobility. Even patients who are independent indoor ambulatory, or who can use a wheelchair indoors, may be unable to manage local community mobility. Some patients may be able to develop this ability if they are provided with sufficient endurance training or relocate to an area where local amenities are close by. Other patients may be taught to maximize their mobility using local transportation options (buses, taxis). Other patients will require some form of outdoor mobility aid. This may be very difficult for the patient (and the staff) to accept, and how to present and train the patient on the use of an aid should be carefully considered.

Driving

Patients are frequently very eager to resume, or if adolescents, begin driving. Jacobs (1988) found that between 1–6 years postinjury, 37% of severely brain-injured patients in his study returned to driving, as compared with 93.7% who were driving preinjury. Neither therapists' clinical judgments nor objective (paper and pencil) tests have been shown to predict on-the-road driving skill (Galski, Ehle, and Bruno, 1990). Van Zomeren, et al. (1988), examined fitness to drive after severe brain injury. Daytime driving was studied in 1) an instrumented car that recorded lateral position control, and 2) in driving the subject's own car with a professional observer. The brain-injured subjects were all at least 3 years postinjury (mean 6.5) and all were driving. In comparison with a control group, the brain-injured subjects performed worse. Five out of nine were classified as incompetent, suggesting that there are many brain-injured individuals who are currently driving who should not be. Of particular interest is the author's suggestion that deficits may not compromise an individual's ability to drive provided that the individual is able to compensate for them. Hence, insight and self-criticism may be a more important determinant for a patient's fitness to drive than the degree of other cognitive deficits. Kewman and coworkers (1985), attempted to improve the performance of postacute traumatically brain-injured patients on behavioral aspects of motor vehicle operation by providing specific training using a small, electrically powered, vehicle. The author's primary interest was whether improvement on these tasks would translate to the functional (and more complex) task of on-the-road automobile driving. A matched traumatic brain injury control group was provided with unstructured experience using the electrically powered vehicle, but were not provided with training. Experimental subjects showed improvements, both on the specific exercises and in performance, on a structured test of on-the-road automobile driving when compared with untrained brain-injured control subjects who did not show improvement. Results suggest a significant therapeutic affect of the specific training program; also that training in specific tasks is more effective than exposure and unstructured experience. The medical branch of the department of motor vehicles can determine whether a brain-injured individual may return to driving. In addition, there are now many specialized centers offering driving instruction and examination to handicapped people.

Shopping and Meal Preparation

Not everybody needs to be able to grocery shop and cook for themselves. Patients who are severely handicapped and are going to remain in an institutional setting or need to be cared for by family members, do not need to be able to purchase and prepare their own food. Many patients will, however, be able to achieve a level of independence where they need to provide themselves with an adequate diet. In addition to shopping and cooking, the individual needs to be able to budget, plan a menu, derive a list of items to purchase from the grocery store, and plan how to get there and back with groceries. Few single people living in the community prepare three cooked meals a day, and this is an unrealistic goal. In initial assessment we prefer to have the individual prepare a cold meal (avoiding the safety issues surrounding stove use). The patient might plan and shop for breakfast or a sandwich. Progress to hot meal preparation may begin with heating a can of soup or a TV dinner. Coordinating the cooking of items which need to be started at different times, and using the stovetop and oven simultaneously, is extremely complicated and is the final stage of assessment. Many patients will need to practice shopping for, and cooking, the same menus repeatedly in order to become proficient.

Social Skills

Social isolation is now recognized as a common long-term consequence of severe brain injury (Thomsen, 1974, 1984). Social skills training has been used in an attempt to ameliorate some of the patient's difficulties in meeting friends and sustaining established relationships. Social skills re-training has been shown to improve the social interactional skills of patients in both psychiatric and nonpsychiatric settings (Plienis, et al., 1987). Evaluative studies of social skills retraining with the brain-injured are few, and results have been inconsistent. Johnson and Newton (1987a) examined 11 severely brain-injured patients attending an occupational therapy day center. The brain-injured patients demonstrated a high level of social anxiety, poor social performance, and low self-esteem. The authors suggest that these are important contributory factors in the poor overall social adjustment of these patients. Johnson and Newton (1987b) attempted to remedy specific problem areas in social interaction by providing social skills retraining once a week for 2 hours, over a 1 year period. The brain-injured group were assessed on a range of measures at the beginning of the study, at 6 months, and at 1 year. In addition, a social performance measure was designed which included videotaping standardized conversation, which was then rated by two observers on 12 aspects of verbal and nonverbal social behaviors. Each training session included a review of the previous meeting and the week's activities, then introduction of the main theme of the meeting, discussion, role play, and feedback. Adjunctive procedures included printed handouts, posters, diaries of activities, and a video system for immediate feedback. After 1 year the changes of the assessment scores were not statistically significant, but the authors suggested that their approach may be a useful starting point from which occupational therapists can develop more effective rehabilitation programs.

Gajar and coworkers (1984), describe the use of feedback and training in self-monitoring on two brain-injured adolescents. Feedback involved providing light signals corresponding to a positive or negative social interaction. Positive responses were those where the client added to a previous group member's statement by making a relevant comment, agreed or disagreed (and provided a rationale), or asked a relevant question. Negative responses were silences following another persons question or statement, statements of three words or less, or if a comment was off the topic, mumbled, a joke, or an interruption. An A1-B1-C1-A2-C2-B2 design was utilized, in which the baseline (A), feedback phase (B) and self-monitoring phase (C) were alternated to control for order effects. The study demonstrated the efficacy of both types of intervention. Helffestein and Weschler (1982) describe the use of Interpersonal Process Recall (IRP) in the remediation of interpersonal and communication skills deficits in the newly brain-injured. Sixteen 17–35-year-old brain-injured adults were randomly assigned to an experimental and a control group. The experimental group received 20 1-hour IRP sessions while the control group received nonspecific attention. The experimental group showed greater improvement in interpersonal skills, as assessed by professional staff ignorant of group placement.

Brotherton, Thomas, Wisotzek, and Milan (1988), described a sessional social skills training approach to social interactional deficits after closed brain-injury. The four patients treated were 2 years postinjury, and were in a coma for at least 7 days. They were nonaphasic, capable of following three stage commands, and were not physically violent. A multiple baseline across behavior design was utilized. The behavioral training package was most effective when applied to simple motoric target behaviors, e.g., self-manipulation or posture. Only the improvements patients made in these domains were retained at 1 year follow-up. Patients were unable to improve or retain improvement on more complex verbal behaviors, possibly because these areas require more linguistic processing ability than was actually present, or because they would only be responsive to long-term behavioral intervention.

Identification of Social Skills Deficits

We have found it useful to consider socially skilled behavior as verbal, including all aspects of speech, e.g., tone of voice, rate of speech, accent, volume, and intonation, and non-verbal, including facial expressions, gestures, and body movements. The aim of social skills training is to alter social behaviors in ways which increase social opportunities. The needs of individual patients are highly variable, so accurate assessment is necessary to ensure a realistic retraining program. In addition, assessment should provide the therapist with information about what is appropriate social behavior for that individual and indicate the environmental demands for social behavior. For example, one patient referred by a group home for treatment could return there if he could stop screaming and not sit so close to the television that he blocked the view of other residents of the home. A higher functioning patient would be able to return to live with his wife and family if he could stop shouting at, and criticizing, his children. Assessment methods include: informal observation data, behavioral observation and role play tests, interviews and self, peer, and family ratings and check lists. Any social situation can be a source of informal observational data, and may be used to assess the brain-injured person's nonverbal and verbal skills. Assessment of the brain-injured in their home environment or in functional social settings, e.g., shops and restaurants, may provide the therapist with an invaluable amount of data on the individual's social behavior.

Behavioral observation employs a more structured approach to data collection, both of the person in natural settings and in structured inter-actions (role plays). A variety of recording methods can be utilized, e.g., ABC recordings, frequency ratings, and behavioral sampling techniques. Although naturalistic observation is the assessment method most advo-cated by behavior therapists (Bellack, Hersen, and Lamparski, 1979), role play tests are frequently used, as they are less time consuming. Repre-sentative of role play tests is the Behavioral Assertiveness Test - Revised (BAT-R) of Eisler, Hersen, Miller, and Blanchard (1975).

Interviews provide information about the brain-injured patient's inter-personal history and provide a setting for informal observation. Inter-views can explore the patient's views of their background, family history, social contacts, understanding of social norms, their own evaluation of their behavior in social interactions, and their view of their present social situation.

Ratings and check list data can be used to categorize patient social skills deficits. To assess the brain-injured individual's level of social con-tact, patients and/or their relatives/friends, can be asked to record spe-cific social activities or interactions in a diary, e.g., the number of friends that visit or the number of times the patient went out socially during a specified period. A number of more general check lists or rating scales, such as the Adaptive Behavior Rating Scale, have sections for rating so-cial skills (Nihara, Foster, Shellhaas, and Leland, 1975).

Training Procedures

Social skills training, developed in psychiatric residential and outpa-tient settings, has tended to adopt a group format of 1–2 hours, 1–2 times per week. Although this format offers many advantages, it is probably not adequate if used in isolation with the severely impaired brain-injured pa-tient. Here we will discuss the use of group social skills training before discussing other aspects of a social skills retraining program.

Group Training Procedures

Group social skills retraining has specific advantages over individual teaching. The group setting provides the opportunity for maladaptive be-haviors to be observed and highlighted, and for patients to learn and prac-tice adaptive behaviors. The social skills group assists the therapist to facilitate the reacquisition and refinement of the basic skills needed for interpersonal communication and social interaction. Groups can provide a sense of belonging, and a safe environment in which to work through problems. The practice of some social skills, e.g., getting to know someone by asking appropriate questions in conversations, conveying verbal and nonverbal interest and attention to a group member, disclosing appropriate information about one's own interests, hobbies and background, and talking about topics that are likely to be of interest to peers, all establish group cohesion. Both group facilitators and group members can provide modelling of appropriate social skills. Participation in group social skills training assists in the identification of real life situations which prove difficult for the brain-injured individual. Patients can work together. This process encourages conversational skill development and assertive behavior.

The use of behavioral rehearsal, practice, and role plays, is facilitated by the group setting. Group rehearsal and practice is more stimulating, and may be more successful in maintaining the individual's attention, than individual work. As in individual sessions, the group requires consistency to ensure learning. The overall aims of retraining need to be reviewed regularly, and the skills practiced within the environment where they are needed.

Individual Programs Using a 24-Hour Approach

In agreement with our more general retraining recommendations, we have suggested (Giles, Fussey, and Burgess, 1988) that 24-hour intervention programs should involve three components: 1) A cognitive overlearning element to ensure that patients know the nature and likely implications of poor social performance; 2) sessional practice of appropriate social interactional skills; and 3) a 24-hour unit operant conditioning procedure. Without additional (highlighting) cues patients frequently do not attend to their social performance. Severely injured patients almost uniformly lack the ability to adopt an "as if" position, so it is not surprising that patients do not understand the impressions they create in others. We advocate multiple methods to increase the salience to the subject of their own social performance. These include unit-based events and reinforcers. In addition, bizarre or funny tokens may be used. On one occasion, in order to highlight to the patient a problem of speaking without pauses, the staff and the client all wore orange colored joke watches to time the patient and (with specific cues and reinforcers) limit her utterances to 90 seconds duration. Targets should be concrete operationalizable and comprehensible to the patient.

Vocational Reentry

Jellinek and Harvey (1982) found that counselling and assistance in pursuing job resources significantly improved the rate of employment in a series of brain-injured patients seen in a medical facility. The patient's premorbid functioning, the extent of individual patient's awareness and acceptance of the disability, and the family support system all influenced the probability for successful rehabilitation.

Appropriate placement and the informed support of employers and co-workers are also vital. Johnson and Gleave (1987) found that both the provision of special work conditions and the maintenance of those conditions over a protracted period were associated with successful return to work. In Johnson and Gleave's (1987) series, no one who changed both employer and type of work had a successful return. Johnson and Gleave (1987) noted that the average duration of work trial, or altered work condition, was longer than the average total work duration in those who lost their jobs (i.e., those patients who returned to work prematurely were terminated in less time than it took for those who returned more gradually to resume a full workload). Employers of those working in professional occupations were more able to provide moderated work conditions. We have found that a trial of work without pay to be of use in persuading employers of workers in more manual employment to rehire a brain-injured individual. Establishing a relationship with the employer is a prerequisite for a good outcome. It is important to know if the employer is committed to the employee returning to work. Educating the employer and coworkers about the difficulties the brain-injured individuals may encounter, and how to help the individual learn to function more effectively, is a central task in ensuring successful vocational reintegration. The therapist also needs to evaluate the feasibility of adjusting the employment to the employment needs, e.g., providing extra supervision, providing more frequent rest periods, providing daytime work shifts or half-days. In our experience, the employer's willingness to be flexible often relates more to the interpersonal climate of the job site and the nature of the job than to the employee's particular work history. Some employers are willing to be extremely flexible to accommodate an employee (even though he or she may have been marginal prior to injury). It is important that employers understand that work reintegration may be lengthy and is best accomplished by on-the-job training, rather than formal classroom instruction. An employer must also be informed that for some individuals change in routine may involve considerable disruption and anxiety until the new routine is learned.

Assessment of Work Skills

Vocational assessment considers the abilities and deficits of the brain-injured individual, their relationship with their previous employer, the degree to which a job can be modified, and the different forms of employment or retraining available. Individual assessment of vocational potential may involve vocational interest inventories, objective tests relating to subskills involved in particular classes of occupation, and work trials. The assessment of work skills varies according to the individual's stage of recovery. Vocational interest inventories are typically administered by a psychologist or a vocational specialist. (These inventories rate interest, not aptitude.) Examples include the Strong Vocational Interest Blank (SVIB) (Hansen, 1985), and the Vocational Preference Inventory (VPI) (Holland, 1985). A language-free vocational interest inventory is available (Becker, 1981), which is made up of 165 pictures of individuals involved in occupations. These are presented in triads and are appropriate for use with the severely impaired.

A number of tests are available which have been used to assess an individual's perceptual-motor ability, as this relates to vocational return. The Purdue pegboard measures finger dexterity and has been used to assist in the selection of employees for industrial (manufacturing) industry. The test-retest reliability is good for the average of three trials. Normative data is available (Mathiowetz, et al., 1986). The use of the Purdue pegboard is based on the premise that a small sample of a specialized and complex manual activity will correlate highly with an individuals ability to perform similar tasks. A number of other tests are available which are intended to perform similar functions (Crawford and Crawford, 1981). Somewhat more extensive tests, referred to as Work Samples, examine, in addition to dexterity, the subject's ability to integrate the performance of subskills into a coherent activity. Frequently, however, the reasons for the brain-injured individual's vocational difficulties are not captured by his or her performance on a "Work Sample." Many patients fail due to an inability to sustain arriving to work on time and in the right place, working with colleagues, and coordinate and plan the day's work. In addition, the brain-injured worker may have difficulty in self-direction and in adjusting behavior when problems arise. By systematically defining the needs of the individual's job, retraining can be directed towards his or her specific areas of deficits. An adequate assessment should take into account the demands of the job, analysis of the task requirements, the expectations of the employers, the individual's present skills, and their ability to adapt to their new situations. Objective tests should never be preferred to observations of real samples of behavior where these are available. Many hospitals have been able to develop volunteer employment sites, in various hospital jobs, which may be used for functional evaluation of clients' work skills.

Retraining Work Skills

Hospital-Based Rehabilitation Model

The standard model of vocational rehabilitation for the brain-injured adult is a medical one. Clients are serially assessed, trained, and placed (often at separate sites). To be effective, this model demands the independent transfer of skills used in one environment to another. Ben-Yishay and coworkers (1987), have reported the results of this method as applied to a group of postacute brain-injured persons. Time from injury to admission ranged from 4–27 months, but all but 2 patients were 12 months postinjury. Severity of injury varied widely (coma duration was 1–120 days). Although none of those admitted to the program was working, the population was otherwise highly selected (18–55 years old; IQ of at least 80; ambulatory; only minimally aphasic; no previous brain injury; no history of alcohol or drug abuse; no psychiatric history). Patients were treated with cognitive rehabilitation followed by a series of graded occupational trials. Results at discharge showed 64% competitively employed and 30% noncompetitively employed. Of those who were 36 months postdischarge at follow-up, 50% were employed competitively and 22% were noncompetitively employed. Patients were able to gain employment for a period, but many patients were unable to maintain employment (i.e., the longer postdischarge, the lower the percentage of people who were found to be employed).

Supported Employment Model

Supported employment involves the provision of on-the-job training and support services to handicapped individuals so as to allow them to hold competitive employment (which they would otherwise be unable to hold). The major emphasis of the supported employment model is on not excluding even the most handicapped in society from employment. Individual placement, enclave, mobile work crew, and small business models are all used. Many centers are now utilizing the supported employment model with various populations, so there is considerable practical experience from which to draw. This "new" approach is really the application of well known principles to a new domain. Supported employment takes the best of behavioral methodology and applies it in the naturalistic work setting. Problems of the transfer of skills are therefore avoided. This highly practical approach represents a significant departure from traditional concepts of vocational rehabilitation in which the attainment of independence and productivity is judged in relation to general society norms. The four major components to the supported employment model are job placement, job site training carried out by a job coach, ongoing client assessment, and the continuing follow along component (Kreutzer, Wehman, Morton, and Stonnington, 1988). On-the-job support may continue for as long as it is required.

Interagency cooperation, educational, and funding issues are particularly important to the approach. It could be argued that the truly novel aspects of supported employment are creative funding options. Wehman, et al. (1988), report a study of the efficacy of supported employment in individuals who have a long history of unemployment or inability to maintain employment. Time in coma averaged 76 days and time since injury 5 years. Of the 32 clients referred, 15 were placed (the reasons for nonplacement are not reported). When followed up 9 months after placement, 11 out of the 15 placed were still employed (73.4%). Staff intervention at the job site declined significantly over the time each client was in work. The initial intervention time averaged 90% of the time that the client was in work. By week 28, however, this had decreased to 10%. Over the entire course of intervention, employment specialists were with the client on the job approximately 50% of the time. Given the size of the sample, these results are not significantly different from the results of those of Ben-Yishay and coworkers (1987), who also used a highly selected sample. In addition, since much of the difficulty with this population is not finding, but retaining employment, an adequate assessment on the intervention requires a considerably longer period of follow-up. The report of Wehman, et al. (1988), describes an encouraging beginning to research into utilization of the supported employment model with the severely handicapped brain-injured population. The stated objective to work with the most profoundly handicapped makes it of special interest. Much further research is required to firmly establish supported employment as a general intervention for the severely brain-injured.

Work Hardening and Endurance

Fatigue is a known consequence of even mild brain-injury and may severely affect work performance. This fact may partially account for the results of Johnson and Gleave (1987) regarding work return. It is known that even apparently subtle neuromuscular changes which follow brain injury, may significantly decrease the efficiency and increase the energy consumption of the brain-injured for a given amount of work. Elements of work hardening programs may therefore be relevant to the brain-injured, although a straightforward work hardening program will fail to meet the needs of most traumatically injured patients.

Returning to College

The central focus of some young people prior to injury was college, and return to college life may, therefore, be the most appropriate option. The existence of college programs for brain-injured adults provides special resources in some locations, but evening or day classes that are offered by community groups offer structured settings for return into community and educational environments. Very similar principles, however, apply to return to college as to work. Return to college should be gradual. Students might begin their return with one class, while in the rehabilitation setting, so as to evaluate fatigue, the need to develop compensatory strategies, and the ability to follow lectures and other class requirements.

SUMMARY

This chapter has developed a model for functional assessment and intervention. The focus on disability and handicap has been maintained. The appropriate selection of functional goals has been emphasized. Retraining approaches to brain-injured individuals have been explored. We have emphasized consideration of the patient's difficulties in learning in the development of retraining programs. Rather than attempt to address the elusive "underlying cause" of a decrement in functional behavior, we have emphasized the advantages of a more direct approach.

References

Becker, R.L. (1981). Reading-free vocational interest inventory. Bellevue, WA: Edmark Corporation.

Bellack, A.S., Hersen, M., and Lamparski, D. (1979). Role-play tests for assessing social skills: Are they valid? Are they useful? Journal of Consulting and Clinical Psychology, 47:335–42.

Ben-Yishay, Y., Silver, S.M., Piasetsky, E., et al. (1987). Relationship between employability and vocational outcome after intensive holistic cognitive rehabilitation. Journal of Head Trauma Rehabilitation, 2:35–48.

Black, P., Markowitz, R.S., and Cianci, S.N. (1975). Recovery of motor function after lesions in the motor cortex of monkey. In: CIBA Foundation Symposium 34. New Series. Outcome of severe damage to the central nervous system. Elsevier Amsterdam.

Brotherton, F.A., Thomas, L.L., Wisotzek, I.E., and Milan, M.A. (1988). Social skills training in the rehabilitation of patients with traumatic head injury. Archives of Physical Medicine and Rehabilitation, 69:827–32.

Cicerone, K.D., Lawar, R.M., and Shapiro, W.R. (1983). Effects of frontal lobe lesions on hypothesis sampling during concept formation. Neuropsychologia, 21:513–24.

Clark-Wilson, J. (1988). The use of a computer in aiding functional skills: A single case study. Cognitive Rehabilitation, 2:199–206.

Cohen, R.E. (1985). Behavioral treatment of incontinence in a profoundly neurologically impaired adult. Archives of Physical Medicine and Rehabilitation, 67:833–34.

Cope, D.N., and Hall, K. (1982). Head injury rehabilitation: Benefits of early intervention. Archives of Physical Medicine and Rehabilitation, 63:433–37.

Crawford, J.E., and Crawford, D.M. (1981). Crawford Small Parts Dexterity Test. New York: Psychological Corporation.

Dolan, M.P. (1979). The use of contingent reinforcement for improving the personal appearance and hygiene of chronic psychiatric in-patients. Journal of Clinical Psychology, 35:140–44.

Dolan, M.P., and Norton, J.C. (1977). A programmed training technique that uses reinforcement to facilitate acquisition and retention in brain damaged patients. Journal of Clinical Psychology, 33:496–501.

Eames, P., and Wood, R. (1985). Rehabilitation after severe brain injury: A follow-up study of a behaviour modification approach. Journal of Neurology, Neurosurgery, and Psychiatry, 48: 613–19.

Eisler, R.M., Hersen, M., Miller, P.M., and Blanchard, E.G. (1975). Situational determinants of assertive behaviour. Journal of Consulting and Clinical Psychology, 43:330–40.

Freedman, P.E., Bleiberg, J., Freedland, K. (1987). Anticipatory behaviour deficits in closed head injury. Journal of Neurology, Neurosurgery and Psychiatry, 50:398–401.

Gajar, A., Schloss, P.J., Schloss, C., and Thompson, C.K. (1984). Effects of feedback and self-monitoring on brain trauma youth's conversational skills. Journal of Applied Behaviour Analysis, 17:353–58.

Galski, T., Ehle, H.T., and Bruno, R.L. (1990). An assessment of measures to predict the outcome of driving evaluations in patients with cerebral damage. The American Journal of Occupational Therapy, 44:709–13.

Giles, G.M., and Clark-Wilson, J. (1993). Occupational therapy for the brain-injured adult: A neurofunctional approach. London: Chapman and Hall.

Giles, G.M., and Clark-Wilson, J. (1988). The use of behavioral techniques in functional skills training after severe brain injury. The American Journal of Occupational Therapy, 42:658–65.

Giles, G.M., and Shore, M. (1989). A rapid method for teaching severely brain-injured adults to wash and dress. Archives of Physical Medicine and Rehabilitation, 70:156–58.

Giles, G.M., Fussey, I., and Burgess, P. (1988). The behavioral treatment of verbal interaction skills following severe head injury: A single case study. Brain Injury, 2:75–81.

Goodman-Smith, A., and Turnbull, J. (1983). A behavioral approach to the rehabilitation of severely brain-injured adults: An illustrated case history. Physiotherapy, 69:393–96.

Hansen, J.I.C. (1985). Manual for the Strong Vocational Interest Blank—Strong-Campbell Interest Inventory. Sanford, CA: Stanford University Press.

Helffestein, D., and Weschler, F. (1982). The use of interpersonal process recall (IPR) in the remediation of interpersonal and communication skill deficits in the newly brain-injured. Clinical Neuropsychiatry, 4:139–43.

Holland, J.L. (1985). Vocational Preference Inventory (VPI) Manual, 1985 Edition. Odessa, FL: Psychological Assessment Resources.

Hooper-Row, J. (1988). Rehabilitation of physical deficits in the post-acute brain-injured: Four case studies. In: Fussey, I., and Giles, G.M. (eds). Rehabilitation of the severely brain-injury adult: A practical approach. London: Croom Helm, 102–16.

Jacobs, H.E. (1988). The Los Angeles head injury survey: Procedures and initial findings. Archives of Physical Medicine and Rehabilitation, 69:425–31.

Jennett, B., and Teasdale, G. (1981). Management of Head Injuries. Philadelphia: F.A. Davis.

Johnson, D.A., and Newton, A. (1987a). Brain-injured persons social interaction group: A basis for social adjustment after brain injury. British Journal of Occupational Therapy, 50:47–52.

Johnson, D.A., and Newton, A. (1987b). Social adjustment and interaction after severe brain injury: 2. Rationale and bases for intervention. British Journal of Clinical Psychology, 26:289–98.

Johnson, R., and Gleave, J. (1987). Counting the people disabled by head injury. Injury, 18:7–9.

Kewman, D.G., Seigerman, C., Kinter, H., Chu, S., Henson, D., and Reeder, C. (1985). Simulation training of psychomotor skills: Teaching the brain-injured to drive. Rehabilitation Psychology, 30:11–26.

Kewman, D.G., Yanus, B., and Kirsch, N. (1988). Assessment of distractibility in auditory comprehension after traumatic brain injury. Brain Injury, 2:131–37.

Kreutzer, J.S., Wehman, P., Morton, M.V., and Stonnington, H.H. (1988). Supported employment and compensatory strategies for enhancing vocational outcome following traumatic brain injury. Brain Injury, 2:205–23.

Lashley, B., and Drabman, R. (1974). Facilitation of the acquisition and retention of sight-word vocabulary through token reinforcement. Journal of Applied Behavioral Analysis, 7:307–12.

Lazarus, C., and Logemann, J. (1987). Swallowing disorders in closed head trauma patients. Archives of Physical Medicine and Rehabilitation, 68:79–84.

Levin, H.S., Goldstein, F.C., High, W.M., and Williams, D. (1988). Automatic and effortful processing after severe closed head injury. Brain and Cognition, 7:283–97.

Lewick, P., Czyzenska, M., and Hoffman, H. (1987). Unconscious acquisition of complex procedural knowledge. Journal of Experimental Psychology: Learning, Memory and Cognition, 13:523–30.

Lewick, P., Hill, T., and Bizot, E. (1988). Acquisition of procedural knowledge about a pattern of stimuli that cannot be articulated. Cognitive Psychology, 20:24–37.

Logemann, J. (1983). Evaluation and treatment of swallowing disorder. Boston: College-Hill Press.

Lorch, E.P., Anderson, D.R., and Well, A.D. (1984). Effects of irrelevant information on speeded classification tasks: Interference is reduced by habituation. Journal of Experimental Psychology: Human Perception and Performance, 10:850–64.

Mathiowetz, V., Rogers, S.L., Dowe-Keval, M., Donahoe, L., and Rennells, C. (1986). The Purdue pegboard: Norms of 14- to 19-year olds. The American Journal of Occupational Therapy, 40:174–79.

Nihara, K., Foster, R., Shellhaas, M., and Leland, H. (1975). Adaptive Behaviour Scale. Manual. Washington, DC: American Association on Mental Deficiency.

Nissen, M.J., and Bullemer, P. (1987). Attentional requirements of learning: Evidence from performance measures. Cognitive Psychology, 19:1–32.

O'Reilly, M.F., and Cuvo, A.J. (1989). Teaching self-treatment of cold symptoms to an anoxic brain-injured adult. Behavioral Residential Treatment, 4:359–75.

Plienis, A.J., Hansen, D.J., Ford, F., Smith, S., Stark, L.J., Kelly, J.A. (1987). Behavioral small group training to improve the social skills of emotionally disordered adolescents. Behaviour Therapy, 18:17–32.

Prigatano, G.P., Fordyce, D.J., Zeiner, H.K., Roueche, J.R., Pepping, M., and Wood, B.C. (1984). Neuropsychological rehabilitation after closed head injury in young adults. Journal of Neurology, Neurosurgery, and Psychiatry, 47:505–13.

Reason, J. (1984). Absent-mindedness and cognitive control. In: Harris, J.E., and Morris, P.E. Everyday memory actions and absent-mindedness. London: Academic Press.

Schneider, W., Dumais, S.T., and Shiffrin, R.M. (1984). Automatic and control processing and attention. In: Parasuraman, R., and Davis, D.R. (eds). Varieties of attention. London: Academic Press.

Shallice, T. (1982). Specific impairment of planning. In: Broardbent, D.E., and Weiskrantz, L. (eds). The neuropsychology of cognitive function. London: The Royal Society, 199–209.

Shallice, T., and Evans, M.E. (1978). The involvement of the frontal lobes in cognitive estimation. Cortex, 14:294–303.

Shaw, L., Brodsky, L., and McMahon, B.T. (1985). Neuropsychiatric intervention in the rehabilitation of head injured patients. The Psychiatric Journal of the University of Ottawa, 10:237–40.

Shriffrin, R.M., and Schneider, W. (1977). Controlled and automatic information processing: II. Perceptual learning, automatic attending, and a general theory. Psychological Review, 84:127–90.

Solokov, E.N. (1963). Perception and the conditioned reflex. Oxford: Pergamon Press.

Squire, L.R. (1986). Mechanisms of memory. Science, 232:1612–19.

Stuss, D.T., Stethem, L.L., Hugenholtz, H., Picton, T., Pivik, J., and Richards, M.T.

(1989). Reaction time after head injury: Fatigue, divided attention, and consistency of performance. Journal of Neurology, Neurosurgery, and Psychiatry, 52:742–48.

Thomsen, I.V. (1974). The patient with severe brain injury and his family: A follow-up of 50 patients. Scandinavian Journal of Rehabilitation Medicine, 6:180–83.

Thomsen. I.V. (1984). Late outcome of very severe blunt head trauma: A 10–15 year second follow-up. Journal of Neurology, Neurosurgery, and Psychiatry, 47:260–68.

Tulving, E. (1972). Episodic and semantic memory. In: Tulving, E., and Donaldson, W. (eds). Organization of memory. New York: Academic Press.

Tulving, E. (1983). Elements of episodic memory. Oxford: Clarendon Press.

Van Zomeren, A.H., Brouner, W.H., Rothengatter, J.A., and Snoek, J.W. (1988). Fitness to drive a car after recovery from severe head injury. Archives of Physical Medicine and Rehabilitation, 69:90–96.

Vilkki, J. (1988). Problem solving after focal cerebral lesions. Cortex, 24:119–27.

Wehman, P., Kreutzer, J.S., Stonnington, H.H., Wood, W., Sherron, P., Diambra, J., Fry, R., and Groah, C. (1988). Supported employment for persons with traumatic brain injury: A preliminary report. Journal of Head Trauma Rehabilitation, 3:82–93.

Wilson, B.A., and Moffat, N. (1984) Clinical Management of Memory Problems. London: Croom Helm.

World Health Organization (1980). International classification of impairment disabilities and handicaps. Geneva: World Health Organization.

Zencius, A.H., Wesolowski, M.D., Burke, W.H., and McQuade, P. (1989). Antecedent control in the treatment of brain-injured clients. Brain Injury, 3:199–205.

8

Assessment and Treatment of Speech, Swallowing, and Communication Disorders Following Traumatic Brain Injury

MARK YLVISAKER
BETH URBANCZYK

It is difficult to overestimate the importance of communication skills in rehabilitation following traumatic brain injury (TBI). The success of an individual's social, vocational, familial, and academic reintegration hinges critically on the recovery of effective communication. This is most obviously true in the case of social, including residential, success, which is directly related to interactive competence (Oddy, 1984; Wood, 1984). It is equally important to recognize that vocational re-entry for individuals with brain injury, as well as for other disability groups, often succeeds or fails as a function of the individual's ability to interact effectively with peers, supervisors, and possibly also customers (Brooks, McKinlay, Symington, Beattie, and Campsie, 1987). Furthermore, families consistently report that it is easier to adjust to physical disability in a loved one than to personality changes, manifested in chronically unsatisfying and stressful interaction patterns (Livingston and Brooks, 1988). Finally, because TBI is largely a young person's disability, many individuals attempt to return to high school or college following their injury. Sophisticated language skills—including auditory and reading comprehension, and verbal and written expression—are indisputably critical to a successful academic career.

Tragically, communication skills are nearly as vulnerable in severe TBI as they are essential to success following the injury. Communication occupies the intersection of motoric, linguistic, cognitive, social, and behavioral functions. Despite the relative infrequency in TBI of aphasic syndromes associated with stroke (Heilman, Safran, and Geschwind, 1971), even in the case of severe TBI (Sarno, 1980, 1984; Sarno, Buonaguro, and Levita, 1986), the complexity and significance of communication functions and the frequency of cognitive, social, and behavioral impairment (Brooks, 1984) necessitate careful attention to communication even in those cases in which speech and language appear to have recovered to pretrauma levels.

Impaired communication is a nearly universal long-term consequence of severe TBI in adults (Sarno, 1980, 1984) and is also common in milder injuries. Although any combination of strengths and weaknesses is possible following TBI, and disability obviously varies with stage of recovery, there is general agreement among investigators that language profiles in head injury differ markedly from those resulting from stroke (Halpern, Darley, and Brown, 1973; Groher, 1990; Hagen, 1982; Luria, 1970; Prigatano, 1986; Sarno, 1984; Ylvisaker, 1992; Ylvisaker and Szekeres, in press). Whereas focal left hemisphere lesions are capable of producing specific constellations of language deficits in the absence of more general cognitive and psychosocial dysfunction, the combination of diffuse and commonly occurring multifocal lesions associated with severe closed head injury results in communication profiles quite different from those of individuals with aphasia. Communication profiles following head injury often include adequate speech and surface language functions (phonology, morphology, syntax, lexicon), but are dominated by socially ineffective language use due in part to generally impaired "executive" functions and by inefficient and concrete language processing due to more general cognitive and psychomotor impairments (Hagen, 1982; Prigatano, 1986; Ylvisaker, 1992; Ylvisaker and Szekeres, 1989, in press). Whereas individuals with aphasia "usually communicate better than they talk, TBI patients frequently talk better than they communicate" (Milton and Wertz, 1986).

Our goal in this chapter is to highlight critical aspects of assessment and treatment in TBI that fall within the scope of practice of speech-language pathologists. There are two dangers in this approach. The first is that in dealing with issues as diverse as swallowing, motor speech, augmentative communication, language, and social communication, we will be unable to go beyond generalities. We have addressed this issue by focusing only on those aspects of speech-language practice that are unique to TBI or particularly critical in the rehabilitation of individuals after TBI. Assessment and treatment themes that apply equally to other types of neurologic disability will not be explored. The second danger is that in addressing issues under the heading of a specific profession, we might inadvertently contribute to professional isolation or territorialism that is not compatible with effective rehabilitation. In all areas of professional practice, the services of speech-language pathologists overlap with those of many other professionals, all of whom must thoughtfully and nondefensively integrate their assessments and treatments.

SPEECH

Following prolonged unconsciousness (coma), most individuals experience a period of recovery during which they respond minimally to environmental events, but do not speak. It is critical at this stage to distinguish between a state of wakeful unresponsiveness (commonly called the "vegetative state"), in which there is little or no intellectual interaction with the environment, and the "locked-in" syndrome, in which adequate intellectual functioning is combined with a near total inability to move any part of the body. The latter, which is an uncommon consequence of TBI, necessitates thorough and creative exploration of expressive communication modalities (e.g., controlling a switch with eye movements or simply shifting eye gaze to indicate requests).

Levin and colleagues (1983) used the term "mutism" to refer to the absence of speech in individuals who are capable of communicating through nonspeech channels, can comprehend at least simple oral commands, and whose lack of speech is not a result of cranial nerve damage. In their cohort of 350 children and adults with moderate-to-severe head injuries, only 9 (3%) were mute in this sense. Speech disorders associated with basal ganglia lesions, more common in the younger patients, carried a better prognosis for functional recovery than did those associated with severe diffuse, including cortical, lesions. Although precise data on persistent severe speech disorders following TBI are not yet available (DeRuyter and Donoghue, 1989), Levin's figures are consistent with the clinical impression that persistent absence of intelligible speech in the presence of good cognitive functioning is a relatively uncommon head injury picture. Yorkston and colleagues (1989) found that 10% of adult TBI patients receiving outpatient treatment following discharge from inpatient rehabilitation continued to have nonfunctional communication because of motor speech disturbance. Recovery of intelligible speech, possibly with considerable effort and intervention, can occur many months and, indeed, years after the injury (Beukelman and Garrett, 1988; Light, Beesley, and Collier, 1988; Workinger and Netsell, 1988).

Frequency and type of dysarthria in TBI have not been well established. Although there is a clinically identifiable "TBI-type" of motor speech disorder that includes articulatory imprecision, phonatory weakness, hypernasality, slow rate, and minimal pitch and loudness variation, any type of dysarthria (flaccid, spastic, ataxic, or mixed; Darley, Aronson, and Brown, 1975) is possible, depending on the location of damage in the central nervous system. Based exclusively on clinical impressions, apraxic disorders seem to be more common early in recovery and in younger patients. Impaired fluency was associated with severe TBI in two small N studies (Hartley, 1990; Penn and Cleary, 1988). In some cases, speech disturbances seem to be related, at least in part, to cognitive (including self-monitoring) weakness. These include excessive or decreased loudness, rapid rate, and monotonous voice.

Motor Speech Assessment

Assessment of dysarthria in TBI is generally indistinguishable from assessment in other etiologies. It includes evaluation of all speech-related motor systems (respiratory, phonatory, resonance, and articulatory) and is essentially an interdisciplinary assessment. Physiatry, physical therapy, occupational therapy, and speech pathology jointly contribute to the assessment of muscle tone (trunk, shoulder girdle, neck, face, and intraoral tone) and muscle control as they affect breathing for speech, vocalization, controlled direction of the air stream through the nose or mouth, and movement of the jaw, lips, tongue, palate, and cheeks for intelligible speech. An otolaryngologist is often consulted to explore phonatory dysfunction, which may be secondary to laryngeal apraxia, unilateral vocal fold paralysis, subglotal stenosis, or granuloma. Velopharyngeal functioning for speech can be examined during the videoradiographic swallowing evaluation.

Speech assessment for clinical purposes generally involves careful description of the perceptual features of speech (e.g., articulatory precision, loudness, rate, voice quality, variation in pitch and loudness, nasality) under a variety of instructions (speech and nonspeech tasks) and of the observable physiologic functions related to speech. A standardized assessment of dysarthria is available, with reportedly adequate reliability and validity (Enderby, 1980, 1983). In addition to identifying the nature of the impairment, speech assessment requires diagnostic intervention designed to identify features that can be modified by means of exercises or compensatory procedures.

Since the purpose of speech is to communicate messages to a listener, evaluation of intelligibility is critical. Factors that impact on intelligibility, in addition to the dysarthric speaker's neuromuscular abilities, include familiarity of the listener, demands of the speaking task, distractions in the environment, and the state of the speaker, including level of medication, fatigue, stress, or depression (see Moore, Yorkston, and Beukelman, 1991). In addition, confusion and tangentiality add to intelligibility challenges by reducing the semantic support for listener interpretation. Yorkston and Beukelman (1981) have standardized the assessment of intelligibility, as it is affected by message length, and of speaking rate. In addition, fatigue level and affective states (e.g., stress, anxiety, depression) are critical variables that must be explored in TBI. Sapir and Aronson (1985) suggested that possible causes for reversible speech disorders following TBI include affective and motivational disorders related to commonly occurring limbic system and frontal lobe disturbances. More recently, Sapir and Aronson (1990) highlighted the importance of evaluating the impact of anxiety and depression on speech production during the first 24 months after TBI.

Cognitive assessment is typically a critical component of all assessments in individuals with TBI. Speech may be monotonous, overly loud or soft, or overly fast or slow, not because of a specific speech disorder, but, rather, as a manifestation of cognitive and self-monitoring impairment. Furthermore, level of cognitive recovery dictates whether new learning, feedback, and self-monitoring techniques can be used in speech intervention. Therefore, careful assessment of cognitive status and differential diagnosis of cognitive and motor-speech contributions to the presenting speech problem are needed (Yorkston and Beukelman, 1991).

Motor Speech Treatment

Intervention options in TBI do not differ from those available to other dysarthric speakers. Procedures are outlined in a variety of valuable textbooks (Berry, 1983; Yorkston and Beukelman, 1991; McNeil, Aronson, and Rosenbek, 1984; Perkins, 1983; Rosenbek and LaPointe, 1985; Yorkston and Beukelman, 1989). Because feedback mechanisms are suspect in cases of widespread diffuse brain injury, TBI speech treatment often includes a considerable focus on mechanisms of feedback. This may include low technology options, such as positioning the patient in front of a mirror during speech exercises, and high technology options, such as microcomputer-based immediate visual display of selected speech characteristics (e.g., loudness, timing, melody, and articulatory accuracy).

Surgical and prosthetic options frequently considered after TBI include vocal fold Teflon, Gelfoam, or collagen injection or thyroplasty to improve phonation in unilateral vocal fold paralysis, and palatal lifts to reduce nasal air flow and associated hypernasality and to improve articulation by increasing intraoral pressure. Palatal augmentation (surgically dropping and recontouring the hard palate to facilitate lingual-palatal contact) has also been used following head injury (Logemann, 1991). We have worked with TBI patients who have benefitted from these procedures. However, the documented fact that significant improvement in motor speech functioning can occur well beyond a year postinjury (Beukelman and Garrett, 1988; Light, Beesley, and Collier, 1988; Workinger and Netsell, 1988) supports a very conservative approach to surgical and prosthetic management, particularly if the surgery is not reversible (Logemann, 1990). We would recommend these options only after at least 1 year of recovery time and intensive speech intervention have failed to produce speech that is reasonably intelligible. Furthermore, palatal lifts may be contraindicated in patients with seizures or behavioral intolerance for irritation (Yorkston and Beukelman, 1991).

Augmentative communication, discussed later in this chapter, is often an integral component of intervention for individuals with severe speech impairment.

SWALLOWING

Most patients in the early acute phase following TBI exhibit both speech and swallowing disorders, as well as severely depressed cognitive functioning. A recent report by Yorkston, Honsinger, Mitsuda, and Hammen (1989) suggested that impaired swallowing (dysphagia) remains a pervasive issue after patients with TBI regain consciousness. In their series, 77.5% of TBI patients in an acute care setting evidenced some degree of swallowing problem, with 45% unable to meet nutritional needs orally. Approximately 67% of the acute rehabilitation patients and 13% of the outpatients continued to evidence impaired swallowing. Interestingly, swallowing disorders occurred without accompanying speech disorder in 39% of the patients, whereas speech disorders occurred without accompanying swallowing disorders in only 2% of the patients. This surprising asymmetry is one of the many contributors to a substantial assessment challenge in TBI swallowing disorders. These data, however, are based largely on evaluation procedures that did not include videoradiography and, therefore, may underestimate the incidence of swallowing disorders following TBI. The extent of the problem was also underscored by Weinstein (1983) who reported a 27% incidence of dysphagia in patients with TBI admitted to a rehabilitation facility, and by Cherney and Halper (1989) who reported a similar rate (26%) in patients admitted to their rehabilitation facility.

TBI can impair any aspect of swallowing, from 1) taking the food into the mouth to 2) preparing a bolus for swallowing to 3) moving the bolus back towards the pharynx to 4) triggering the pharyngeal swallow to 5) moving the food efficiently through the pharynx to 6) protecting the airway to 7) moving the food into and through the esophagus. Possible swallowing disorders are thoroughly explained by Logemann (1983) and in the textbook edited by Groher (1992).

Lazarus and Logemann (1987) examined types of swallowing disorders in a consecutive series of 53 head trauma patients referred for videofluoroscopic swallowing evaluation. Their findings are reproduced in Table 8.1. Of the 9 swallowing motility disorders identified by videofluorographic study, difficulty triggering the pharyngeal swallow was by far the most frequent (81% of the patients). It is possible that this large percentage would be reduced somewhat if a larger amount of food had been used. Forty-seven percent of the patients had a two-component problem, of which the most frequently occurring were reduced tongue control combined with delayed or absent pharyngeal swallows (22%) and delayed

Table 8.1.
Frequency of Swallowing Motility Disorders in 53 Closed-Head Trauma Subjects[a]

SWALLOWING MOTILITY	NUMBER OF SUBJECTS	PERCENTAGE OF TOTAL
Problem with triggering pharyngeal swallow	43	81
Delayed swallow	37	70
Absent swallow	6	11
Reduced lingual control	28	53
Reduced peristalsis	17	32
Reduced laryngeal closure	3	6
Reduced laryngeal elevation	2	4
Spasm in larynx	2	4
Cricopharyngeal dysfunction	3	6
Esophageal stricture	1	2
Normal swallow	1	2
Could not test	1	2

[a]From Lazarus, C. (1989). Swallowing disorders after traumatic brain injury. Journal of Head Trauma Rehabilitation, 4(4):34–41. Reproduced with permission.

pharyngeal swallow combined with reduced pharyngeal peristalsis (17%). Twenty of the 53 patients (38%) aspirated during the swallow study, with the most common etiology of aspiration being delayed or absent pharyngeal swallow. Clinicians must also be alert to the possibility in head injury patients of direct neck trauma, which may negatively affect swallowing function.

Most individuals with TBI who have severe oral intake and swallowing disorders also have severe cognitive, behavioral, and communicative disorders (Cherney and Halper, 1989). Agitation, impaired attention, reduced impulse control, reduced initiation, memory deficits, inability to follow directions, and impaired judgment all impact significantly on treatment and general management decisions.

Swallowing Assessment

The complexity of possible physiologic disorders of swallowing following TBI combined with the influence of complex cognitive and behavioral disturbances, necessitates thorough assessment and careful management (Logemann, 1989). Assessment combines bedside evaluation of the feeding/swallowing mechanism, videofluorographic evaluation of the anatomic and physiologic aspects of swallowing that cannot be visualized at bedside, and evaluation of related cognitive, behavioral, and communicative functioning. Bedside and radiographic procedures are described in detail by Logemann (1983, 1986), Miller (1992), and Ekberg (1992), and will not be reviewed here. Bedside evaluation should be used in part as preparation for radiographic evaluation, especially in physically involved and minimally responsive patients. Responses to handling, intraoral stimulation, taste, temperature, and consistency can be explored without feeding the patient. Armed with this information, the clinician can make effective use of limited feeding trials under radiographic conditions.

The videofluorographic assessment of swallowing, or modified barium swallow test, has become a routine component of evaluation following severe TBI. Because "silent aspirators" are frequently missed during bedside swallowing evaluation (Lazarus, 1989; Logemann, 1983), the radiographic procedure provides information needed by the attending physician to determine if the patient can eat safely. Of equal importance, it provides critical management information to the feeding/swallowing specialist (often a speech-language pathologist). Possible physiologic disorders of feeding and swallowing can be precisely identified, the safest and most effective feeding arrangements (including food consistency, method of intake, head and body position, compensatory swallowing procedures, and instructions or self-cues) can be discovered, possible effects of intervention techniques (e.g., thermal stimulation) can be explored, and information critical to family counseling and training is obtained. In effect, the videoradiographic procedure is trial therapy and should be conducted by the professional responsible for designing feeding and swallowing treatment.

In addition to the feeding/swallowing therapist who may be a speech-language pathologist, the dysphagia evaluation and intervention team includes the attending physician and relevant medical subspecialists, occupational and physical therapists who contribute to decisions about positioning and self-feeding, and the psychologist. A family therapist is often needed to help family members accept an approach that in their judgment may proceed too slowly and cautiously in the direction of oral intake.

Swallowing Treatment

Appendix A (from Ylvisaker and Logemann, 1985) includes a wide variety of treatment procedures, organized according to the functional physiologic disorder they address. Procedures were taken from the adult dysphagia literature (e.g., Logemann, 1983) and the pediatric neurodevelopmental treatment literature (e.g., Morris, 1977, 1982). As with any clinical decision, specific procedures should not be used prior to a careful identification of the disorder. Of the variables that impact on feeding/swallowing success, one of the most critical and the easiest to control is food consistency. Thin liquids are often the most difficult for TBI patients with swallowing disorders, because it is difficult to manipulate a thin liquid bolus and liquids move too quickly through a system that is slow to respond (Lazarus, 1989). Pureed consistencies that are not sticky (e.g., well pureed apple sauce) are frequently the easiest to swallow safely.

Controlled consistencies of various foods are now commercially available (e.g., Magic Menu, Indianapolis, IN). Additional treatment strategies have been presented by Lazarus (1991) and Castelli-Linden (1991).

Figure 8.1 represents a model of progression for the management of patients with severe feeding and swallowing problems. We have found this representation of the steps involved in recovery useful in family counseling. Family members often want to feed their loved one, even before it is safe to do so. Mothers of severely injured adolescents and young adults may reassume a nurturing role, a critical component of which is feeding. With this as background, sensitive and clear presentation of information and reasons for a cautious approach is critical. An explanation of the progression outlined in Figure 8.1, together with a guided viewing of the video swallow study, helps family members accept team decisions and play a cooperative role in re-establishing oral feeding.

Following recovery of adequate swallow physiology, patients with TBI may remain a management challenge because of cognitive and behavioral or self-regulatory disorders. Individuals who are agitated, extremely impulsive, or highly distractible may require ongoing one-on-one supervision to eat safely. Patients who lack initiation may not feed themselves despite hunger and the presence of food. Patients with episodic memory disorders may forget to eat or, more likely, forget that they have eaten and therefore eat far too often. Patients who lack organizational skills or sound judgment may not be capable of following a treatment regimen that includes compensatory techniques. In each of these cases, the problem must be approached not as a specific feeding problem, but as a cognitive or behavioral problem. In rehabilitation facilities, behavioral and cognitive psychologists are important members of the dysphagia team.

Individuals who are discharged from rehabilitation still unable to eat safely by mouth should be followed at regular intervals for an extended period of time. In some cases, normal swallowing is recovered more than a year after the injury, even in cases in which intensive treatment over the first year did not result in functional swallowing (Logemann, 1989).

AUGMENTATIVE AND ALTERNATIVE COMMUNICATION

Augmentative communication encompasses all modalities of communication other than speech, including eye gaze, facial expression, nonspeech vocalization, natural gestures, manual signs, writing, typing, communication boards (consisting of photos, pictures, visual symbols, letters, or words), and electronic systems, including powerful computer-based devices with synthesized speech output. These are the options open to any person who lacks intelligible speech, temporarily or permanently. Augmentative communication assessment and intervention for individuals with TBI must particularly consider issues of emotional acceptance of

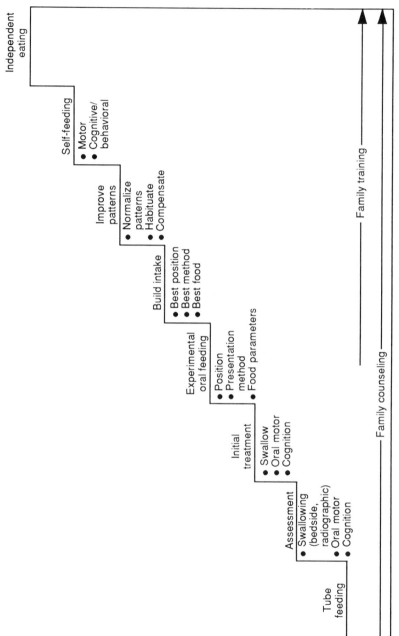

Figure 8.1. Stages of progression from tube feeding to oral feeding.

communication other than speech, behavioral tolerance for slow and cumbersome communication, and cognitive skills related to learning and using a new means of communicating. Critical areas of cognition include visual perceptual skills, organizational ability, memory and new learning skills, initiation, and ability to transfer new skills to functional settings and tasks.

Augmentative Communication Assessment

Augmentative communication assessment is necessarily interdisciplinary. It includes identification of 1) the best motor movement for pointing, gesturing, or operating a switch, 2) cognitive potential to learn a new communication system, 3) academic skills (e.g., reading, writing) related to communication options, 4) visual-perceptual skills related to the type and number of pictures, symbols, or words that may be displayed on a board or device, 5) emotional and behavioral ability to accept a new means of communicating and tolerate the frustration that inevitably accompanies communicating slowly and laboriously, 6) potential to recover speech, and 7) family willingness to accept and promote an augmentative communication environment. Principles that guide assessment include the following:

1. All expressive modalities should be explored. Even if an individual is capable of learning and using a sophisticated electronic device, there will always be situations (e.g., bath, swimming pool, automobile) in which communication without a device is mandatory.
2. Form follows function. It is rare for a person who does not try to communicate in some way with behavior under his or her control to become an active communicator with the provision of a communication aid. Assessment must identify the scope and level of the individual's unaided communicative function and only then explore how communication may be augmented. Furthermore, communication systems must be selected in light of the individual's specific communication needs and situations, both current and projected. Generally, that system is best which combines simplicity with the ability to meet most of the patient's goals. Options closest to natural communication should be explored first.
3. Individuals change frequently and rapidly during the early weeks and months after the injury. Therefore, flexibility must be built into augmentative options.
4. The period of recovery following severe TBI can extend well beyond 1 year. It is not uncommon for individuals whose speech is unintelligible at 1 year postinjury to ultimately recover intelligible speech, often with considerable effort and therapeutic intervention. Therefore, expensive

devices must be avoided until it is certain that recovery of function is at an end.

5. The complexity and technologic sophistication of a communication should be no greater than needed to meet the individual's communication requirements. If a simple homemade letter board is sufficient, it makes little sense to exhaust resources (time, energy, and money) on anything more elaborate.

6. Given the complexity of the issues and the rapid rate at which the field of augmentative communication continues to develop, referral to a specialized rehabilitation technology evaluation center is often in the interest of the patient.

Specific procedures for functional augmentative communication assessment of adults with TBI are outlined by DeRuyter and Kennedy (1991), Ladtkow (1993), Beukelman, Yorkston, and Lossing (1984), and Bray and colleagues (1987).

Augmentative Communication Treatment

Speech pathologists are often presented with the challenge of equipping nonspeaking patients who are just emerging from coma with a consistent yes/no response signal. In this context, augmentative communication decisions enter rehabilitation early in recovery. For example, the ability to communicate yes and no would enable patient's to participate in their medical and nursing care. Furthermore, staff members who follow the patient's cognitive function have an understandable desire to assess cognitive return by using yes/no questions. Finally, family members desperately want to know to what extent their loved one recognizes, comprehends, and remembers, and, therefore, they begin early to explore yes/no signals.

For patients who recover slowly, this process frequently carries great frustration for all involved. For example, different parties may independently encourage the individual to use different signals (e.g., hand squeezing, eye blinking, hand raising). In addition to the confusion that results from inconsistent signals, the chosen signal may be a reflexive movement (e.g., hand squeezing, eye blinking) and therefore very unreliable.

More fundamentally, this approach to establishing early communication is insensitive to the cognitive complexity involved in communicating "yes" and "no" in the sense of affirmation and denial. Normal cognitive development in infants, which often serves as a window on cognitive complexity, sheds light on this issue. Normally developing babies do not signal "yes" and "no" in the sense of affirmation and denial until months after they have been actively and consistently signaling other intentions, such as rejection (e.g., by turning away or pushing away), want (e.g., by looking, reaching, and vocalizing), pleasure (e.g., by smiling and laughing), and discomfort (e.g., by whining and crying). It makes sense, therefore, in the very early stages of recovery to focus on promoting and responding to natural communication acts of this sort and to work actively at establishing yes/no only when the patient gives evidence of readiness for this level of cognitive demand. Simple natural gestures can be encouraged by routinely interpreting the patient's behavior and responding as though it were communicative, and by offering choices (e.g., foods, clothes, activities) and taking any of the developmentally early forms of communication as adequate signals.

To be effective, a yes/no response should be at the same time unambiguous and easy to produce. Unfortunately these goals are often in conflict. The easiest movements—such as eye blinks and hand squeezes—are also the most ambiguous because they occur reflexively. Unambiguous movements—such as thumbs up versus thumbs down or clear up-down versus side-side head movements—often require substantial energy and motor planning skill, and may not be consistently available to the individual because of fatigue. There is no generally applicable resolution of this dilemma. Team and family members should negotiate a signal system with which they are all comfortable and that comes as close to meeting both goals (easy and unambiguous) as possible.

There is also value in introducing remote switches to very severely injured patients early in recovery. Physical and occupational therapists are typically involved in selecting the easiest and least problematic movement capable of triggering a switch. The switch is connected to something that family members agree the patient would like to control if he or she were capable of such control (e.g., a VCR playing videos of home and friends; a tape recorder playing favorite music). If the arrangement can be set up in the patient's room, family members and nursing staff can prompt the switch controlling movement many times every day.

This approach serves a variety of purposes. First, it can play a role in family education and counseling. At this stage of recovery, there is frequently conflict between family members and staff regarding the patient's level of awareness. This conflict is rarely resolved with words. Family members may, however, acquire a more accurate perception of the patient's level of functioning through daily switch interaction of this sort. Second, switch programs can serve an assessment purpose. For example, the team may discover that there is greater awareness and interactive capability than they had assumed. Finally, physical and cognitive treatment purposes may be served by engaging the patient in this activity many times a day. In any case, switch control over interesting events enables individuals to "wake up" in a world in which they are *acting* and not simply being acted upon. Furthermore, if sophisticated electronic communication devices are indicated later in recovery, a great deal of the preparatory work will have been done.

If patients continue to be unable to speak during the alert but confused stages of recovery (Rancho Los Amigos Levels 5 and 6), communication boards (using letters, words, symbols, or photographs) are useful. Because patients change rapidly during this phase, the boards should be simple and easily modified. Cognitive and visual-perceptual simplicity is also required by the patient's level of cognitive and perceptual functioning at this stage. Additional words or symbols can be added as recovery permits. At this stage of recovery, patients are likely to have difficulty learning an essentially new system of communication and may not initiate communication even if they have a communication need and have demonstrated potential to use the new system. Furthermore, it is unlikely that they will generalize its use from one setting to another (Beukelman and Yorkston, 1989). Despite these limitations, the board can serve three valuable purposes. First, it can be the context for functional cognitive and perceptual exercises. Second, the presence of a communication board on a lap tray promotes communication by informing others in the environment that the patient is capable of communicating and by offering topics for conversation. Finally, even if a communication act is prompted by others, it is still a communication act and gives the individual the important opportunity to express feelings and desires.

Communication boards tend to be limiting in the content that they make available to the patient. Inevitably, family members and staff resort to a guessing game to enable the patient to express additional thoughts, feelings, and desires. If unsystematic, these guessing games are the source of great frustration. One way to reduce the frustration and increase efficiency of communication is to structure the 20 questions-type guessing game according to an agreed upon set of message categories (e.g., "Is it about food or drink? A person? A feeling? Something to do? Something about home? Something you want me to do?") and specific messages. Family members and staff can work with the patient to create a customized and well organized system of message categories and specific messages. With this set of categories and messages always available with the patient, communication partners are not left to guess in a vacuum, but can proceed systematically through the set of categories until the correct category is found, and then through a set of frequently occurring preselected messages. At the same time, all forms of communication, including gesture, eye gaze, vocalization, and others, should be encouraged.

A relatively small percentage of individuals with TBI remain nonspeaking despite good recovery of cognitive functioning (Levin, Madison, Bailey, et al., 1983; Yorkston, Honsinger, Mitsuda, and Hammen, 1989).

Because recovery of intelligible speech may be achieved well over a year after the injury (13 years postinjury reported by Workinger and Netsell, 1988; 9 years by Beukelman and Garrett, 1988; 7 years by DeRuyter and Kennedy, 1991; and 3 years by Light, Beesley, and Collier, 1988) and accurate projection of recovery rate is impossible given the current state of research (Beukelman and Garrett, 1988), staff should avoid a premature recommendation for purchase of an expensive electronic communication system. In addition, it should be anticipated that very long-term followup will be required to ensure that an individual's communication system remains optimally functional and efficient over time.

Beyond the confused stages of recovery, primary obstacles to functional use of an augmentative system are often in the domain of emotional acceptance and behavioral tolerance. It is easy for the patient and family alike to assume that using a device is tantamount to admitting that speech is no longer a reasonable goal. It is critical that speech-language pathologists and other support staff help patients and families understand that, far from interfering with the recovery of speech, nonspeech systems often promote speech recovery (Light, Neesley, and Collier, 1988; Silverman, 1980) by reducing the frustration and stress associated with communication. In addition, family members require education and training to be in a position to communicate most effectively with their loved one using the augmentative system (Beukelman and Yorkston, 1989).

Behavioral issues should also be anticipated. Unlike individuals with congenital neuromuscular disorders, those with TBI are accustomed to communicating effortlessly and at a rapid rate. Even the best augmentative devices involve considerable effort and are extremely slow relative to standards of normal verbal interaction. Furthermore, frustration tolerance is often reduced in TBI. For these reasons, intervention must be structured to enhance success and reduce the behavioral and emotional burdens as much as possible. Engaging patients in decisions about the device, about the type and amount of practice, and about the transition to functional use helps reduce the behavioral and emotional threats. Furthermore, extensive practice with a device before it is used for functional interactive communication may help to reduce frustration. Bray and colleagues (1987) presented a useful decision tree as well as other assessment and treatment considerations related to augmentative communication following head injury.

LANGUAGE AND COMMUNICATION

In the introduction to this chapter, we emphasized the pervasiveness in severe TBI (especially in *closed* head injury) of language and communication disorders unlike those associated with traditional aphasic syndromes following left hemisphere stroke. Although specific persisting language disturbances in the phonologic, morphologic, and syntactic domains of language may occur (particularly under cognitive or social stress; Campbell and Dollaghan, 1990), they are not common. In contrast, open head injuries associated with penetrating missile wounds often result in nonfluent aphasic disorders similar to those secondary to left hemisphere stroke (Newcombe, 1969).

Despite general agreement on the existence of "nonaphasic" language disturbances following severe closed head injury, investigators do not agree on their best characterization. Sarno used the term "subclinical aphasia" to refer to verbal impairments that are not evident in everyday conversation but are revealed by careful testing. These symptoms include impaired confrontation naming, word fluency, and comprehension of complex oral commands. In two separate studies of patients with TBI admitted to an inpatient rehabilitation facility, Sarno found that 100% had language disturbances, although only a relatively small minority were classifiable as aphasic (Sarno, 1980, 1984).

Halpern, Darley, and Brown (1973) highlighted the "language of confusion" typically seen in patients with TBI during the acute phase of recovery. Symptoms include "reduced recognition and understanding of and responsiveness to the environment, faulty short-term memory, mistaken reasoning, disorientation in time and space, and behavior which is less adaptive and appropriate than normal" (p. 163). Hagen (1982) described "cognitive-language" disturbances that often persist beyond the confused stages of recovery and are a product of underlying cognitive disorganization, including impaired attention and perception, disorientation, poor memory, disorganized thinking, and reduced judgment. Cognitive-language symptoms that coexist with adequate speech and grammar include word retrieval problems, decreased auditory and reading comprehension, and expressive language characterized by confabulation, circumlocution, lack of relevance, tangentiality, and a general lack of verbal organization.

In this chapter, we will use the term "cognitive-communicative" impairment to include the nonaphasic communication disturbances described by Halpern and colleagues, Sarno, and Hagen. However, we wish to collect under this heading an additional set of communication challenges not highlighted by these investigators. It makes clinical sense to include in this category those problems that are a likely result of cognitive weakness as well as those associated with behavioral and psychosocial deficits frequently seen in TBI. "Cognitive-communicative" impairment is the label used in the American Speech, Language, and Hearing Association's scope of practice statement that addresses the speech-language pathologist's role with TBI patients. These problems may include:

- Confused language, including confabulation and irrelevant, bizarre, perseverative, and socially awkward language;
- Difficulty retrieving specific words, particularly under time pressure or social stress;
- Difficulty understanding spoken or written language under time pressure, or given significant amounts of language to organize and comprehend, or in the presence of environmental distractions;
- Difficulty organizing expressive language in conversation (e.g., rambling, tangential, unconnected conversational turns) and in extended descriptions and narratives (spoken or written);
- Difficulty comprehending and producing abstract language (e.g., metaphors, figures of speech);
- Difficulty learning new concepts and associated words;
- Unconventional and awkward social interactive behavior, including social disinhibition as well as social withdrawal;
- Specific violations of pragmatic rules and conventions, including reduced conversational initiation, unrelated turns, excessive pause time, unspecific reference, inappropriate prosody, and excessive laughter;
- Inadequate use of language for reasoning and problem solving.

It is generally assumed that these difficulties are not specific to language and communication, but rather are the manifestation of more general cognitive and psychosocial disruption. Hartley and Jensen (1985) suggested that there may be three subtypes of individuals with TBI in relation to these general cognitive-communicative variables: Those with generally confused discourse (typically early in their recovery), those with excessive and disorganized language, and those with very little spontaneous language.

Speech-language pathologists who work with these patients must be skilled in identifying communicative consequences of cognitive and psychosocial weakness. Attentional problems, for example, may be associated with impaired word retrieval, reduced comprehension in group settings, unconnected discourse, inability to shift topic, and other communication problems. Perceptual weakness can reduce perception of social cues and result in awkward interaction. Memory problems not only depress new language learning, but may result in irritating repetition of thoughts and may contribute to difficulty staying on topic in conversation. Organizational weakness can negatively affect word retrieval, precision of expression, comprehension of extended text (e.g., grasping main ideas and relationships among ideas), organized expression of complex ideas in speaking and writing, and coherent conversation. Impaired reasoning and concrete thinking results in difficulty interpreting abstract language (e.g., metaphors, figures of speech, humor), drawing inferences and seeing connections, generalizing newly acquired skills, and assuming the perspective of others. Impaired executive functions may result in impulsive and socially inappropriate language, perseveration, lack of initiation, poor monitoring of conversational flow and reactions of partners, and failure to use available strategies to find words and organize responses.

Cognitive-Communicative Assessment

Standardized batteries of aphasia tests are appropriately used with that minority of individuals who have aphasic deficits after closed head injury. Furthermore, some of the specific tasks included in aphasia batteries are particularly useful in identifying language challenges associated with TBI. For example, the Word Fluency subtest of the Neurosensory Center Comprehensive Evaluation of Aphasia (Spreen and Benton, 1977) is a sensitive index of word retrieval skill, particularly as it is affected by time pressure. In general, however, standardized aphasia batteries are not well suited to the task of identifying communication strengths and weaknesses following TBI.

Used with individuals with aphasia following stroke, aphasia tests often underestimate communicative competence in real world communication tasks. Used with individuals with cognitive-communicative impairment following TBI, aphasia tests typically overestimate the individual's ability to maintain effective communication in demanding real-world settings. To the extent that communication is negatively affected by attentional, perceptual, organizational, and executive system dysfunction, language testing by its very nature may compensate for the underlying weakness. For example, the controlled testing environment reduces attentional challenges; clear instructions and well defined tasks help to ensure orientation to task and reduce the effects of cognitive inflexibility; test items that include only relatively small amounts of language compensate for organizational weakness; the deliberate rate at which information is presented compensates for difficulties with speeded performance; the supportive and encouraging manner of the examiner may compensate for an inability to cope with interpersonal stress; and commonly used tests fail to measure the individual's ability to learn new information and skill and to generalize new skills from one setting or task to another. Most importantly, existing aphasia batteries fail to identify communication strengths and weaknesses as they are affected by the communication context. Contextual variables, including partner, place, topic, and level of cognitive and social stress, are believed to have a powerful impact on overall communication effectiveness following TBI.

Hartley (1990, 1992) presented a clinically useful and thorough discussion of functional communication assessment for individuals with TBI. In this section we will simply highlight some of the key questions that should be asked about communication following TBI and give selected procedures that are useful in answering these questions. Most of these procedures are not standardized or norm-referenced; for this reason, only extreme results (positive or negative) may have clinically interpretable significance. The focus and depth of the assessments vary with the individual's overall level of recovery and also with the communication demands of the setting to which he or she returns. Evaluating the language competence of a student returning to college requires a level of depth that may be unnecessary for an individual returning to a less demanding setting.

Receptive Language

Key Question: What is the individual's receptive vocabulary level and how is comprehension affected by increasing language processing demands? Vocabulary baseline can be established with the *Peabody Picture Vocabulary Test: Revised* (Dunn and Dunn, 1981). To determine the effects of speeded performance, tape recorded Token Test commands can be presented at rapid and slow rates of speech. Similarly, timed versus untimed reading comprehension levels should be determined. The effects of organizational demands can be determined by systematically comparing comprehension of sentence-length material with longer texts (both auditory and reading comprehension). The larger units of language can be taken from textbooks and lectures for students, and from newspapers and newscasts for others. Effects of abstraction can be determined by comparing comprehension of narratives or descriptions that include only literal meaning with texts that include a variety of nonliteral uses of language. Effects of environmental interference can be determined by comparing comprehension in a controlled environment with comprehension in a distracting environment.

Expressive Language

Key Question: What is the individual's unstressed expressive vocabulary level and how is expression affected by increasing processing demands? An expressive vocabulary or naming test can be used to establish baseline levels and to compare with receptive vocabulary levels. Effects of speed demands can be determined using the Word Fluency test for word retrieval and by comparing timed versus untimed spoken and written narratives. Effects of organizational deficits may be evident in extended descriptions or narratives (spoken and written) which should be analyzed for coherence (Is the information logically connected?), cohesion (Are appropriate linguistic ties used?), general organization (e.g., Are main ideas followed by supporting detail?), accuracy, detail, and appropriate presuppositions.

Social Interaction

The Pragmatic Protocol of Prutting and Kirchner (1987) is useful for describing a variety of pragmatic behaviors, including conversational competencies, speech acts, and paralinguistic and nonverbal aspects of communication. Because interactive performance following TBI varies across contexts (Mentis and Prutting, 1987; Milton, Prutting, and Binder, 1984), it is critical to sample spontaneous interaction in a variety of settings, including socially demanding settings, and with a variety of partners.

Additional aspects of the language evaluation may be shared with other members of the interdisciplinary team. For example, assessment of verbal learning and long-term retention of verbal information may be included in the evaluations of the neuropsychologist, educational specialist, and speech-language pathologist. For well-recovered students returning to high school or college, teaching new academic content and examining the student's learning rate and style (e.g., dependent/independent; strategic/nonstrategic; impulsive/deliberate) are critical components of the assessment and must supplement traditional memory assessment.

In the final analysis, an evaluation that proves to be useful in treatment planning not only identifies intact and disrupted skills, but more importantly sorts out which specific factors contribute to failure to perform a task well and identifies ways in which tasks can be modified or strategies used to turn failure into success. Exploration of this type of detective work is beyond the scope of this chapter. Ylvisaker and colleagues (1990, in press) presented procedures for systematic investigation of cognitive-communicative functioning in children and adolescents with TBI.

COGNITIVE-COMMUNICATIVE INTERVENTION

Acute Stages of Recovery

Environmental Intervention

For most individuals with TBI, the period of recovery characterized by confusion, agitation, and generally inappropriate behavior occurs in a hospital or rehabilitation center. During this stage, communication management largely coincides with general behavior management which includes environmental procedures designed to promote adaptive behavior, facilitate successful communication, reduce confusion and behavioral manifestations of confusion, and prevent the evolution of learned maladaptive behavior. Environmental procedures include consistency in schedule and staff, ample orientation cues (e.g., clearly printed schedule, photographs of staff), task expectations consistent with the ability to perform, a full and varied schedule of meaningful activities, elimination of events known to elicit confusion and agitation, and interaction with the patient that is positive and therapeutic.

Environmental management presupposes that significant people in the environment are oriented to principles and procedures of environmental intervention. In hospital and rehabilitation settings, speech-language pathologists, often working with behavioral psychologists, provide regular training to staff (direct care staff and others) and family members in techniques of communication and therapeutic interaction with significantly confused patients. The goal of this training is to ensure that everybody who interacts regularly with patients 1) communicates in a way that is as easy as possible for the patient to comprehend (appropriate simplification of form and content); 2) encourages patients to communicate in natural contexts; 3) creates an environment in which the likelihood of successful communication is increased; 4) actively communicates respect for patients; 5) knows how to prevent or diffuse behavioral outbursts; 6) can redirect agitated or perseverative patients without reinforcing maladaptive behavior; and 7) refrains from personalizing hostile comments or aggressive acts that are the product of confusion. Ylvisaker, Feeney, and Urbanczyk (1993) describe in detail a communication training program designed to meet these goals.

Specific Interventions

During the acute phase of recovery, language intervention is rarely directed at specific linguistic targets (e.g., phonology, grammar, or specific lexical items). There is value, however, in therapeutic activities which systematically challenge the patient's cognitive processing skills and promote reorganization of the semantic knowledge base. Semantic feature analysis developed by Szekeres (Ylvisaker, Szekeres, Henry, Sullivan, and Wheeler, 1987) is one example of a treatment procedure designed to meet these goals. A word representing a familiar object, person, or event is placed in the center box in the feature analysis guide (Fig. 8.2). The individual or group then systematically search semantic memory—proceeding clockwise around the Guide—for relevant information about the object or event, filling the boxes with as much information as possible. The information collected is then put to functional use in writing descriptive paragraphs, doing problem solving exercises, or some other functional task to which the information about the object or event is relevant.

At this stage of recovery, there are several goals that might be achieved by means of this activity. Initially, focused and sustained attention to language tasks may be the primary objective. For individuals with severely impaired word retrieval associated with a disorganized semantic knowledge base or with weak divergent thinking, the exercise helps to reorganize the conceptual base and create a map for searching semantic memory. For individuals with adequate divergent thinking (or divergent thinking that is out of control) but inadequate convergent thinking, insist-

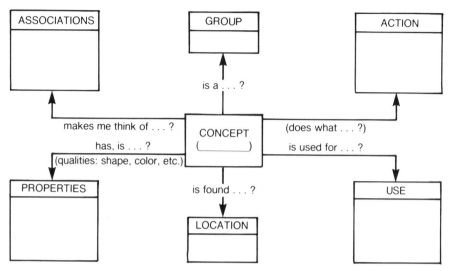

Figure 8.2. Feature analysis guide. (From Ylvisaker, M., and Szekeres, S.F. (1986). Management of the patient with closed head injury. In: Chapey, R. (ed). Language intervention strategies in adult aphasia (2nd ed). Baltimore: Williams & Wilkins, 481. Reprinted with permission.)

ing on only directly relevant information in each box helps to harness associations and recreate a sense of relevance. Later in recovery, individuals who have persistent word retrieval problems may use the Guide as a word search strategy.

Postacute Stages of Recovery

Individuals with persisting cognitive-communicative deficits following resolution of confusion and disorientation may profit from targeted exercises designed to improve specific verbal functions or related cognitive skills. However, there is considerable controversy about the effectiveness of remedial cognitive exercises, particularly if the treatment tasks bear little resemblance to real world tasks (Ben-Yishay and Prigatano, 1990; Schacter and Glisky, 1986). In most cases of persisting deficit, there is little hope of restoring the individual's cognitive and language processing abilities to their preinjury status. The remaining rehabilitative options include 1) helping individuals to acquire procedures that they can use deliberately to compensate for persisting deficits, 2) making changes in the environment and in the behavior and expectations of significant people in the environment so that communication can be as effective and satisfying as possible despite residual deficits, and 3) helping the individual to adjust emotionally to the changes caused by ongoing disability.

Elsewhere, we have discussed principles and procedures of strategy intervention for individuals with TBI (Ylvisaker, Szekeres, Henry, Sullivan, and Wheeler, 1987; Ylvisaker, Szekeres, and Hartwick, 1992). In this section, our goal is simply to highlight some of the critical aspects of this intervention. Strategies for compensating for language weakness include procedures such as 1) asking speakers to slow their rate, repeat themselves, or write important information down (for auditory processing deficits), 2) using study guides, self-questions, imagery, outlining, and elaboration techniques (for weakness in comprehending text), 3) using outlines and script guides (for disorganized language expression), and 4) using circumlocution, self-cuing gestures, sentence completion, free association, or structured association (for word retrieval problems).

A critical component of strategy intervention is the selection of individuals who are good candidates for this approach. Patients who remain confused and very concrete in their thinking may be taught to use external aids (e.g., a schedule card, pictures and printed names of staff, a memory book), but are unlikely to learn to use internal or complex compensatory procedures. In addition to general level of cognitive recovery, a set of variables must be considered in selecting candidates and in setting goals:

1. *Goals*: Since strategic behavior is essentially goal directed, individuals who lack goals are weak candidates for this intervention.
2. *Metacognitive Knowledge*: Good strategy users know that their performance needs to be enhanced, that strategic procedures will enhance performance, that they are capable of using the procedure, and that the procedure is relevant to a specific set of circumstances. If metacognitive awareness of this sort is weak, it must become a direct target of intervention if strategy instruction is to succeed.
3. *Self-Monitoring*: Individuals must be capable of monitoring their performance to recognize that it is effective or ineffective, with or without a strategy.
4. *Working Memory*: There must be enough "space" in working memory to allow the individual to think about strategic procedures and the task at hand at the same time.
5. *Impulsiveness*: Individuals who are extremely impulsive are likely to act before they think to use their strategy.
6. *Initiation*: Individuals with minimal initiation of activity will likely also not initiate strategic activity.
7. *Anxiety*: Individuals who are extremely anxious are often so concerned about failure that they forget to use procedures designed to prevent failure.
8. *Environmental Support*: If family members, teachers, or employers are

not supportive of compensatory procedures, it is unlikely that they will be generalized to functional settings.

Selection of specific strategies requires equally thoughtful decision making. The commonplace clinical practice of selecting procedures based on test performance and then simply instructing the patient in the procedure is unwise for many reasons. Strategic behavior is essentially problem solving behavior. In denying the patient a role in the problem solving, the clinician is essentially undercutting the ultimate goal of strategy intervention. In addition, it is most unlikely that individuals will have an investment in procedures that they did not participate in choosing.

The following considerations merit attention in selecting compensatory procedures:

1. *Negotiation*: It is critical to involve the individual in brainstorming about the need for compensatory behavior and the specific procedures that may be useful.
2. *Spontaneous use*: Other things being equal, procedures that an individual uses spontaneously are more likely to be generalized and used functionally.
3. *Complexity and abstractness*: Concrete, external aid strategies are useful for individuals with substantial cognitive impairment. Internal procedures (e.g., elaboration of information) presuppose good cognitive recovery.
4. *Domain of applicability*: Customized task-specific strategies (e.g., procedures for outlining college texts) are often best for specific problems. General strategies (e.g., writing down information that must be remembered) may be useful for some individuals with pervasive functional deficits.
5. *Personality fit*: Sensitive negotiation is required to ensure that strategies are acceptable emotionally. Compensatory behavior may be stigmatizing or just plain difficult and therefore presupposes commitment to its use.

Again, the most critical component of strategy intervention is active involvement of the patient, including identification of the problem and of the procedure designed to compensate for the problem. Ylvisaker and Szekeres (in press), and Ylvisaker, Szekeres, and Hartwick (1992), outlined an intervention program designed to help individuals with TBI become more effective in identifying their problems and possible solutions to those problems.

In many ways, strategy instruction is like other types of instruction and falls under many of the same guidelines and principles. These include: 1) careful task analysis; 2) systematic progression from simple, easy-to-master components to more complex procedures; 3) gradual fading of cues and prompts which were designed specifically at each stage to ensure success; 4) limited goals, so the individual can see the task as manageable and experience success; 5) reasonable criterion levels; and 6) a bit of fun. Components of strategy instruction that deserve particular attention include promoting general strategic thinking, facilitating generalization and maintenance, and overcoming resistance.

General Strategic Thinking

Effective use of compensatory procedures presupposes adequate awareness of the deficit and its effect on functional activities, and appreciation of the value of the strategy. Procedures designed to enhance this awareness include: 1) "Product monitoring" tasks: Patients are asked to perform a functional task with and without the use of a strategic procedure. The "products" (measures of performance) are then carefully compared and the strategy evaluated in relation to important goals for the individual. For example, a student may read chapters in a text with and without the use of an organized outlining procedure. Test results on the two chapters can then be compared. 2) Self-viewing on videotape: Patients with adequate emotional strength can observe their performance on video to heighten their appreciation of the need to do "something special." 3) Group role playing and modeling: Role playing of successful and unsuccessful language activities with and without strategies can be followed by group discussion of the usefulness of these procedures.

Generalization and Maintenance

As is the case with most clinical interventions, the touchstone of success for strategy intervention is generalization (transfer) from clinical to functional settings and activities, and maintenance over time. One way to deal with the issue of transfer is to make it a nonissue by providing the training using the setting and activities in which functional use is targeted. For example, this approach would apply to individuals who need to use special procedures to understand and remember work instructions in a sheltered workshop situation. It is far more effective to provide situationally precise training in that context than to provide it elsewhere and hope for generalization.

Generalization procedures for less severely impaired individuals include 1) role-playing and in other ways practicing situational discrimination so that it is amply clear under what circumstances the strategy is to be used; 2) varying the activity, place, and participants during strategy practice; 3) rehearsing the strategy to the point of automaticity; 4) making generalization an explicit goal of the individual, including having him or her keep a log of success in real world contexts; and 5) ensuring that the strategy has a sufficiently beneficial effect on performance that the motivation to use it will be strong.

Overcoming Resistance

Compensatory strategies can be time consuming (e.g., outlining, taking notes) or stigmatizing (e.g., asking speakers to repeat themselves or to speak slowly). Therefore, resistance is expected and may need to be addressed by a clinical psychologist or social worker as part of adjustment to disability. Within language therapy sessions, testimonials from other patients are useful, as is discussion of the pervasive use of "tricks" of one sort or another by individuals who are not brain-injured. Customized images and metaphors can also be effective. For example, one young man refused to use a memory book until it was compared to a "back-up" truck (to be used in the event of a breakdown) at his former work place. Another started to use an outlining procedure only after it was likened to the back brace that Joe Montana wore after his injury. A young woman with language processing weakness felt foolish asking speakers to clarify their messages until she recalled that one of her heroines, Gloria Steinum, did exactly the same thing routinely in her work as a journalist.

SUMMARY

The scope of practice of speech-language pathologists is broad in brain injury rehabilitation. The goal of this chapter was to highlight areas of particular concern in working with this population. Inevitably, much has been omitted. For example, there was no discussion of procedures for helping individuals recover social interactive competence (see Chapters 7 and 13). In postacute head injury rehabilitation centers, this is often the dominant intervention focus of speech-language pathologists. Ylvisaker, Urbanczyk, and Feeney (1992) presented a perspective on social skills intervention for individuals with TBI. Ylvisaker, Szekeres, Haarbauer-Krupa, Urbanczyk, and Feeney (in press) recently summarized available literature on social skills intervention as it applies to adolescents with TBI.

We wish that we could appeal to editorial constraints as the explanation for limited comments in this chapter on treatment effectiveness. With the exception of isolated reports on efficacy studies related to social skills training following TBI (e.g., Eames and Wood, 1985; Giles, Fussey, and Burgess, 1988; Helffenstein and Wechsler, 1982), there is little reported data on the effects of communication-related services for individuals with TBI (Ylvisaker and Urbanczyk, 1990). It is our hope that textbooks on head injury rehabilitation published at the turn of the century will be supported by a considerably deeper knowledge base.

References

Ben-Yishay, Y. and Prigatano, G.P. (1990). Cognitive remediation. In: Rosenthal, M., Griffith, E., Bond, M., and Miller, J.D. (eds). Rehabilitation of the adult and child with traumatic brain injury. Philadelphia: F.A. Davis, 393–409.

Berry, W.R. (ed). (1983). Clinical dysarthria. San Diego: College-Hill Press.

Beukelman, D.R., and Garrett, K. (1988). Augmentative and alternative communication for adults with acquired severe communication disorders. Augmentative and Alternative Communication, 4:104–21.

Beukelman, D.R., and Yorkston, K.M. (1989). Augmentative and alternative communication application for persons with severe acquired communication disorders: An introduction. Augmentative and Alternative Communication, 5:42–48.

Beukelman, D.R., and Yorkston, K.M. (1991). Communication disorders following traumatic brain injury: Management of cognitive, language, and motor impairments. Austin, TX: Pro-Ed.

Beukelman, D.R., Yorkston, K.M., and Lossing, C. (1984). Functional communication assessment of adults with communication disorders. In: Halper, A., and Fuhrer, M. (eds). Functional assessment in rehabilitation Baltimore: Paul H. Brooks, 101–15.

Bray, L.J., Carlson, F., Humphrey, R., Mastrilli, J.P., and Valko, A.S. (1987). Physical rehabilitation. In: Ylvisaker, M. (ed). Community re-entry for head injured adults. Austin, TX: Pro-Ed, 25–85.

Brooks, N. (ed). (1984). Closed head injury: Psychological, social, and family consequences. Oxford, England: Oxford University Press.

Brooks, N., McKinlay, W., Symington, C., Baettie, A., and Campsie, L. (1987). Return to work within the first seven years of severe head injury. Brain Injury, 1:5–19.

Campbell, T.F., and Dollaghan, C.A. (1990). Expressive language recovery in severely brain-injured children and adolescents. Journal of Speech and Hearing Disorders, 55(3):567–81.

Castelli-Linden, P. (1991). Treatment strategies for adult neurogenic dysphagia. Seminars in Speech and Language, 12:255–61.

Cherney, L.R., and Halper, A.S. (1989). Recovery of oral nutrition after head injury in adults. Journal of Head Trauma Rehabilitation, 4(4):42–50.

Darley, F.L., Aronson, A.E., and Brown, J.R. (1973). Motor speech disorders. Philadelphia: W.B. Saunders.

DeRuyter, F., and Donoghue, K.A. (1989). Communication and traumatic brain injury: A case study. Augmentative and Alternative Communication, 5:49–54.

DeRuyter, F., and Kennedy, M.T.R. (1991). Augmentative communication following traumatic brain injury. In: Beukelman, D.R., and Yorkston, K.M. (eds). Communication disorders following traumatic brain injury: Management of cognitive, language, and motor impairments. Austin, TX: Pro-Ed, 317–65.

Dunn, L., and Dunn, L. (1981). Peabody picture vocabulary test—revised. Circle Pines, MN: American Guidance Service.

Eames, P., and Wood, R.I. (1985). Rehabilitation after severe brain injury: A follow-up study of a behavior modification approach. Journal of Neurology, Neurosurgery, and Psychiatry, 48:613–619.

Eckberg, O. (1992). Radiographic evaluation of swallowing. In: Groher, M.E. (ed). Dysphagia diagnosis and management (2nd ed). Boston: Butterworth-Heinemann, 163–95.

Enderby, P. (1980). Frenchay dysarthria assessment. British Journal of Communication Disorders, 15:165–73.

Enderby, P. (1983). The standardized assessment of dysarthria is possible. In: Berry, W.R. (ed). Clinical dysarthria. San Diego: College-Hill Press.

Giles, G.M., Fussey, I., and Burgess, P. (1988). The behavioural treatment of verbal interaction skills following severe head injury: A single case study. Brain Injury, 2:75-79.

Groher, M.E. (1990). Communication disorders in adults. In: Rosenthal, M., Griffith, E.R., Bond, M.R., and Miller, J.D. (eds). Rehabilitation of the adult and child with traumatic brain injury (2nd ed). Philadelphia: F.A. Davis Co., 148-62.

Groher, M.E. (1992). Dysphagia diagnosis and management (2nd ed). Boston: Butterworth-Heinemann

Hagen, C. (1982). Language disorders in head trauma. In: Holland, A.L. (ed). Language disorders in adults. San Diego: College-Hill Press, 245-281.

Halpern, H., Darley, F.L., and Brown, J.R. (1973). Differential language and neurologic characteristics in cerebral involvement. Journal of Speech and Hearing Disorders, 38:162-73.

Hartley, L.L. (1990). Assessment of functional communication. In: Tupper, D.E., and Cicerone, K.D. (eds). The neuropsychology of everyday life: Assessment and basic competencies. Boston: Kluwer Academic Publishers, 125-68.

Hartley, L.L. (1992). Assessment of functional communication. Seminars in Speech and Language, 13:264-79.

Heilman, K.M., Safran, A., and Geschwind, N. (1971). Closed head trauma and aphasia. Journal of Neurology, Neurosurgery, and Psychiatry, 34:265-69.

Helffenstein, D., and Wechsler, F. (1982). The use of interpersonal process recall (IPR) in the remediation of interpersonal and communication skill deficits in the newly brain-injured. Clinical Neuropsychology, 4:139-43.

Ladtkow, M. (1993). Traumatic brain injury and severe expressive communication impairment: The role of augmentative communication. Seminars in Speech and Language, 14:61-73.

Lazarus, C. (1989). Swallowing disorders after traumatic brain injury. Journal of Head Trauma Rehabilitation, 4(4):34-41.

Lazarus, C.L. (1991). Diagnosis and management of swallowing disorders in traumatic brain injury. In: Beukelman, D.R., and Yorkston, K.M. (eds). Communication disorders following traumatic brain injury: Management of cognitive, language, and motor impairments. Austin, TX: Pro-Ed, 367-417.

Lazarus, C., and Logemann, J. (1987). Swallowing disorders in closed head trauma patients. Archives of Physical Medicine and Rehabilitation, 68:79-84.

Levin, H.S., Madison, C.F., Bailey, C.B., et al. (1983). Mutism after closed head injury. Archives of Neurology, 40:601-06.

Light, J., Beesley, M., and Collier, B. (1988). Transition through multiple augmentative communication systems: A three-year case study of a head-injured adolescent. Augmentative and Alternative Communication, 4:2-14.

Livingston, M.G., and Brooks, D.N. (1988). The burden on families of the brain-injured: A review. Journal of Head Trauma Rehabilitation, 3(4):6-15.

Logemann, J. (1983). Evaluation and treatment of swallowing disorders. San Diego: College-Hill Press.

Logemann, J.L. (1986). Manual for the videofluorographic study of swallowing. Boston: College-Hill Press.

Logemann, J. (1989). Evaluation and treatment planning for the head-injured patient with oral intake disorders. Journal of Head Trauma Rehabilitation, 4(4):24-33.

Logemann, J. (1990). Dysphagia. Seminars in Speech and Language, 11:157-64.

Logemann, J. (1991). Evaluation and treatment of dysphagia in brain injury. Presented at the conference International Brain Injury Symposium, New Orleans, March 8, 1991.

Luria, A.R. (1970). Traumatic aphasia: Its syndromes, psychology, and treatment. The Hague: Mouton.

McNeil, M., Aronson, A., and Rosenbek, J. (eds). (1984). The dysarthrias: Physiology, acoustics, perception, management. Austin, TX: Pro-Ed.

Mentis, M., and Prutting, C. (1987). Cohesion in the discourse of normal and head-injured adults. Journal of Speech and Hearing Research, 30:88-98.

Miller, R.M. (1992). Clinical examination for dysphagia. In: Groher, M.E. (ed). Dysphagia diagnosis and management (2nd ed). Boston: Butterworth-Heinemann, 143-62.

Milton, S., Prutting, C., and Binder, G. (1984). Appraisal of communicative competence in head injured adults. In: Brookshire, R. (ed). Clinical aphasiology conference proceedings. Minneapolis: BRK Publishers, 114-23.

Milton, S.B., and Wertz, R.T. (1986). Management of persisting communication deficits in patients with traumatic brain injury. In: Uzzell, B.B., and Gross, Y. (eds). Clinical neuropsychology of intervention. Boston: Martinus Nijhoff Publishing, 223-56.

Moore, C.A., Yorkston, K.M., and Beukelman, D.R. (1991). Dysarthria and apraxia of speech: Perspectives on management. Baltimore: Paul H. Brookes Publishing Co.

Morris, S. (1978). Oral-motor problems and guidelines for treatment. In: Wilson, J.M. (ed). Oral-motor function and dysfunction in children. Chapel Hill, NC: University of North Carolina.

Morris, S. (1982). The normal acquisition of oral feeding skills: Implications for assessment and treatment. New York: Therapeutic Media, Inc.

Newcombe, F. (1969). Missile wounds of the brain. London: Oxford University Press.

Oddy, M. (1984). Head injury and social adjustment. In: Brooks, N. (ed). Closed head injury: Psychological, social, and family consequences. New York: Oxford University Press, 108-92.

Penn, C., and Cleary, J. (1988). Compensatory strategies in the language of closed head injured patients. Brain Injury, 2:3-17.

Perkins, W.H. (1983). Dysarthria and apraxia. New York: Thieme-Stratton, Inc.

Prigatano, G.P. (1986). Neuropsychological rehabilitation after brain injury. Baltimore: Johns Hopkins University Press.

Prutting, C., and Kirchner, D. (1987). A clinical appraisal of the pragmatic aspects of language. Journal of Speech and Hearing Disorders, 52:105-19.

Rosenbek, J.C., and LaPointe, L.L. (1985). The dysarthrias: Description, diagnosis, and treatment. In: Johns, D.F. (ed). Clinical management of neurogenic communicative disorders (2nd ed). Boston: Little, Brown and Co.

Sapir, S., and Aronson, A.R. (1985). Aphonia after closed head injury: Aetiologic considerations. British Journal of Disorders of Communication, 20:289-96.

Sapir, S., and Aronson, A.R. (1990). The relationship between psychopathology and speech and language disorders in neurologic patients. Journal of Speech and Hearing Disorders, 55:503-09.

Sarno, M.T. (1980). The nature of verbal impairment after closed head injury. Journal of Nervous and Mental Disease, 168:685-92.

Sarno, M.T. (1984). Verbal impairment after closed head injury: Report of a replication study. Journal of Nervous and Mental Disease, 172:475-79.

Sarno, M.T., Buonaguro, A., and Levita, E. (1986). Characteristics of verbal impairment in closed head injury patients. Archives of Physical Medicine and Rehabilitation, 67: 400-05.

Schacter, D.L., and Glisky, E.L. (1986). Memory remediation: Restoration, alleviation, and the acquisition of domain-specific knowledge. In: Uzzell, B., and Gross, Y. (eds). Clinical neuropsychology of intervention. Boston: Martinus Nijhoff Publishing, 257-82.

Silverman, F. (1980). Communication for the speechless. Englewood Cliffs, NJ: Prentice Hall.

Spreen, O., and Benton, A. (1977). Neurosensory Center Comprehensive Examination for

Aphasia: Manual of directions (rev ed). Victoria, BC: Neuropsychology Laboratory, University of Victoria.

Weinstein, C. (1983). Neurogenic dysphagia: Frequency, progression, and outcome in adults following head injury. Physical Therapy, 63:1992–96.

Wood, R. (1984). Behavior disorders following severe head injury: Their presentation and psychological management. In: Brooks, N. (ed). Closed head injury: Psychological, social, and family consequences. New York: Oxford University Press, 195–219.

Workinger, M., and Netsell, R. (1988). Restoration of intelligible speech 13 years post-head injury [Unpublished manuscript].

Ylvisaker, M. (1992). Communication outcome following traumatic brain injury. Seminars in Speech and Language, 13:239–50.

Ylvisaker, M., Chorazy, A., Cohen, S., Mastrilli, J., Molitor, C., Nelson, J., Szekeres, S., Valko, A., and Jaffe, K. (1990). Rehabilitative assessment following head injury in children. In: Rosenthal, M., Griffith, E., Bond, M., and Miller, J.D. (eds). Rehabilitation of the adult and child with traumatic brain injury (2nd ed). Philadelphia: F.A. Davis.

Ylvisaker, M., Feeney, T., and Urbanczyk, B. (1993). Developing a positive communication culture in rehabilitation: Communication training for staff and family members. In: Durgin, C., Schmidt, N., and Fryer, J. (eds). Staff development and clinical intervention in brain injury rehabilitation. Gaithersburg, MD: Aspen Publishers.

Ylvisaker, M., and Logemann, J. (1985). Therapy for feeding and swallowing disorders following head injury. In: Ylvisaker, M. (ed). Head injury rehabilitation: Children and adolescents. San Diego: College-Hill Press, 195–215.

Ylvisaker, M., and Szekeres, S. (1989). Metacognitive and executive impairments in head-injured children and adults. Topics in Language Disorders, 9:34–49.

Ylvisaker, M., and Szekeres, S. (in press). Closed head injury. In: Chapey, R. (ed). Language intervention strategies in adult aphasia (3rd ed). Baltimore: Williams and Wilkins, 474–90.

Ylvisaker, M., Szekeres, S., and Hartwick, P. (1992). Cognitive rehabilitation following traumatic brain injury in children. In: Tramontana, M., and Hooper, S. (eds). Advances in child neuropsychology (Vol. 1). New York: Springer Verlag.

Ylvisaker, M., Szekeres, S., Haarbauer-Krupa, J., Urbanczyk, B., and Feeney, T. (in press). Language intervention. In: Savage, R., and Wolcott, G. (eds). Educational programming for children and young adults with acquired brain injury. Austin, TX: Pro-Ed.

Ylvisaker, M., Szekeres, S., Henry, K., Sullivan, D., and Wheeler, P. (1987). Topics in cognitive rehabilitation therapy. In: Ylvisaker, M., and Gobble, E.M.R. (eds). Community re-entry for head injured adults. Austin, TX: Pro-Ed.

Ylvisaker, M., and Urbanczyk, B. (1990). The efficacy of speech-language pathology intervention: Traumatic brain injury. Seminars in Speech and Language, 11:215–26.

Ylvisaker, M., Urbanczyk, B., and Feeney, T.J. (1992). Social skills following traumatic brain injury. Seminars in Speech and Language, 13:308–21.

Ylvisaker, M., and Weinstein, M. (1989). Recovery of oral feeding after pediatric head injury. Journal of Head Trauma Rehabilitation, 4(4):51–63.

Yorkston, K.M., and Beukelman, D.R. (1981). Assessment of intelligibility of dysarthric speech. Tigard, Oregon: C.C. Publications.

Yorkston, K.M., and Beukelman, D.R. (1989). Recent advances in clinical dysarthria. Boston: Little, Brown, and Co.

Yorkston, K.M., and Beukelman, D.R. (1991). Motor speech disorders. In: Beukelman, D.R., and Yorkston, K.M. (eds). Communication disorders following traumatic brain injury: Management of cognitive, language, and motor impairments. Austin, TX: Pro-Ed, 251–315.

Yorkston, K.M., Honsinger, M.J., Mitsuda, P.M., and Hammen, V. (1989). The relationship between speech and swallowing disorders in head-injured patients. Journal of Head Trauma Rehabilitation, 4(4):1–16.

9

Neuropsychologic Assessment and Cognitive Rehabilitation: Issues of Psychologic Validity

DAVID J. FORDYCE

A "traditional" neuropsychologic evaluation usually entails a clinical interview and the administration and interpretation of psychologic tests. Such an assessment can be used to indicate the type and severity of the injury, the current "stage" of recovery, and to delineate each individual's cognitive deficits and assets. The same data can be utilized to make important predictions about future recovery (magnitude or rate), and to establish rehabilitation targets and guide intervention strategies. The neuropsychologic evaluation is not sufficient, however, for any of these enterprises. As is clear from examining the table of contents of this volume, as well as most other recent comprehensive texts on brain injury rehabilitation (e.g., Beukelman and Yorkston, 1991; Christensen and Uzzell, 1988; Meier, Benton, and Diller, 1987; Prigatano, etal., 1986; Rosenthal, Griffith, Bond, and Miller, 1983; Uzzell and Gross, 1986), an adequate understanding of the consequences of brain injury, and the implementation of appropriate interventions, must involve multiple professionals employing, at least to some extent, unique methods. It might also be remembered that a few hours of testing, while yielding useful information, is not a substitute for extended contact with patients and families during the first few weeks of rehabilitation (Prigatano and Others, 1986).

There has been an explosion in the size of the professional literature and the number of brain injury rehabilitation programs in the 1980's. Unfortunately, the relevant literature has grown so fast that practicing professionals are largely unable to keep up with it (Diller, 1988). The growth in brain injury rehabilitation programs has placed rehabilitation specialists, including neuropsychologists, in central roles determining how scarce clinical resources and sometimes large sums of money are to be allocated. Given this responsibility, it seems important to review general issues of psychologic validity as they relate to our current practices. Neuropsychologic evaluation and rehabilitation are probably more art than science. The specific tests and techniques employed vary among practitioners. In the rehabilitation setting a neuropsychologic evaluation should assist in understanding a patient's level of cognitive, emotional, and interpersonal functioning. It should also provide information concerning such issues as motivation, malleability, and probable psychologic response to intervention attempts. In the following section a context for understanding and practicing neuropsychologic evaluation and cognitive rehabilitation is elaborated. While some specific instruments and practices are briefly described, more general issues related to psychologic measurement are reviewed to provide a context for current practices and to set the stage for future development.

EARLY ASSESSMENT

Most sudden onset neurologic conditions, particularly traumatic head injury, have characteristic recovery patterns with considerable implications for neuropsychologic evaluation and rehabilitation. In general, initial injury is followed by relatively severe cognitive impairment which tends to improve with time. The rapidly changing early clinical picture makes the use of adequate experimental controls crucial in assessing treatment efficacy. In addition, significant disturbances in consciousness greatly limit the kind of early assessments and interventions possible. Yet, objective measurement of coma, disorientation, and posttraumatic amnesia serve as a starting point for recovery and rehabilitation planning.

Glasgow Coma Scale

The Glasgow Coma Scale (GCS) provides a reliable and objective measure of the degree of disturbed consciousness in neurologically impaired patients (Teasdale and Jennett, 1974, 1976). Scores range from 3–15, based on the maximum performance over three domains of behavior: Eye opening, best verbal response, best motor response. While GCS scores do tend to fluctuate (Braakman, Gelpke, Habbema, Maas, and Minderhoud, 1980; Jennett, Teasdale, Braakman, Minderhoud, Heiden, and Kurze, 1979), and it is not clear when the optimal initial coma assessment should occur (Eisenberg and Weiner, 1987), GCS scores have been employed frequently as an index of injury severity after head trauma. Some have adapted components of the GCS in their efforts to find a more stable index of initial injury severity. Sureyya Dikmen, and her colleagues at the University of Washington Medical School (Dikmen, Machamer, Temkin, and McLean, 1990; Dikmen, McLean, Temkin, and Wyler, 1986), have found that the time from injury (hours/days) to when patients can follow commands is a useful index of length of coma.

The period of posttraumatic amnesia (PTA) is characterized by disorientation and significant problems in new learning and memory (Russell, 1932; Smith, 1961). While there has been some debate about how to assess

PTA (Levin, Benton, and Grossman, 1982; Russell, 1971; Schacter and Crovitz, 1977), it continues to serve as another useful measure of injury severity. PTA assessment in the early stages of recovery may need to be repetitive. Traditional tests of new learning and memory are of limited value given their length, complexity, and the relative absence of multiple equivalent forms. The Galveston Orientation and Amnesia Test (GOAT) provides an objective and repeatable measure of disorientation (Levin, O'Donnell, and Grossman, 1979). While it emphasizes assessment of orientation, two questions asking the patient for retrospective reports of retrograde and anterograde amnesia are also included. The GOAT has been shown to reliably track the reemergence of orientation in individual subjects, and to covary in a regular fashion with independent measures of injury severity and outcome (Levin, et al., 1982). The GOAT does not assess short-term memory, however, and some alternative method must be utilized to more completely evaluate this aspect of PTA.

Ranchos Los Amigos

The Level of Cognitive Functioning Scale developed at Ranchos Los Amigos Hospital (Hagen, Malkmus, and Durham, 1979; Malkmus, Booth, and Kodimer, 1980) provides an observational approach for assessing those who are untestable. The Rancho scale offers a common vocabulary and conceptual framework, guiding appropriate intervention efforts for the major cognitive and behavioral stages of recovery. It would seem to be of greatest utility for rehabilitation professionals working with comatose, grossly disoriented, or agitated patients. Unfortunately, the absence of operationally defined measurement methods, with the accompanying lack of reliability and validity data, limits the usefulness of the Ranchos scale for those not well versed in its characteristics.

It makes little sense to subject a patient to an extended neuropsychologic evaluation in the acute stages of recovery. Even if the level of confusion were such that formal testing were possible, the rapid cognitive improvements typically seen in the early stages of recovery would quickly render the results obsolete. Lezak (1983) has suggested delaying formal testing for 6–8 weeks after onset. Instruments such as the GOAT might well assist decisions about when the patient is capable of more comprehensive assessment.

VALIDITY ISSUES IN COMPREHENSIVE NEUROPSYCHOLOGIC EVALUATIONS
Diagnostic Heritage

The traditional neuropsychologic evaluation, in nearly all its forms, developed from the largely independent enterprises of the medical/

neurologic examination, and the psychologic assessment of individual differences in human abilities (Ben-Yishay and Diller, 1983a; Hart and Hayden, 1986; Russell, 1986). Its validity heritage is predominantly one of predictive "criterion" validity (American Psychological Association, 1954; Cronbach and Meehl, 1955), with the criterion of interest being the presence or absence of brain impairment. Simultaneously, clinical and more basic research has attempted to elucidate the nature of specific cognitive skills and their relationship to underlying brain structures (construct validity). Diagnostic criterion validity has been repeatedly demonstrated for the Halstead-Reitan Neuropsychological Test Battery (HRB) (Boll, 1981; Reitan, 1986), as well as for the Luria-Nebraska Neuropsychological Test Battery (LNNB) (e.g., Golden, Kane, Sweet, Moses, Cardellino, Templeton, Vincente, and Graber, 1981), and many other tests (Lezak, 1983). Construct validation has proceeded less efficiently. This has seemingly resulted from the tendency to employ instruments developed for diagnostic purposes (Loring and Papanicolaou, 1987), as well as the historical separation of the disciplines of clinical neuropsychology and cognitive psychology. The diagnosis of brain impairment, or the demonstration that a particular test appears to have some valid meaning with respect to a specific cognitive process, are events with only indirect relevance for the rehabilitation setting.

It initially appeared that the development of sophisticated radiographic techniques, such as CT and MRI scanning, reduced the need for diagnostic neuropsychologic evaluations (Costa, 1983; Kohn, 1986; Loring and Papanicolaou, 1987). Yet, two coincident forces seemed to offset such a trend. First, there was a shift in diagnostic emphasis to more subtle conditions such as mild head injury or neurotoxin exposure. The initial excitement over this focus (Boll, 1985) appears to have been tempered, however, by subsequent analyses of the complexity of the diagnostic issues (Binder, 1986; Hawkins, 1990). The demonstration of diagnostic criterion validity is naturally much more difficult when the independent measures of the criterion are elusive or unavailable. Secondly, the value of a comprehensive description of a patient's cognitive strengths and impairments for intervention purposes began to be promoted. Most contemporary presentations of neuropsychology extol the benefits of the expanded psychologic profile obtained from a comprehensive evaluation. This notion, coupled with recent interest in rehabilitating cognitive impairments, have acted to cement the neuropsychologist to the rehabilitation setting. Unfortunately, the potential benefits of the neuropsychologic evaluation in rehabilitation has sometimes been expressed with insufficient consideration of the fact that validity studies designed to establish the association between test behavior and other behavioral criteria are largely lacking. It appears in clinical practice that a test score is assumed to reflect a "sign" of a cognitive attribute, with the latter similar to the notion of a trait in personality theory (Wiggins, 1973). A particular score is thought to allow meaningful inferences about, or extrapolations to, other behaviors or situations. For example, people are reported as having limitations in attention, abstraction, or short-term memory which are felt to have functional consequences. While this conceptualization seems preferable to the alternative notion that test scores are a "sample" of behavior, given the rather artificial nature of the testing setting, confirming rehabilitation-relevant validity studies are not available.

Impairments and Disabilities

Diller (Ben-Yishay and Diller, 1983a; Diller, 1987, 1988) has noted that neuropsychologists deal with *impairments* in operationally defined underlying cognitive "structures or functions." These impairments are the attributes (constructs) noted above. Rehabilitation specialists, on the other hand, are concerned with *disabilities, handicaps*, or alterations in *status*. Disabilities reflect problems in daily living that may in some way relate to underlying impairments. Handicaps refer to problems in functioning in specific psychosocial environments, and statuses can be seen as an individual's major life roles. It is important to note that impairments and disabilities are not the same. A particular level of cognitive impairment does not imply a specific level of cognitively-related disability (Diller, 1987; Hart and Hayden, 1986; Mayer, Keating, and Rapp, 1986). With but a few exceptions (Wilson, Cockburn, Baddeley, and Hiorns, 1989), there have been no attempts to design tests that might maximize predictive criterion validity for important rehabilitation targets (disabilities). The item content of nearly all traditional neuropsychologic measures has little to do with the thinking demands of day-to-day living. Those studies that have assessed the predictive or concurrent validity of traditional neuropsychologic measures have demonstrated generally modest relationships. Finally, as will be reviewed later, a construct of remediable cognitive impairment has yet to be validated. This is of particular concern in the head-injured patient population, especially with respect to generating meaningful changes in disabilities.

Qualitative/Quantitative Distinction

Kohn (1986) noted that Kurt Goldstein, the patriarch of neuropsychologic rehabilitation, cautioned about the inherent limitations in test scores or other categorical measures of impairment. He felt that the processes by which patients solved problems were more important for rehabilitation than the test scores themselves. Others have certainly echoed this view (Cicerone and Tupper, 1986; Christensen, 1979; Milberg, Hebben, and

Kaplan, 1986). Quantitative fixed batteries are touted, on the other hand, as increasing the likelihood that a broad range of cognitive *strengths* and impairments will be identified (Goldstein, 1987). In addition, quantitative assessment techniques can certainly direct rehabilitation efforts, although test data are often augmented with other behavioral measures (Alfano and Finlayson, 1987; Goldstein, 1987). While quantitative and qualitative methods are sometimes seen as antagonistic, it seems that most practicing clinical neuropsychologists combine both strategies. Both are likely appropriate and necessary for comprehensive assessment (Lezak, 1983).

Qualitative methods seem to reflect an attempt to obtain a more fine grained analysis of test performance. Most neuropsychologic measures are complex, requiring a number of subroutines or component skills for successful solution (Luria, 1980; Milberg, et al., 1986). The propensity for individuals to employ a unique set of processes is masked by a single test score. Edith Kaplan, and her colleagues at the Boston VA Hospital (Milberg, et al., 1986), have developed scoring methods which allow some quantification of the process approach. It certainly seems intuitive that a careful analysis of the strategies people employ during testing would provide a rich source of hypotheses about how to maximize performance. "Testing to the limits" (Lezak, 1983) exemplifies one example of this approach. Luria (Luria and Tsvetkova, 1964) has shown how an analysis of problem solving process impairments can generate specific intervention strategies. A similar, somewhat more empirical, literature has been provided by the rehabilitation psychologists from the New York University Medical School (Ben-Yishay, Diller, Gerstman, and Gordon, 1970; Diller, Ben-Yishay, Gerstman, Goodkin, Gordon, and Weinberg, 1974; Diller and Weinberg, 1977; Weinberg, Diller, Gordon, Gerstman, Lieberman, Lakin, Hodges, and Ezrachi, 1977, 1979). With the exception of a few studies from NYU, neither the construct nor concurrent validity of more qualitative neuropsychologic measures has been established (Newcombe, 1987).

Predictive Criterion Validity

The neuropsychologic literature is by no means devoid of analyses of criterion validity for predicting everyday functioning. These are generally, however, *post hoc* efforts that compare traditional test measures with some global status (i.e., employment) or some other index of function such as a measure of self-care skills. Several comprehensive reviews of this topic are available (Acker, 1986; Chelune, 1985; Heaton and Pendleton, 1981). Virtually all of these studies employ group parametric statistical methods to indicate the degree of average relationship between individual or multivariate test scores, and some measure of disability or psychosocial function. Gratifyingly, most of these studies do indicate some degree of shared variance between the two domains of information. Not surprisingly, given the complexities of human behavior and the environments in which we live, multiple regression coefficients are more powerful predictors of status than individual test scores. The obtained relationships tend to be modest in scope, R's ranging from .4–.7 are common, and the test score distributions for different outcome criterion groups almost always have some degree of overlap. Rehabilitation planning is concerned with how specific impairments may relate to specific problems in complex psychosocial function. The criterion studies noted above tell us some relationships might exist, but they do not detail what these might be.

For example, survivors of traumatic head injury, with different levels of gross outcome as assessed by the Glasgow Outcome Scale (GOS) (Jennett and Bond, 1975), can be statistically differentiated on the basis of overall neuropsychologic test performance (Brooks, Hosie, Bond, Jennett, and Aughton, 1986; Levin, Grossman, Rose, and Teasdale, 1979). The relationship between levels of cognitive impairment and GOS outcome appears to diminish, however, with time (Brooks, et al., 1986). Also, residual cognitive impairments are present even with "Good Outcome" (Stuss, Ely, Hugenholtz, Richard, LaRochelle, Poirer, and Bell, 1985).

In addition, more unemployment is associated with greater levels of neuropsychologic impairment (Bayless, Varney, and Roberts, 1989; Dikmen and Morgan, 1981; Fraser, Dikmen, McLean, Miller, and Temkin, 1988; Heaton, Chelune, and Lehman, 1978; Newman, Heaton, and Lehman, 1978), and initial severity of injury (Fahy, Irving, and Milac, 1967; Gronwall and Wrightson, 1974; Minderhoud, Boelens, Huizenga, and Saan, 1980; Rimel, Giordani, Barth, Boll, and Jane, 1981). Yet, there is tremendous variability in vocational outcome, regardless of initial injury severity or level of neuropsychologic impairment. In addition, not all researchers have found that employed and unemployed groups are clearly distinguishable on the basis of a single neuropsychologic evaluation (Prigatano, Fordyce, Zeiner, Roueche, Pepping, and Wood, 1984). Finally, it should be noted that measures of emotional or personality functioning also discriminate between employed and unemployed groups at least as well as neuropsychologic test scores (Heaton, et al., 1978; Prigatano, et al., 1984). It is perhaps sobering to note that a relatively simple assessment of anosmia (perhaps suggesting frontal lobe impairment) discriminates employment status at levels similar to most studies utilizing neuropsychologic test scores (Varney, 1988). Stronger relationships would probably exist between specific neuropsychologic measures and more circumscribed measures of work performance. Newman, et al. (1978), for example, present data suggesting that neuropsychologic test performance relates better to the cognitive requirements of a job than to motor/perceptual demands. That there is no consistent relationship between general neuropsychologic function and employment should not be surprising. WAIS IQ values in uninjured individuals, while bearing some relationship to level of occupational attainment, relate minimally to actual job success (Chelune, 1985; Matarazzo, 1972).

Finally, the criterion validity of traditional neuropsychologic methods has been examined by looking at how test scores relate to measures of ambulation, self-care, or higher order activities of daily living (Acker, 1986; Baird, Brown, Adams, Shatz, McSweeny, Ausman, and Diaz, 1987; Ben-Yishay, Gerstman, Diller, and Haas, 1970; McCue, Rogers, and Goldstein, 1990; Torkelson, Jellinek, Malec, and Harvey, 1983), self-report measures of independence following hospital discharge (Sundet, Finset, and Reinvang, 1988), or instruments measuring level of psychosocial function (Fordyce and Roueche, 1986; McSweeney, Grant, Heaton, Prigatano, and Adams, 1985). Again, parametric correlational methods predominate these analyses, yielding positive results of modest magnitude and unknown specificity.

In summary, traditional neuropsychologic tests have been developed to diagnose brain injury or to operationally define certain cognitive skills (impairments). Whether more qualitative or quantitative techniques are employed, the traditional validity literature does not directly relate to rehabilitation guidance or outcome prediction. Those predictive criterion studies available yield modest average relationships between multivariate test indices and gross status. It is not clear that these general results have much application to individual patients.

EMOTIONAL AND PERSONALITY FUNCTIONING
MMPI

The Minnesota Multiphasic Personality Inventory (MMPI) has long been included in the HRB. This reflects an understanding that the assessment of personality and emotional state provides a unique set of data of great clinical importance. The dichotomization of human functions into cognitive and affective domains is somewhat arbitrary (Hart and Hayden, 1986). As George Prigatano has noted in many of his writings (Prigatano, 1987a; Prigatano and Others, 1986; Prigatano, Pepping, and Klonoff, 1986), there are complex relationships between brain function, affect and personality, cognition, and level of psychosocial functioning, that have tremendous importance for assessment and rehabilitation. The concept of executive function, including the capacity to set goals, initiate action, monitor and correct performance, and to have self-awareness, is a good example of how personality and cognition are sometimes hard to distinguish. Emotional and interpersonal problems, some more "neurologic" and some more "psychologic," abound after brain injury. Changes in emotional and personality function must be understood from within the framework of premorbid personality, much as altered neuropsychologic status needs to be represented within the context of probable premorbid intellectual endowment. It is well known, for example, that certain psychosocial characteristics increase the likelihood that head injuries may occur (Fahy, et al., 1967; Rimel, et al., 1982; Gruvstad, Kebbon, and Gruvstad, 1958). The Diagnostic and Statistical Manual for Mental Disorders (DSM-III) (American Psychiatric Association, 1980) attempts to distinguish long-standing personality characteristics from more immediate emotional reactions. While its objective diagnostic criteria are to be commended, there remain some problems in applying the DSM-III system to brain injured individuals (Grant and Alves, 1987).

Like neuropsychologic evaluation, personality assessment still remains more an art than a science. Several discussions of personality and emotional assessment for neurologically impaired patients are available (Prigatano, 1987a; Grant and Alves, 1987). It is extremely difficult to objectify the relationship between premorbid personality and postmorbid emotional reactions (Kozol, 1945, 1946). Extended contact with patients and families during rehabilitation and psychotherapy, however, can provide useful information about how coping styles, temperament, or problems in functioning prior to the injury may relate to adjustment difficulties afterwards. Such information seems necessary to establish realistic rehabilitation goals. Extended contact also provides an opportunity to comprehend psychosocial influences coincident, but not directly related, to the neurologic illness or injury. Financial disincentives, coincident unrelated stresses, or early posttraumatic learning, may also impact on emotional functioning, motivation, or general adjustment. The recent enthusiasm over the potential of neuropsychologic measures to have diagnostic utility in cases of mild acquired brain impairment seems to have generated a rather constricted understanding of the origins of long-term disability in such cases (Fordyce, 1989).

The MMPI remains the more commonly employed instrument to objectively assess emotion and personality after brain injury. There has been long-standing concern that the length and linguistic complexity of the MMPI (perhaps improved with the MMPI2) precludes valid assessment of confused brain-injured patients. While specific concurrent or predictive psychosocial criterion validity studies are largely lacking, there are many published studies that have given the MMPI to brain-injured patients. For example, there were early attempts to use the MMPI to diagnose brain injury. These efforts were generally unsuccessful and have been largely abandoned (Lezak, 1983). More recently there have been reports that the neurologic content of many MMPI items may yield artificially elevated profiles (false positives), not reflective of the patient's actual emotional state (Cripe, 1989, Alfano, Finlayson, Stearns, and Nelson, 1990). Not unexpectedly, removal of these items usually lowers profile elevations and can also change profile configuration. This kind of concern seems to be based on the presumption of a one-to-one correspondence between the verbal endorsement of a symptom and that symptom's actual presence.

The MMPI was originally constructed with the understanding that the relationship between a test item response and an internal state (the item's referent) was complex and not directly knowable (Dahlstrom and Welsh, 1960; Wiggins, 1973). There is a large body of data, in fact, that suggests neurologically impaired patients do not demonstrate any consistent tendency to endorse a particular set of items (remember, again, the failed diagnostic efforts). Furthermore, there is no consistent relationship between injury severity and levels of posttraumatic emotional distress assessed in a variety of ways (Bond, 1975; Levin and Grossman, 1978; Levin, High, Goethe, Sisson, Overall, Rhoades, Eisenberg, Kalisky, and Gary, 1987; Ruesch and Bowman, 1945; Keshavan, Channabasavanna, and Reddy, 1981; Van Zomeren and Van Den Burg, 1985), including through use of the MMPI (Fordyce, Roueche, and Prigatano, 1983). There is some evidence, in fact, that more mildly injured patients may express more emotional distress at some points in the recovery process compared to those more severely injured (McLean, Dikmen, Temkin, Wyler, and Gale, 1984; Levin, et al., 1987; Ruesch and Bowman, 1945). The absence of a "severity gradient" makes it difficult to accept the logic that a patient's reaction to a more neurologic MMPI item has some special significance. The fact that levels of emotional distress on the MMPI correlate significantly with independent measures of personal awareness (Fordyce and Roueche, 1986; Heaton and Pendleton, 1981) highlight the complex relationships existing between injury, personality, cognition, and affect. It would seem reasonable, given the size of the general MMPI literature, to proceed with additional validation studies on neurologically impaired groups with the original instrument intact. Like some psychiatric patients, some brain-injured patients will not be able to take the MMPI. As in the case of all other psychologic tests, it is up to the clinician to decide when it should be used, and how to interpret the results within the context at hand. Some validity data are available. Fordyce, et al. (1983), for example, demonstrated that time since injury, not obvious differences in injury severity or levels of neuropsychologic impairment, was related to MMPI elevations among a group of traumatic head injury patients. More importantly, independent ratings of emotional dysfunction using the KATZ Adjustment Scale paralleled the MMPI results. Finally, multivariate analyses suggested an item correlational structure which, in some ways, paralleled that noted for other clinical groups (Dahlstrom and Welsh, 1960).

REHABILITATION

The excitement generated by new brain injury rehabilitation techniques during the 1980's was substantial, as were the accompanying controversies and pressures. The excitement derived, in part, from the rediscovery of a large clinical population (victims of traumatic head injury) with a number of sometimes devastating physical, emotional, intellectual, and social problems. It was also observed that these people, and their families, often received inadequate assistance in managing permanent disabilities. Simultaneously, animal research began to suggest that underlying brain structure could be directly modified by postinjury experiences (Rosenzweig, 1984). The field of neuropsychology grew with emphasis on elaborating the cognitive consequences of acquired brain injury. Early rehabilitation programs were developed by bright and dynamic individuals such as Yahuda Ben-Yishay and George Prigatano. Their ideas were presented internationally in an articulate and passionate manner to interested professionals. The excitement has been further supported through the National Head Injury Foundation, and the several excellent annual national conferences on head injury rehabilitation. All of these forces, plus the perceived profitability of head injury rehabilitation activities, led to an explosion in the number of treatment programs available.

The accompanying pressures were of equal magnitude. Brain injury rehabilitation is extremely demanding work. The impairments are perplexing and difficult to treat. The scope of disability for the patient, their families, and society is distressingly broad. The newly developed brain injury rehabilitation techniques were based on the realization that the cognitive and behavioral impairments serving as the targets of rehabilitation also acted as "barriers" to rehabilitation (Ben-Yishay and Diller, 1983b). As a result, treatment would need to occur with great intensity, repetition, duration, and organization (Ben-Yishay and Diller, 1983b; Prigatano and Others, 1986). These intense models create unique demands on staff, with transference and countertransference dynamics becoming quite powerful. The amount of time spent with patients and families may erode the boundaries separating staff from clients. Therapists may find it hard to leave their work at work, and staff burnout and turnover continue to be issues of great importance (Prigatano and Others, 1986).

The controversies are also many. The intensity of treatment noted above is done at some considerable cost. It is not uncommon to find outpatient postacute rehabilitation programs costing over $30,000, excluding follow-up. While the cost of services has risen, the same insurance reimbursement pressures so traumatically experienced in acute medical care recently, have begun to be felt in brain injury rehabilitation settings. It seems that the unknown proportion of survivors of head injury that currently have access to rehabilitation services may shrink in the future. Programs are also coming under more scrutiny by third-party payers, with accompanying demands to demonstrate efficacy and to cut costs. Environmental pressures may be forcing greater flexibility and a reduction in intensity. Some programs may not yet have experienced these forces. It is suspected that this reflects a temporary respite, as national trends unequivocally indicate a movement towards cost accounting and containment, with service delivery practices being dictated by nonclinicians. Most head injury rehabilitation professionals take issues of outcome measurement seriously. Unfortunately, the current pressures for demonstrations of efficacy are being applied to a clinical enterprise that is only 10–15 years old. This early developmental stage will likely limit the number of quality clinical outcomes.

Contemporary brain injury rehabilitation practices attempt to help human beings feel and function better. They are conceptually similar to older clinical activities such as psychotherapy and speech and language therapy. It is important to note that even though both these practices have existed for a relatively longer period of time, controversy over issues of efficacy and outcome remain considerable (Basso, 1987; American Psychologist, 1986). As Strupp (1986) has recently noted, third-party reimbursement for psychotherapy developed from its medical heritage and allowed more individuals to receive help. It has also led, however, to reimbursement agencies examining psychotherapy outcome research to establish criteria for reimbursement. By and large, outcome research in psychotherapy was not designed with such purposes in mind. While demonstrations of clinical efficacy remain extremely important for all helping professions, the complexities of human behavior and their accompanying environments, coupled with the immaturity of our current practices, suggests demonstrations of clear patterns of clinical efficacy may currently be difficult. In addition, some aspects of human interaction may have benefits which are extremely difficult to objectify (Strupp, 1986). Public policy must play a role in determining what kind of, and how much, future brain injury rehabilitation activities individuals will have access to. Unfortunately, there is concern that the marketing of brain injury rehabilitation programs and techniques, being sometimes driven by forces of economic profit, have implied a state of development more apparent than real. This seems to be true for some comprehensive programs where patients are sometimes selected on the basis of their level of funding, rather than with respect to clinical issues or prognosis. In addition, cognitive rehabilitation practices, in some settings, continue to be marketed and practiced with an enthusiasm suggesting a degree of efficacy not yet established.

COGNITIVE REHABILITATION

Rehabilitation practices for cognitively impaired patients rest securely on the fact that even the most severely brain-injured individuals often maintain the capacity to learn some information. Procedural knowledge (learning how to do things) may occur as efficiently in amnestic individuals as in normals (Squire and Butters, 1984). Declarative information can also be learned, albeit inefficiently, by individuals with memory impairments (e.g., Kovner, Mattis, and Goldmeirer, 1983; Kovner, Mattis, and Pass, 1985; Schacter, Rich, and Stampp, 1985). Behavioral methods have been shown to be useful in helping brain-injured individuals acquire a wide range of complex skills (McGlynn, 1990). Even unrealistic self-appraisal appears to be modifiable in some cases (Fordyce and Rouche, 1986; McGlynn, 1990; Youngjohn and Altman, 1989). Of critical importance, however, is determining whether changes in clinical measures suggest that underlying cognitive impairments have been remediated, or whether specific behavioral skills have been trained. This is a question of considerable importance in determining what rehabilitation activities should occur to whom and for how long. The controversy is strengthened by observing that many brain-injured individuals, particularly those with severe traumatic injuries or with more localized frontal lobe injuries, may have considerable difficulty transferring a skill learned in one setting to another.

Space limitations preclude as comprehensive an analysis of the cognitive rehabilitation literature as it deserves. Many well-designed studies of tremendous scientific merit have been published. An admittedly critical and theoretical appraisal is offered with the understanding that cognitive rehabilitation techniques may seldom be employed in isolation of other rehabilitation interventions. A conservative approach to cognitive rehabilitation is strongly indicated at this time. A general appreciation of this fact will insure that brain injury interventions are reasonable, rational, and will withstand the present and future rigors of third-party scrutiny.

Definition

As has been noted (Sohlberg and Mateer, 1989a), the term cognitive rehabilitation is used in many ways. For the purposes of the present discussion it will be narrowly defined as any therapeutic activity which seeks to directly restore or improve an acquired cognitive impairment through means other than the use of some external physical aid. The purpose of cognitive rehabilitation is to minimize important disabilities for brain-injured individuals by reducing the impact of cognitive impairments underlying such disabilities. Thus, it promotes the possibility of a savings in rehabilitation resources through the modification of a general cognitive attribute. This would be more efficient than attempting to modify the multitude of setting-by-response interactions important to each patient (Bracy, 1984).

Heritage

The historical roots of cognitive rehabilitation are extensive and cannot be reviewed here. A feature of considerable importance, however, would seem to be the fact that current practices derive mainly from the study of individuals recovering from focal brain injury. This is reflected in Luria's work (Luria, Naytin, Tsvetkova, Vinarskaya, 1969; Luria and Tsvetkova, 1964) based on his theories of cortical organization (Luria, 1980). It is also represented in the extensive speech and language therapy literature on the rehabilitation of linguistic deficits following dominant hemisphere CVA, and in the rehabilitation of visual-spatial deficits following non-dominant CVA as reported by the rehabilitation psychologists from the NYU Medical School (Diller and Weinberg, 1986). Practices developed on individuals with focal brain injury may not generalize to cases of diffuse brain injury (Gordon, 1987). This possibility was raised some time ago by Zangwill (1947), and continues to remain a critical issue. Those surviving severe traumatic brain injury, for example, appear to have specific problems in attention and concentration, speed of information processing, memory functioning, and a variety of executive skills. Coupled with the inherent differences in age and premorbid psychologic characteristics, these impairments would seem to strongly suggest the need for a unique set of intervention strategies.

Conceptual and Logic Issues

One type of cognitive rehabilitation takes the form of repetitive practice on materials chosen because they appear to elicit behavior phenomenologically similar to the impairment of interest (Fordyce, 1991). Whether computer programs or paper and pencil instruments are employed, patients tend to practice on materials that seem to have some face validity. Sometimes these materials also reflect a particular theoretical orientation (e.g., Ben-Yishay and Diller, 1983b; Sohlberg and Mateer, 1989a). While training data are seldom provided, most outcome studies of cognitive rehabilitation imply improved performance on cognitive tasks repetitively practiced. These data do not necessarily imply, however, that some underlying cognitive impairment has been remediated. A more parsimonious explanation might be that a specific behavioral skill (i.e., taking tests of attention) has been learned. The necessary requirements for demonstrating the effectiveness of cognitive rehabilitation practices are known (e.g., Gordon, 1987; Seron, 1987). These are perhaps best conceptualized within a construct validity framework. At the most basic level, a cognitive rehabilitation technique could be said to be valid if, under specified conditions, it was shown to lead to improved performance on a behavior conceptually related to the targeted cognitive process, as assessed by some alternative methodology. Furthermore, it should be demonstrated that other unrelated cognitive processes assessed by the same methods, or conceptually unrelated behaviors assessed by some other methodology, do not demonstrate similar improvements. These are the basic steps in establishing convergent and discriminant validity in support of construct validation efforts (Campbell and Fiske, 1959). By demonstrating the impact of cognitive rehabilitation interventions on everyday disabilities we are also assessing the criterion validity or generalizability of these techniques. Most published cognitive rehabilitation studies, especially those employing head injured patients, test efficacy on psychometric instruments often similar to the training materials themselves. There is little, if any, attempt at analysis of generalization to day-to-day functions. Improvement on a neuropsychologic test measure of attention, following the completion of a cognitive rehabilitation program of attentional skills, does not imply that the underlying impairment has been remediated. Such a finding may simply indicate the degree to which the training and testing materials share "method variance" (Campbell and Fiske, 1959), with the patient manifesting improved facility in the taking of psychometric tests.

Cognitive rehabilitation, especially in the early stages of treatment, often takes place in a quiet room with limited distractions. This situation is similar to that in which neuropsychologic tests are typically administered, again raising the possibility that improvements in test scores may be relatively situation (and instrument) specific. While it makes some conceptual sense to begin cognitive rehabilitation in a quiet, controlled environment (Ben-Yishay and Diller, 1983b), unless some active attempt is made to promote generalization, the problems with abstraction, planning, and self-awareness accompanying more serious diffuse injuries would suggest it unlikely that transfer of training would spontaneously occur (Lezak, 1987). In reviewing several of the more sophisticated studies of cognitive rehabilitation, it is this author's opinion that a gradient of generalizability is suggested, such that those dependent variables most psychometrically similar to the training materials show the greatest improvements after training (e.g., Ben-Yishay, Piasetsky, and Rattok, 1987; Rattok, Ben-Yishay, Ross, Lakin, Silver, Thomas, and Diller, 1982; Sohlberg and Mateer, 1987; Weinberg, et al., 1977, 1979). In the case of traumatic head injury, there are few methodologically sound papers that have even attempted to measure transfer to more functional behaviors.

A second form of the conservatively defined cognitive rehabilitation enterprise discussed here, involves teaching the patient a new cognitive operation that, when utilized, promotes enhanced performance on tests measuring the targeted skill. The most common examples involve the teaching of verbal or visual association strategies (e.g., Binder and Schreiber, 1980; Gasparrini and Satz, 1979; Gianutsos and Gianutsos, 1979; Gianutsos, 1981; Goldstein, McCue, Turner, Spanier, Malec, and Shelly, 1988; Kovner, et al., 1983; Kovner, et al., 1985), or an internalized problem solving strategy (Webster and Scott, 1983; Lawson and Rice, 1989), to enhance new learning and memory performance. In almost all cases there is some improvement in a memory task, usually word list learning, but no direct attempt to demonstrate generalization to natural settings. In fact, such generalization is unexpected among those individuals with such significant information processing deficits that the use of these internal strategies overloads an already taxed system (O'Connor and Cermak, 1987; Sohlberg and Mateer, 1989a).

CURRENT PRACTICES AND FUTURE DIRECTIONS

Neuropsychologic evaluation and rehabilitation has grown tremendously in the 1980's. As we begin a new decade it is appropriate to appreciate the difference between what we can do, and what we wish we could do. It is also important to develop and research new techniques so that the former can better approach the latter. The following is offered in support of both these endeavors.

Predictive Criteria

Issues of predictive criterion validity for important cognitively based disabilities need to be emphasized before neuropsychologic rehabilitation can proceed and effective outcome demonstrations produced. First, important criterion disabilities need to be more clearly specified through the development of valid and reliable measurement systems. Secondly, new neuropsychologic tests should be developed which demonstrate more clearly the relationship between cognitive impairments and associated disabilities. A few efforts are underway in both arenas. For example, reliable, naturalistic, and multifactorial behavioral performance scales have been developed to measure automobile driving skill (Kewman, Seigerman, Kintner, Chu, Hensen, and Reeder, 1988), wheelchair driving skill (Webster, Cottam, Gouvier, Blanton, Biessel, and Wofford, 1989), general work skills (Lewis, Hinman, and Roessler, 1988), and specific work task performance (Butler, Anderson, Furst, Namerow, and Satz, 1989) in brain injury. Another example of such work is seen in the development of new tools to assess the pragmatic communication deficits often found in patients with traumatic head injury (see Kennedy and Deruyter, 1989, for a review). These more refined and specific measures of disability allow much greater opportunity to demonstrate the functional consequences of brain injury, as well as the relative efficacy of a host of rehabilitation techniques. Behavioral rating scales may permit more natural analysis of the emotional and interpersonal characteristics of brain-injured individuals (Levin, et al., 1987). It should be noted that the application of behavioral observation principles to the task of refining criterion disability measures has obvious merit.

Less is being done in the area of more traditional neuropsychologic test development. The Rivermead Behavioral Memory Test (RBMT) is a good recent example of a psychometric instrument developed with greater face validity for day-to-day memory problems than our more traditional measures (Wilson, et al., 1989). Some recent data have indicated, not surprisingly, that the RBMT relates better to measures of disability following brain injury than more conventional tests of memory skill (Wilson, 1990). The Goldman-Fristoe-Woodcock Auditory Skills Test Battery (Goldman, Fristoe, and Woodcock, 1974) includes an attentional task with a variety of naturally occurring distracting noises as background.

Construct-Valid Neuropsychologic Tests

The development of construct-valid neuropsychologic tests also needs to continue, a process that might proceed more dramatically with new materials relatively uncontaminated by our diagnostic tradition (Loring and Papanicolaou, 1987). Effective demonstrations of cognitive rehabilitation may await this important groundwork. Interestingly, there has been considerable recent debate about whether valid principles of human memory are determinable outside of naturalistic settings (Banaji and Crowder, 1989; American Psychologist, 1991). Putting this question aside, it is clear that construct validation operations have little importance unless they have some reference to everyday function. Our heritage is difficult to modify, however. Some recommended construct validation procedures would have the demonstration of criterion validity as the last step of a multistep process (Mapou, 1988).

Cognitive Rehabilitation Practices

Cognitive rehabilitation practices should continue for some patients in some programs. It is essential, however, that these not be undertaken with the naive view that a core cognitive impairment is being remediated. If this is the presumed purpose, those practicing cognitive rehabilitation have an obligation to demonstrate treatment efficacy, particularly transfer of training to important areas of disability. A knowledge of experimental methods, perhaps particularly single case design, becomes crucial. Otherwise, repetitive practice during cognitive rehabilitation can be a preferred way of teaching a specific skill, or imparting specific knowledge, that may serve to reduce important disabilities. An example would be instruction in microprocessor operation (Schachter and Gliskey, 1986). Finally, the cognitive rehabilitation setting can provide a powerful psychotherapeutic medium. When supervised by a skilled therapist, such activities can provide a relatively nonconfrontational interaction for helping patients become more aware of their impairments (Prigatano, 1987), as well as better appreciating their skills (Fordyce and Roueche, 1986). Similarly, the cognitive rehabilitation setting can provide a ground school in which patients can first learn how to employ compensations that may have functional utility in daily life (Sohlberg and Mateer, 1989).

Intervention

Effective rehabilitation programs will intervene directly at the levels of impairments, disabilities, handicaps, and statuses. Generalization of cognitive rehabilitation practices must be formally promoted through specific therapeutic activities which ultimately take individuals into natural settings (Sohlberg and Mateer, 1989). Rehabilitation planners must be aware of cost efficiency issues in determining which level of intervention to emphasize. Psychosocial adjustment, social skill training, family intervention, and directed vocational rehabilitation all remain crucial components of brain injury rehabilitation.

Program Flexibility

Program flexibility should be emphasized. Few can afford full-time day treatment or residential rehabilitation programs. Some more limited interventions may be helpful in some cases, however. Varying severities, chronicities, levels of psychiatric dysfunction, degrees of physical impairment, or presence of unique symptoms such as chronic pain, all demand differing strategies and intensities.

References

Acker, M., (1986). Relationships between test scores and everyday life functioning. In: Uzzell, B., and Gross, Y. (eds). Clinical neuropsychology of intervention. Boston: Martinus Nijhoff Publishing, 85–118.

Alfano, D., and Finlayson, A. (1987). Clinical neuropsychology in rehabilitation. The Clinical Neuropsychologist, 1:105–23.

Alfano, D., Finlayson, A., Stearns, G., and Nelson, P. (1990). The MMPI and neurologic dysfunction: Profile configuration and analysis. The Clinical Neuropsychologist, 4:69–79.

American Psychiatric Association (1980). Diagnostic and statistical manual of mental disorders, 3rd ed. Washington DC: APA.

American Psychological Association, American Educational Research Association, and National Council of Measurement Used in Education (Joint Committee) (1954). Technical recommendations for psychological tests. Psychological Bulletin, 51:201–38.

American Psychologist (1986). Special issue: Psychotherapy research, 41(2).

American Psychologist (1991). Science watch, 46:1185-93.

Baird, A., Brown, G., Adams, K., Shatz, M., McSweeny, A., Ausman, J., and Diaz, F. (1987). Neuropsychological deficits and real world dysfunction in cerebral revascularization candidates. Journal of Clinical and Experimental Neuropsychology, 9:407-22.

Banaji, M., and Crowder, R. (1989). The bankruptcy of everyday memory. American Psychologist, 44:1185-93.

Basso, A. (1987). Approaches to neuropsychological rehabilitation: Language disorders. In: Meier, M., Benton, A., and Diller, L. (eds). Neuropsychological rehabilitation. New York: The Guilford Press, 294-314.

Bayless, J., Varney, N., and Roberts, R. (1989). Tinker toy test performance and vocational outcome in patients with closed head injuries. Journal of Clinical and Experimental Neuropsychology, 11:913-17.

Ben-Yishay, Y., and Diller, L. (1983a). Cognitive deficits. In: Rosenthal, M., Griffith, E.R., Bond, M.R., and Miller, J.D. (eds). Rehabilitation of the head injured adult. Philadelphia: F.A. Davis Company, 167-84.

Ben-Yishay, Y., Diller, L., Gerstman, L.J., and Gordon, W.A. (1970). Relationships between initial competence and ability to profit from cues in brain damaged individuals. Journal of Abnormal Psychology, 75:248-59.

Ben-Yishay, Y., Gerstman, L., Diller, L., and Haas, A. (1970). Prediction of rehabilitation outcomes from psychometric parameters in left hemiplegics. Journal of Consulting and Clinical Psychology, 34:436-41.

Ben-Yishay, Y., Piasetsky, E.B., and Rattok, J. (1987). A systematic method for ameliorating disorders of basic attention. In: Meier, M., Benton, A., and Diller, L. (eds). Neuropsychological rehabilitation. New York: The Guilford Press, 165-81.

Beukelman, D., and Yorkston, K. (eds) (1991). Communication disorders following brain injury. Austin: Pro Ed.

Binder, L. (1986). Persisting symptoms after a mild head injury: A review of the postconcussive syndrome. Journal of Clinical and Experimental Neuropsychology, 8:323-46.

Binder, L., and Schreiber, V. (1980). Visual imagery and verbal mediation as memory aids in recovering alcoholics. Journal of Clinical Neuropsychology, 2:71-74.

Boll, T. (1981). The Halstead-Reitan neuropsychological battery. In: Filskov, S., and Boll, T. (eds). Handbook of clinical neuropsychology: Vol. 1. New York: John Wiley and Sons, 577-607.

Boll, T. (1985). Developing issues in clinical neuropsychology. Journal of Clinical and Experimental Neuropsychology, 7:473-85.

Bond, M. (1975). Assessment of psychological outcome after severe head injury. CIBA Foundation Symposium, 34:141-53.

Braakman, R., Gelpke, G., Habbema, J., Maas, A., and Minderhoud, J. (1980). Systematic selection of prognostic features in patients with severe head injury. Neurosurgery, 6:362-70.

Bracy, O. (1984). Editor's note. Cognitive Rehabilitation, 2:2.

Brooks, D., Hosie, J., Bond, M., Jennett, B., and Aughton, M. (1986). Cognitive sequelae of severe head injury in relation to the Glasgow Outcome Scale. Journal of Neurology, Neurosurgery, and Psychiatry, 49:549-53.

Bulter, R., Anderson, L., Furst, C., Namerow, N., and Satz, P. (1989). Behavioral assessment in neuropsychological rehabilitation: A method for measuring vocational-related skills. The Clinical Neuropsychologist, 3:235-43.

Campbell, D.P., and Fiske, D.W. (1959). Convergent and discriminant validity in the multitrait-multimethod matrix. Psychological Bulletin, 56:81-105.

Chelune, G. (1985). Neuropsychology and vocational behavior. Paper presented at the American Psychological Association Convention, Los Angeles, CA.

Christensen, A., and Uzzell, B. (eds) (1988). Neuropsychological rehabilitation. Boston: Kluwer Academic Publishers.

Cicerone, K., and Tupper, D. (1986). Cognitive assessment in the neuropsychological rehabilitation of head injured adults. In: Uzzell, B., and Gross, Y. (eds). Clinical neuropsychology of intervention. Boston: Martinus Nijhoff Publishing, 59-84.

Costa, L. (1983). Clinical neuropsychology: A discipline in evolution. Journal of Clinical Neuropsychology, 5:1-11.

Cronbach, L.J., and Meehl, P.E. (1955). Construct validity in psychological tests. Psychological Bulletin, 52:281-302.

Dahlstrom, W., and Welsh, G. (1960). An MPI handbook (Vol. 1: Clinical interpretation, revised edition). Minneapolis: University of Minnesota Press.

Dikmen, S., Machamer, J., Temkin, N., and McLean, A. (1990). Neuropsychological recovery in patients with moderate to severe head injury: Two-year follow-up. Journal of Clinical and Experimental Neuropsychology, 12:507-19.

Dikmen, S., McLean, A., Temkin, N., and Wyler, A. (1986). Neuropsychological outcome at one month postinjury. Archives of Physical Medicine and Rehabilitation, 67:507-13.

Dikmen, S., and Morgan, S. (1980). Neuropsychological factors related to employability and occupational status in persons with epilepsy. The Journal of Nervous and Mental Disease, 168:236-40.

Diller, L. (1987). Neuropsychological rehabilitation. In: Meier, M., Benton, A., and Diller, L. (eds). Neuropsychological rehabilitation. New York: The Guilford Press, 3-17.

Diller, L. (1988). Rehabilitation in traumatic brain injury—Observations on the current U.S. scene. In: Christensen, A., and Uzzell, B. (eds). Neuropsychological rehabilitation. Boston: Kluwer Academic Publishers, 53-68.

Diller, L., Ben-Yishay, Y., Gerstman, L.J., Goodkin, R., Gordon, W., and Weiberg, J. (1974). Studies in cognition and rehabilitation in hemiplegia. Rehabilitation Monograph 50. New York: New York University Medical Center.

Diller, L., and Weinberg, J.M. (1977). Hemi-inattention in rehabilitation: The evolution of a rational remediation program. In: Weinstein, E.A., and Friedland, R.P. (eds). Advances in neurology. New York: Raven Press.

Diller, L., and Weinberg, J. (1986). Learning from failures in perceptual cognitive retraining in stroke. In: Uzzell, B., and Gross, Y. (eds). Clinical neuropsychology of intervention. Boston: Martinus Nijhoff Publishing, 283-93.

Eisenberg, H., and Weiner, R. (1987). Input variables: How information from the acute injury can be used to characterize groups of patients for studies of outcome. In: Levin, H., Grafman, J., and Eisenberg, H. (eds). Neurobehavioral recovery from head injury. New York: Oxford University Press, 13-29.

Fahy, T., Irving, M., and Milac, P. (1967). Severe head injuries: A six-year follow-up. Lancet, 475-79.

Fordyce, D. (1989). Chronic disability following mild head injury. Paper presented at the Pacific Northwest Neuropsychological Society Conference. Seattle, WA.

Fordyce, D. (1991). Conceptual issues in cognitive rehabilitation. In: Beukleman, D., and Yorkston, K. (eds). Communication disorders following brain injury. Austin: Pro Ed, 57-73.

Fordyce, D., and Roueche, J.R. (1986). Changes in perspectives of disability among patients, staff, and relatives during rehabilitation of brain injury. Rehabilitation Psychology, 31:217-29.

Fordyce, D., Roueche, J., and Prigatano, G. (1983). Enhanced emotional reactions in chronic head trauma patients. Journal of Neurology, Neurosurgery, and Psychiatry, 46:620-24.

Fraser, R., Dikmen, S., McLean, A., Miller, B., and Temkin, N. (1988). Employability of head injury survivors: First year postinjury. Rehabilitation Counseling Bulletin, 31:276-88.

Gasparrini, B., and Satz, P. (1979). A treatment for memory problems in left hemisphere CVA patients. Journal of Clinical Neuropsychology, 1:137-50.

Gianutsos, R. (1981). Training in short- and long-term verbal recall of a postencephalitic amnesia. Journal of Clinical Neuropsychology, 2:143-53.

Gianutsos, R., and Gianutsos, J. (1979). Rehabilitating the verbal recall of brain injury patients by mnemonic training: An experimental demonstration using single case methodology. Journal of Clinical Neuropsychology, 1:117-35.

Golden, C., Kane, R., Sweet, J., Moses, J., Cardellino, J., Templeton, R., Vincente, P., and Graber, B. (1981). Relationship of the Halstead-Reitan neuropsychological test battery to the Luria-Nebraska battery. Journal of Consulting and Clinical Psychology, 49:410-17.

Goldman, R., Fristoe, M., and Woodcock, R. (1974). Goldman-Fristoe-Woodcock auditory skills test battery. Minnesota: American Guidance Services, Inc.

Goldstein, G. (1987). Neuropsychological assessment for rehabilitation: Fixed batteries, automated systems, and nonpsychometric methods. In: Meier, M., Benton, A., and Diller L. (eds). Neuropsychological rehabilitation. New York: The Guilford Press, 18-40.

Goldstein, G., McCue, M., Turner, S., Spanier, C., Malec, E., and Shelly, C. (1988). An efficacy study of memory for patients with closed-head injury. The Clinical Neuropsychologist, 2:251-59.

Gordon, W.A. (1987). Methodological considerations in cognitive remediation. In: Meier, M., Benton, A., and Diller, L. (eds). Neuropsychological rehabilitation. New York: The Guilford Press, 111-31.

Grant, I., and Alves, W. (1987). Psychiatric and psychosocial disturbances in head injury. In: Levin, H., Grafman, J., and Eisenberg, H. (eds). Neurobehavioral recovery from head injury. New York: Oxford University Press, 232-61.

Gronwall, D., and Wrightson, P. (1974). Delayed recovery of intellectual function after minor head injury. Lancet, 605-09.

Gruvstad, M., Kebbon, L., and Gruvstad, S. (1958). Social and psychiatric aspects of pretraumatic personality and posttraumatic insufficiency reactions in traumatic head injuries. Acta Soc. Med. Uppsal., 63:101-13.

Hagen, C., Malkmus, D., and Durham, P. (1979). Levels of cognitive functioning. In: Rehabilitation of the head-injured adult: Comprehensive physical management. Professional Staff Association of Ranchos Los Amigos Hospital. Downey, CA. Hart, T., and Hayden, M.E. (1986). The ecological validity of neuropsychological assessment and remediation. In: Uzzell, B., and Gross, Y. (eds). Clinical neuropsychology of intervention. Boston: Martinus Nijhoff Publishing, 21-50).

Hawkins, K. (1990). Occupational neurotoxicology: Some neuropsychological issues and challenges. Journal of Clinical and Experimental Neuropsychology, 12:664-80.

Heaton, R., Chelune, G., and Lehman, R. (1979). Using neuropsychological and personality tests to assess the likelihood of patient employment. Journal of Nervous and Mental Disease, 166:408-16.

Heaton, R., and Pendleton, M. (1981). Use of neuropsychological tests to predict adult patients' everyday functioning. Journal of Consulting and Clinical Psychology, 49:807-21.

Jeannett, B., and Bond, M. (1975). Assessment of outcome after severe brain damage: A practical scale. Lancet, 480-84.

Jeannett, B., Teasdale, G., Braakman, R., Minderhoud, J., Heiden, J., and Kurze, T. (1979). Prognosis of patients with severe head injury. Neurosurgery, 4:283-89.

Kennedy, M., and DeRuyter, F. (1991). Cognitive and language bases for communication disorders. In: Beukleman, D., and Yorkston, K. (eds). Communication disorders following brain injury. Austin: Pro Ed, 123-90.

Keshavan, M., Channabasavanna, S., and Reddy, G. (1981). Posttraumatic psychiatric disturbances: Patterns and predictors of outcome. British Journal of Psychiatry, 138:157-60.

Kewman, D., Seigerman, C., Kintner, H., Chu, S., Hensen, D., and Reeder, C. (1985). Simulation training of psychometric skills: Teaching the brain injured to drive. Rehabilitation Psychology, 30:11-27.

Kohn, H. (1986). Qualitative neuropsychological assessment: Kurt Goldstein revisited. In: Uzzell, B., and Gross, Y. (eds). Clinical neuropsychology of intervention. Boston: Martinus Nijhoff Publishing, 51-58.

Kovner, R., Mattis, S., and Goldmeier, E. (1983). A technique for promoting robust free recall in chronic amnesia. Journal of Clinical Neuropsychology, 5:65-71.

Kovner, R., Mattis, S., and Pass, R. (1985). Some amnesic patients can freely recall large amounts of information in new contexts. Journal of Clinical and Experimental Neuropsychology, 7:395-411.

Kozol, H. (1945). Pretraumatic personality and psychiatric sequelae of head injury, I. Archives of Neurology and Psychiatry, 53:358-64.

Kozol, H. (1946). Pretraumatic personality and psychiatric sequelae of head injury, II. Archives of Neurology and Psychiatry, 57:245-75.

Lawson, M., and Rice, D. (1989). Effects of training in use of executive strategies on a verbal memory problem resulting from closed head injury. Journal of Clinical and Experimental Neuropsychology, 11:842-54.

Levin, H.S., Benton, A.L., and Grossman, R.G. (1982). Neurobehavioral consequences of closed head injury. New York: Oxford University Press.

Levin, H., and Grossman, R. (1978). Behavioral sequelae of closed head injury. Archives of Neurology, 35:720-27.

Levin, H., Grossman, R., Ross, J., and Teasdale, G. (1979). Long-term neuropsychological outcome of closed head injury. Journal of Neurosurgery, 50:412-22.

Levin, H.S., High, W., Goethe, K., Sisson, R., Overall, J., Rhoades, H., Eisenberg, H., Kalisky, Z., and Gary, H. (1987). The neurobehavioral rating scale: Assessment of the behavioral sequelae of head injury by the clinician. Journal of Neurology, Neurosurgery, and Psychiatry, 50:183-93.

Levin, H., O'Donnell, V., and Grossman, R. (1979). The Galveston orientation and amnesia test: A practical scale to assess cognition after head injury. Journal of Nervous and Mental Disease, 167:675-84.

Lewis, F., Hinman, S., and Roessler, R. (1988). Assessing TBI clients' work adjustment skills: The work performance assessment (WPA). Rehabilitation Psychology, 4:213-20.

Lezak, M. (1983). Neuropsychological assessment. New York: Oxford University Press.

Lezak, M. (1987). Assessment for rehabilitation planning. In: Meier, M., Benton, A., and Diller, L. (eds). Neuropsychological rehabilitation. New York: The Guilford Press, 41-58.

Loring, D., and Papanicolaou, A. (1987). Memory assessment in neuropsychology: Theoretical considerations and practical utility. Journal of Clinical and Experimental Neuropsychology, 9:340-58.

Luria, A.R. (1980). Higher cortical functions in man. New York: Basic Books, Inc.

Luria, A., Naytin, V., Tsvetkova, L., and Vinarskaya, E. (1969). Restoration of higher cortical function following local brain damage. In: Vinekin, P., and Bruyn, G. (eds). Handbook of clinical neurology, Vol. 3. New York: American Elsevier, 368-433.

Luria, A., and Tsvetkova, L. (1964). The programming of constructive activity in local brain injuries. Neuropsychologia, 2:95-107.

Malkmus, D., Booth, B., and Kodimer, C. (1980). In: Rehabilitation of the head-injured adult: Comprehensive cognitive management. Professional Staff Association of Ranchos Los Amigos Hospital. Downey, CA.

Mapou, R. (1988). Testing to detect brain damage: An alternative to what may no longer be useful. Journal of Clinical and Experimental Neuropsychology, 10:271-78.

Matarazzo, J. (1972). Wechsler's measurement and appraisal of adult intelligence (5th ed). Baltimore: Williams and Wilkins.

Mayer, N., Keating, D., and Rapp, D. (1986). Skills, routines, and activity patterns of daily living: A functional nested approach. In: Uzzell, B., and Gross, Y. (eds). Clinical neuropsychology of intervention. Boston: Martinus Nijhoff Publishing, 205–22.

McCue, M., Rogers, J., and Goldstein, G. (1990). Relationships between neuropsychological and functional assessment in elderly neuropsychiatric patients. Rehabilitation Psychology, 35:91–99.

McGlynn, S. (1990). Behavioral approaches to neuropsychological rehabilitation. Psychological Bulletin, 108:420–41.

McLean, A., Dikmen, S., Temkin, N., Wyler, A., and Gale, J. (1984). Psychosocial functioning at one month after head injury. Neurosurgery, 14:393–99.

McSweeney, A., Grant, I., Heaton, R., Prigatano, G., and Adams, K. (1985). Relationship of neuropsychological status to everyday functioning in healthy and chronically ill persons. Journal of Clinical and Experimental Neuropsychology, 7:281–91.

Meier, M., Benton, A., and Diller, L. (eds.). (1987). Neuropsychological Rehabilitation. New York: The Guilford Press.

Milberg, W., Hebben, N., and Kaplan, E. (1986). The Boston process approach to neuropsychological assessment. In: Grant, I., and Adams, K. (eds). Neuropsychological assessment of neuropsychiatric disorders. New York: Oxford University Press, 65–86.

Minderhoud, J., Boelens, M., Huizenga, J., and Saan, R. (1980). Treatment of minor head injuries. Clinical Neurology and Neurosurgery, 82:127–40.

Newcombe, F. (1987). Psychometric and behavioral evidence: Scope, limitations, and ecological validity. In: Levin, H., Grafman, J., and Eisenberg, H. (eds). Neurobehavioral recovery from head injury. New York: Oxford Press, 129–45.

Newman, O., Heaton, R., and Lehman, R. (1978). Neuropsychological and MMPI correlates of patients' future employment characteristics. Perceptual and Motor Skills, 46:635–42.

O'Connor, M., and Cermak, L.S. (1987). Rehabilitation of organic memory disorders. In: Meier, M., Benton, A., and Diller, L. (eds). Neuropsychological rehabilitation. New York: The Guilford Press, 260–79.

Prigatano, G. (1987a). Personality and psychosocial consequences after brain injury. In: Meier, M., Benton, A., and Diller, L. (eds). Neuropsychological rehabilitation. New York: The Guilford Press, 355–78.

Prigatano, G.P. (1987b). Recovery and cognitive retraining after craniocerebral trauma. Journal of Learning Disabilities, 20:603–13.

Prigatano, G.P., Fordyce, D.J., Zeiner, H.K., Roueche, J.R., Pepping, M., and Wood, B.C. (1984). Neuropsychological rehabilitation after closed head injury in young adults. Journal of Neurology, Neurosurgery, and Psychiatry, 47:505–13.

Prigatano, G.P., et al. (1986). Neuropsychological rehabilitation after brain injury. Baltimore: John Hopkins University Press.

Prigatano, G., Pepping, M., and Klonoff, P. (1986). Cognitive, personality, and psychosocial factors in neuropsychological assessment. In: Uzzell, B., and Gross, Y. (eds). Clinical neuropsychology of intervention. Boston: Martinus Nijhoff Publishing, 135–66.

Rattok, J., Ben-Yishay, Y., Ross, B., Lakin, P., Silver, S., Thomas, L., and Diller, L. (1982). A diagnostic remedial system for basic attention disorders in head trauma patients undergoing rehabilitation: A preliminary report. In: Ben-Yishay, Y. (ed). Working approaches to remediation of cognitive deficits in brain damaged persons. New York University Medical Center, Rehabilitation Monograph 66, 177–87.

Reitan, R. (1986). Theoretical and methodological bases of the Halstead-Reitan neuropsychological test battery. In: Grant, I., and Adams, K. (eds). Neuropsychological assessment of neuropsychiatric disorders. New York: Oxford University Press, 3–30.

Rimel, R., Giordani, B., Barth, J., Boll, T., and Jane, J. (1981). Disability caused by minor head injury. Neurosurgery, 9:221–28.

Rosenthal, M., Griffith, E.R., Bond, M.R., and Miller, J.D. (eds). (1983). Rehabilitation of the head injured adult. Philadelphia: F.A. Davis Company.

Rosenzweig, M.R. (1984). Experience, memory, and the brain. American Psychologist, 39:365–76.

Ruesch, J., and Bowman, K. (1945). Prolonged posttraumatic syndromes following head injury. American Journal of Psychiatry, 100:480–96.

Russell, E. (1986). The psychometric foundation of clinical neuropsychology. In: Filskov, S., and Boll, T. (eds). Handbook of clinical neuropsychology: Vol. 2. New York: John Wiley and Sons, 45–80.

Russell, W. (1932). Cerebral involvement in head injury. Brain, 55:549–603.

Russell, W. (1971). The traumatic amnesias. New York: Oxford University Press.

Schacter, D., and Crovitz, H. (1977). Memory function after closed head injury: A review of the quantitative research. Cortex, 13:150–76.

Schachter, D.L., and Glisky, E.L. (1986). Memory remediation: Restoration, alleviation, and the acquisition of domain-specific knowledge. In: Uzzell, B., and Gross, Y. (eds). Clinical neuropsychology of intervention. Boston: Martinus Nijhoff Publishing, 257–82.

Schacter, D., Rich, S., Stampp, M. (1985). Remediation of memory disorders: Experimental evaluation of the spaced-retrieval technique. Journal of Clinical and Experimental Neuropsychology, 7:79–96.

Seron, X. (1987). Operant procedures and neuropsychological rehabilitation. In: Meier, M., Benton, A., and Diller, L. (eds). Neuropsychological rehabilitation. New York: The Guilford Press, 132–62.

Smith, A. (1961). Duration of impaired consciousness as an index of severity in closed head injuries. Diseases of the Nervous System, 22:69–74.

Sohlberg, M., and Mateer, C. (1987). Effectiveness of an attention training program. Journal of Clinical and Experimental Neuropsychology, 9:117–30.

Sohlberg, M., and Mateer, K. (1989a). Introduction to cognitive rehabilitation: Theory and practice. New York: The Guilford Press.

Sohlberg, M., and Mateer, K. (1989b). Training use of compensatory memory books: A three-stage behavioral approach. Journal of Clinical and Experimental Neuropsychology, 11:871–91.

Squire, L.R., and Butters, N. (eds). (1984). Neuropsychology of Memory. New York: The Guilford Press.

Strupp, H. (1986). Psychotherapy: Research, practice, and public policy (how to avoid dead ends). American Psychologist, 41:120–30.

Stuss, D., Ely, P. Hugenholtz, H., Richard, M., LaRochelle, S., Poirer, C., and Bell, I. (1985). Subtle neuropsychological deficits in patients with good recovery after closed head injury. Neurosurgery, 17:41–47.

Sundet, K., Finset, A., and Reinvang, J. (1988). Neuropsychological predictors in stroke rehabilitation. Journal of Clinical and Experimental Neuropsychology, 10:363–79.

Teasdale, G., and Jennett, B. (1974). Assessment of coma and impaired consciousness. Lancet, 81–84.

Teasdale, G., and Jennett, B. (1976). Assessment and prognosis of coma after head injury. Acta Neurochirurgica, 34:45–55.

Torkelson, J., Jellinek, H., Malec, J., and Harvey, R. Traumatic brain injury: Psychological and medical factors related to rehabilitation outcome. Rehabilitation Psychology, 28:196.

Uzzell, B., and Gross, Y. (eds). (1986). Neuropsychology of intervention. Boston: Martinus Nijhoff Publishing.

Van Zomeren, A., and Van Den Burg, W. (1985). Residual complaints of patients 2 years after severe head injury. Journal of Neurology, Neurosurgery, and Psychiatry, 48:21-28.

Varney, N. (1988). Prognostic significance of anosmia in patients with closed head trauma. Journal of Clinical and Experimental Neuropsychology, 10:250-54.

Webster, J., Cottam, G., Gouvier, W., Blanton, P., Beissell, G., and Wofford, J. (1989). Wheelchair obstacle course performance in right cerebral vascular accident victims. Journal of Clinical and Experimental Neuropsychology, 11:295-310.

Webster, J., and Scott, R. (1983). The effects of self-instructional training on attentional deficits following head injury. Clinical Neuropsychology, 4:69-74.

Weinberg, J., Diller, L., Gordon, W., Gerstman, L., Lieberman, A., Lakin, P., Hodges, G., and Ezrachi, O. (1977). Visual scanning training effect on reading-related tasks in acquired right brain damage. Archives of Physical Medicine and Rehabilitation, 58:479-86.

Weinberg, J., Diller, L., Gordon, W., Gerstman, L., Lieberman, A., Lakin, P., Hodges, G., and Ezrachi, O. (1979). Training sensory awareness and spatial organization in people with right brain damage. Archives of Physical Medicine and Rehabilitation, 60:491-96.

Wiggins, J. (1973). Personality and prediction: Principles of personality assessment. Reading, MA: Addison-Wesley.

Wilson, B. (1990). Do amnesic people remember the lessons they've learned? Paper presented at the International Neuropsychological Society Meeting, Kissimmee, FL.

Wilson, B., Cockburn, J., Baddeley, A., and Hiorns, R. (1989). Development and validation of a test battery for detecting and monitoring everyday memory problems. Journal of Clinical and Experimental Neuropsychology, 11:855-70.

Youngjohn, R., and Altman, I. (1989). A performance-based group approach to the treatment of anosognosia and denial. Rehabilitation Psychology, 34:217-22.

Zangwill, O. (1947). Psychological aspects of rehabilitation in cases of brain injury. British Journal of Psychology, 37:60-69.

10

Innovative Approaches
to Frontal Lobe Deficits

DONALD T. STUSS, CATHERINE A. MATEER, and M.M. SOHLBERG

Rehabilitation, to be effective, must be matched with the nature of the underlying neuropsychologic impairment. This direction of rehabilitative efforts is dependent upon knowledge of the underlying disorder. We argue that the most significant impairment following traumatic brain injury (TBI) involves the executive control functions of the brain, related most frequently to the frontal lobes. Based on this premise, the emphasis in brain injury rehabilitation treatment should be directed toward the executive psychologic processes. This chapter is divided into two major sections. The first section presents the psychologic and anatomic rationale that should focus rehabilitative efforts. Specific approaches to rehabilitation and management of these disorders are suggested in section two.

A RATIONALE FOR REHABILITATION DIRECTION

The vast structure and complex neuroanatomic connections of the frontal lobes testify to their importance. The frontal lobes constitute between 1/4 and 1/3 of the total cortical surface. Based on both phylogenetic and ontogenetic evolution, it is one of the last brain areas to develop, suggesting a prominent status on the developmental ladder (Stuss, 1992). The reciprocal connections of the frontal lobes with cortical, subcortical, and limbic brain regions provide the basis for understanding their essential role in so many levels of information processing (Luria, 1973; Nauta, 1971; Pandya and Barnes, 1987). The term "frontal functions" is frequently used in this chapter to refer to a set of behaviors that have been associated with a defined structural region, the frontal and prefrontal cortex. It is nevertheless acknowledged that the term must extend beyond a strict localizationist association. As will be seen, this is particularly true in brain injury.

A Model of Brain Functioning

Many models of frontal lobe functioning have been proposed (see Stuss and Benson, 1986, for a review). Fuster (1989), Goldman-Rakic (1987), Grafman (1989), and Shallice (1988), provide examples of contemporary proposals. In this chapter, we combine concepts extracted from certain of these models with the idea of a feedback loop (Carver and Scheir, 1982; Miller, Galanter, and Pribram, 1960; Powers, 1973; Pribram, 1971). This feedback loop was added for the following reasons: it is compatible in various respects with published explanations of frontal lobe functions (Fuster, 1989; Stuss and Benson, 1986; Stuss, 1991a, b; Teuber, 1964); it has been used in social psychology (Carver and Scheir, 1982), suggesting that it has a broader range of application; it outlines a framework to understand the possibility of behavior modification through rehabilitation; and it provides a rationale for the decision on a bottom-up, top-down, or combined approach to rehabilitation.

The proposed model (Fig. 10.1) is based on the premise that there is a hierarchy of functions. The interaction of these levels of functioning is complex, and certain levels appeared to be fractionated into independent processes. While only three levels are described, other levels may be possible, as well as subsystems within levels. For the purpose of our argument, the three levels depicted will provide the outline for understanding rehabilitative decisions.

Each level is organized as a feedback control system and consists of three primary components: Incoming information, which can differ either in domain (content) specificity or according to the level of representation of information; a comparator, which analyzes the information in relation to the subject's reference points which may be inherently present or have been acquired; and an output mode, which translates the results of the comparative evaluation into some type of response. If the comparison indicates a homeostatic balance, no response is required. If the incoming information and comparator values are not equivalent, the following may be required: An action to change or respond to the input; a call for more information from the environment or input source; or, where appropriate, a petition to higher processing levels, even to the point of altering the template upon which the comparisons are made. In addition, a feedforward system may preset the system to anticipate change in action or to alter the sensitivity to incoming information.

First Level: Sensory/Perceptual Information

The input at the first level described relates to sensory/perceptual information, and is domain or module specific. While operations may be

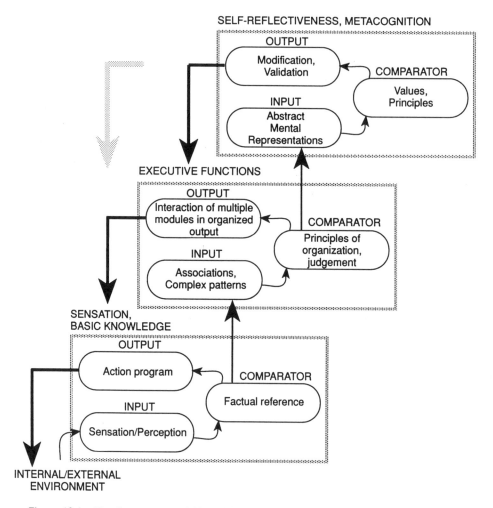

Figure 10.1. The three proposed hierarchical and interactive representations of self: Sensory-perceptual, executive control, and self-reflectiveness. Monitoring, control, and change are possible by means of a feedback loop at each level.

simple or complex, they are overlearned, automatic, and rapid. From an anatomic point of view, these processes, the basis of daily routine behavior, tend to be related more to nonfrontal brain regions (Mesulam, 1981; Stuss and Benson, 1986). "Contention scheduling" is the term used to describe the process of routine selection of routine actions or thought processes (Norman and Shallice, 1986; Shallice, 1988).

Second Level: Executive Control

The next two levels proposed are related to the functions of the frontal lobes. The second level, associated with the executive control or supervisory function of the frontal lobes, receives its input as elaborated level 1 sensory/perceptual information. This second level adjusts and directs the ongoing automatic behaviors of lower modules (Shallice, 1988; Stuss and Benson, 1986). The well-recognized reciprocal connections of anterior brain regions with the posterior and limbic zones are the neural bases of these interactions. The comparator at the second level has been divided conceptually and experimentally into specific subfunctions, such as anticipation, goal articulation, and plan formulation (Petrides, 1987; Shallice and Burgess, 1991; Stuss and Benson, 1986).

Since neither routine responses nor knowledge is available at this second level, the processing of the feedback loop is slower and effortful. With time and repetition, however, the new complex behaviors requiring selective deliberation and monitoring may become automatic in ordinary circumstances. Eventually, control of such behaviors is transferred to the lower level.

Third Level: Self-Reflectiveness

Self-reflectiveness is the comparator of the third and highest level described. Defined as the ability to be aware of oneself and the ability to reflect on any process itself, this metacognitive ability appears to be intimately represented in the prefrontal region (Stuss, 1991a, b; Stuss and Benson, 1986). Inputs to this level are presumably the abstract mental representations deriving from the two lower levels. Output, including a feedforward system, goes primarily to level 2 in order to establish the principles by which executive control is maintained.

The feedback loop, working at each level, should be viewed as one component of an information processing system that works within this hierarchical and interactive model. From a rehabilitative perspective, it is important to know what level is impaired, in order to define the appropriate treatment and management. We emphasize that the approach will vary for different patients. In some patients, a bottom-up approach will be emphasized, even to the point of focusing primarily on modifying the patient's environment. The metacognitive level is often addressed only in selective patients.

Closed Head Injury and Frontal Lobe Trauma

In this section, we offer evidence that frontal dysfunction is perhaps the most prominent disturbance following TBI (Stuss and Gow, 1992).

Data from clinical descriptions, neuropsychologic investigations, and studies of the neuropathology of head injury are reviewed.

Neuropsychologic studies of the effects of TBI have, until recent years, emphasized dysfunction in abilities such as memory, as well as those tapped by measures of I.Q. Clinical descriptions, however, have alluded to the resemblance of the symptoms present after TBI to the symptoms observed following focal frontal lobe damage. Jefferson (1933) hypothesized that frontal lobe contusion may be at the root of the symptoms in TBI. Lambooy, Van der Zwan, and Fossen (1965), described the effects of severe head injury as "more or less a frontal-lobe syndrome combined with brainstem abnormalities" (p. 441). The parallel between the effects of focal frontal damage and closed head injury is perhaps most striking in the common description of the emotional disturbances and personality changes suffered in both instances. Disinhibition, tactlessness and jocularity, aggressive outbursts, emotional instability, decreased tolerance to noise and distracters, "depression" and withdrawal, or disinhibition and euphoria have been described in both disorders (Blumer and Benson, 1975; Bond, 1984; Fisher, 1985; Jarvie, 1954; Slater and Roth, 1969; Stuss and Benson, 1986). Alexander's (1982) description of three distinct behavioral syndromes observable in the recovery from severe TBI presents a notable similarity between the effects of TBI and the effects of focal frontal dysfunction at each of the three stages. Neuropsychologic studies also suggest frontal dysfunction in TBI. There is evidence to link self-reflectiveness and evaluative abilities with the frontal lobes (McGlynn and Schacter, 1989; Stuss, 1991a, b; Stuss and Benson, 1986). A very similar impairment appears to be significant in patients with brain injury. Prigatano (1987) compared the patient's judgments with the judgment of the patient's significant others with respect to the effects of the brain injury. The patients were unrealistic in their self-appraisal, overestimating their level of recovery. Levin and colleagues (1987) described four major neurobehavioral factors in patients with brain injury. One of these factors, the ability to self-evaluate, monitor, regulate, and plan, was related to the severity of the injury and was most prominent when frontal contusions or hematomas were present. This "frontal lobe syndrome" was considered to be the major neurobehavioral impairment in these patients. A disorder of self-reflectiveness and monitoring, supposedly related to frontal lobe damage, appears to be a prominent dysfunction in patients with brain injury.

Other "frontal deficits" have been demonstrated in patients with brain injury. Stuss and colleagues (Stuss, et al., 1985; Stuss, 1987) hypothesized that, if frontal regions are most damaged after TBI, then these patients should be most impaired on "frontal" tests. Impairment of psychologic functions related to nonfrontal regions should be minimal or nonexistent.

This should hold true, particularly if the patients' recovery, as measured by the Glasgow Outcome Scale, was positive. The hypothesis was experimentally confirmed.

Levin and Goldstein (1986) assessed the organization of verbal memory, and concluded that "traumatic injury involving the frontotemporal regions results in a deficient separation of various memory stores and difficulty in screening out irrelevant information" (p. 653). Using a semantic encoding paradigm, a similar deficit has been found in patients with focal frontal lobe damage (Zatorre and McEntee, 1983).

One hypothesized function of the frontal lobes is anticipation (Luria and Homskaya, 1964; Nauta, 1971; Robinson and Freeman, 1954; Stuss and Benson, 1986). Patients with TBI are similarly impaired in their ability to regulate their behavior in anticipation of consequences, again suggesting a strong parallel between the effects of brain injury and focal frontal lobe damage. For example, the contingent negative variation, an electrophysiologic negative shift of slow potentials that has been associated with the psychologic construct of anticipation, has been demonstrated to be reduced in patients with brain injury and in those with focal frontal lobe damage (Luria, 1973; Rizzo, et al., 1978; Tecce, 1977, Walter, 1973). Similar findings have also been demonstrated using a behavioral task. Tanaka (1973, 1974) had reported that monkeys with frontal lobe lesions had intact escape behavior (a nonanticipatory task) but were impaired on avoidance learning (an anticipation task, related to the ability to foresee consequences). When patients with brain injury were assessed using adapted tasks, a similar dissociation was revealed (Freedman, Bleiberg, and Freedland, 1987). Patients with TBI were significantly impaired in the task assessing anticipation.

The attentional disorder in patients with TBI is similar at least in certain respects to that of patients with frontal lesions. Frontal lobe patients have impaired focused attention (Luria, 1973; Perret, 1974) and also frequently lack consistency in performance (Arnot, 1952; Fuster and Bauer, 1974). Patients with varying severity of brain injury, including mildly concussed patients, also show impairment in both focused and sustained (i.e., consistent) attention (Stuss, et al., 1989). These two deficits appeared to be interactive in at least some individuals with brain injury. The patients could not maintain the "top-down" control necessary for repeated successful completion of the task, resulting in an intermittent impairment in focused attention.

In summary, clinical descriptions and neuropsychologic studies support the presence of "frontal dysfunction" in patients who have suffered TBI. Are these disorders related exclusively to *focal* frontal lobe damage after brain injury? Certain evidence suggests that such a conclusion is not feasible. Traumatic brain injury is aptly characterized by heterogeneity in both the pathophysiology and psychologic consequences (Alexander, 1982, 1987; Eisenberg and Weiner, 1987). Newcombe (1982) stated "it is not plausible to think in terms of a discrete locus of damage after closed head injury" (p. 112). A brief review of the neuropathology leads to a possible compromise solution.

Traumatic brain injury does frequently result in focal frontal lobe damage. Lacerations, contusions, and hemorrhages are prominent in the frontal and temporal regions after brain injury, as demonstrated in human clinical and animal and human experimental research (Courville, 1937; Holbourn, 1943; Nevin, 1967; Ommaya and Gennarelli, 1974; Ommaya, Grubb, and Naumann, 1971). This occurs independently of the site of impact (Clifton, et al., 1980; Cullum and Bigler, 1986; Gentry, Godersky, and Thompson, 1988; Gentry, Godersky, Thompson, and Dunn, 1988; Papo, Caruselli, Scarpelli, and Luongo, 1982; Sekino, et al., 1981). An extensive postmortem histologic analysis of 434 head-injured patients led to the following conclusion: "The selectively severe involvement of the frontal and temporal lobes in a nonmissile head injury is even more apparent than in our earlier publication . . ." (Adams, et al., 1985, p. 303). While not denying that pathology may be diffuse, these data suggest that frontal (and temporal) damage is a common and relatively more severe consequence of TBI.

Diffuse axonal injury (DAI) is the diffuse degeneration of the cerebral white matter after brain injury. This common mechanism of brain injury after trauma may vary in severity. While almost any fiber tract may be damaged, there is a predisposition for dysfunction to several areas. The frontal lobes are usually involved (Gentry, et al., 1988 a; Nevin, 1967). In addition, DAI may occur in the brainstem with degeneration throughout the brainstem, including the reticular and raphé core (Jane, Steward, and Gennarelli, 1985; Povlishock, Becker, Cheng, and Vaughan, 1983). Such brainstem pathology may disrupt major biochemical systems. For example, the dopamine system, which has its origin in the ventromedial mesencephalic tegmentum, is the major transmitter to prefrontal cortex (Glowinski, Tassin, and Thierry, 1984). The major serotonergic neurons lie in the dorsal and medial central raphé nuclei. Serotonergic deficiencies tend to be maximal in the hippocampus and frontal cortex (Agid, Ruberg, Dubois, and Pillon, 1987).

In addition to focal frontal lobe damage, the deficits in TBI labelled as "frontal dysfunction" may be attributable to other pathology. Diffuse white matter pathology itself may hinder efficient brain functioning, the end result being impairment in "frontal" tests (Alexander, 1982; Kinsbourne, 1977). The incomplete nature of this diffuse white matter pathology could affect less frequently used higher level abilities, while overlearned activities would be less impaired. The shearing, tearing, and stretching of axons may also result in a true disconnection between pre-frontal, limbic, and association cortices (Levin, et al., 1987). In addition, brainstem damage, either directly or due to biochemical alterations, may lead to disturbances of attention, perhaps due to disturbed brainstem arousal, or to a frontal brainstem control dysfunction (Barth, et al., 1983; Herscovitch, Stuss, and Broughton, 1980; Mason, 1981; Mindenhoud, van Woerkom, and van Weerden, 1976; Pisa and Fibiger, 1983; Simon, 1981).

Another possible cause of "frontal dysfunction" may be very indirectly related to the pathology, if at all. Executive control functions can be viewed as the highest of psychologic abilities, and most susceptible to any type of dysfunction (Goldberg and Bilder, 1987). Factors such as pain, fatigue, and general medical problems are common after head injury. These may be secondary causes of executive control dysfunction.

"The pre-eminent role of the frontal lobes in the organization of brain abilities based on its anatomical connections, as well as the position of the executive control functions in the hierarchy of psychological functions, makes executive control abilities extremely susceptible to many disturbances. The nature of traumatic brain injury, both pathological and psychological, puts these particular human abilities at more significant risk than other behavioral functions" (Stuss and Gow, 1992).

In summary, we propose that executive dysfunction in TBI is common. The underlying cause of the deficits, however, may vary from focal brain lesions in the frontal lobe to an inability to mobilize higher resources for any reason. Consequently, a term emphasizing the dysfunction rather than the anatomic location, such as "executive control dysfunction," may be more appropriate as it has a more general applicability.

Assessment

The assessment of the frontal lobes and executive abilities is not an easy task (Lezak, 1983; Walsh, 1987). Appropriate and comprehensive assessment, however, is essential to the selection of rehabilitative goals and procedures. Due to space limitation, this section primarily presents cautions to be exercised in three modes of examination—neurologic, neuro-psychologic, and real life procedures.

Large areas of the frontal lobes may be damaged and not be detected by a routine neurologic examination (Brickner, 1936; Hebb and Penfield, 1940). Even widely used measures such as the frontal motor and release signs may reflect pathology in areas other than the frontal lobes or be absent even when major frontal pathology is present (Benson and Stuss, 1982). Conjugate eye deviation, although seen with frontal eye field damage, is not an absolute frontal sign (DeRenzi, Colombo, Faglioni, and Gibertoni, 1982). Of more value is the neurobehavioral portion of the neurologic exam, such as the examination of language disturbance

(Alexander, Benson, and Stuss, 1989). This, however, demands specific knowledge of the particular syndrome and its manifestation after focal frontal lobe damage. Routinely, a neuropsychologic examination is required to provide more quantified data.

The neuropsychologic assessment has been helpful in detecting frontal lobe abnormalities. There are, however, several possible problems in the use and interpretation of neuropsychologic measures. First, it is possible for the examiner to administer a test in a structured manner such that he/she "becomes the frontal lobes" of the patient (Stuss, Benson, Kaplan, Weir, and Della Malva, 1981). The essence of standardized testing procedures is the elimination of uncontrolled variables. The executive behavioral disturbance, perhaps present in unstructured situations, may not be obvious in organized circumstances. Second, the experience of the examiner in dealing with such patients is an important factor. For example, awareness of the enhanced capacity of the patient in the structured setting would identify potentially effective rehabilitation procedures. In addition, observations of qualitative performance may provide helpful clues to the presence and nature of frontal dysfunction (see Table 10.1) (Kaplan, 1983). Third, many neuropsychologic tests do not assess frontal function adequately, if at all. The advances achieved in recent years with

Table 10.1.

FUNCTIONAL LEVEL	TREATMENT STRATEGY	REFERENCE
Self-reflectiveness/ Metacognition	Self-appraisal training	Ylvisaker & Szekeres, 1989
	Self-instructional strategies	Cicerone & Wood, 1987
	Metacognition strategy training	Lawson & Rice, 1987 Kirbey & Grimley, 1986
Executive functions	Improving initiation (practice portion of training)	Sohlberg, et al., 1988 Wood, 1987
	Higher level attention	Mateer, in press Mateer, et al., 1990
	Training use of compensatory aids (memory books/ books/organizers)	Sohlberg & Mateer, 1989b
	Training prospective memory	Sohlberg, et al., 1991a, b
	Planning and scheduling exercises	Sohlberg & Mateer, 1989a
	Route finding tasks	Boyd, et al., 1987
	Problem solving training	von Cramon & Matthes-von Cramon, 1990
Basic knowledge/ Sensation	Teaching task specific routines	Craine, 1982

experimental research, albeit still limited, have not yet been translated into clinical practice. Fourth, it must be recognized that even widely accepted frontal lobe tests are not uniquely sensitive to frontal lobe damage. Because of reciprocal interconnections with other brain regions, and the fact that these functions are supramodel to other abilities, impairment on traditional "frontal lobe measures" can be found with lesions virtually anywhere in the brain. It is the relative differences among spared and impaired abilities that are important in the diagnosis and understanding of frontal dysfunction. Finally, there is variability in performance on frontal lobe tests both across and within patients with frontal lobe disturbance. That is, at times certain patients may be significantly impaired on tests, and at other times perform reasonably well. Moreover, different frontal lobe patients may be impaired on different tests, likely reflecting lesion location.

An insufficiently utilized assessment procedure is that of real-life observation (Eslinger and Damasio, 1985). Sohlberg and Mateer (1989a) described an Executive Function Rating Scale which attempts to focus observations made in natural settings with a view to evaluating capacity for executive functioning in everyday life. In the use of real-life assessment techniques, one must be aware of the considerable range in the use of executive abilities amongst the normal population. Indeed, there is notable variation even within the same individual, depending upon the context. Even though the variation of frontal abilities amongst the more normal population has yet to be extensively studied, the psychosocial approach can still be a powerful adjunct in the assessment of executive behavioral disturbances.

In summary, the first section has suggested that executive control dysfunction is frequently present after traumatic brain injury. In the following section, the application of this knowledge to the development and implementation of rehabilitative procedures is proposed.

REHABILITATION OF FRONTAL LOBE DEFICITS

Individuals with executive function compromise can be among the most baffling and sometimes frustrating patients that rehabilitation specialists encounter. These individuals may demonstrate average or even above average intellectual functions, have seemingly adequate recall of information, and apparently have knowledge when a verbal response is requested; yet, they fail to accomplish goals or complete even the simplest of tasks in the absence of cuing or structure. In the remainder of this chapter, we will discuss various approaches to rehabilitation of patients with frontal system compromise. The various treatment approaches will be organized and presented in relation to the 3-level hierarchy described earlier. It is recognized, however, that this is a conceptual division. Training tasks such as memory book and initiation training frequently involve all three levels: Teaching knowledge (level 1), providing practice in executive tasks (level 2), and facilitating awareness and generalization (level 3).

Sensation and Basic Knowledge (Level 1)

At this level, the rehabilitation specialist focuses on reinstituting basic and routine lower level processes, even at the level of structuring of the environment to control input and output processes. In some instances, the therapist "becomes the frontal lobes" of the patient. In other instances (e.g., attention training), the therapist attempts to improve the patient's basic information processing capacity.

Compensatory Strategies

If the patient is very acute in the rehabilitation process and/or is demonstrating very severe executive function disturbance, it may be profitable to focus initially on teaching task specific routines. The assumption here is that the patient will not be capable of a wide variety of different action plans in different settings because of stimulus boundedness, perseveration, severe related cognitive disorders of attention or memory, or extremely limited insight and awareness. In such individuals, it may not be reasonable to facilitate flexible individually determined sequences, but training of particular sequences for standard highly repetitive functional activities may be possible (Craine, 1982). Included here would be a variety of grooming and dressing routines such as showering, taking care of one's toilet, or dressing. Routines could be written and trained using a step-by-step format. Another common task-specific routine that might be taught is preparation of a very simple meal. If executive functions are severely impaired, there should probably be a limited number of food items utilized and an avoidance of potential dangers, such as use of the stove or waste disposers. The patient might be taught a simple sequence (e.g., 4 steps) for preparing juice, toast, and cereal. Although initially varying little from day to day, certain variations could be introduced over time in sequence with the patient's improvement.[a]

In some patients even this level of structured support is not adequate. In such patients a compensatory approach would include environmental restructuring. This might involve organizing the environment to reduce distractions or potentially dangerous situations. Additionally, the provision of specific labels in the environment, (e.g., identifying the contents in kitchen cupboards or bathroom drawers) might be a useful modification.

---

[a]A handbook on the teaching of task specific routines was prepared by staff of the Good Samaritan Hospital, Puyallup, WA (Geyer, 1988).

Visual cues posted within the home listing task-specific routines (e.g., a morning grooming sequence on the bathroom mirror) can also compensate for executive control dysfunction.

Training Automatic Attentional Skills

Attention may be divided into basic categories such as automatic and effortful or routine and directed (Shiffrin and Schneider, 1977; Shallice, 1988). At this first level, the therapist addresses the more basic and routine attentional functions such as the ability to sustain tonic attention and to have adequate phasic attentional capabilities to orient attention appropriately. Even when more complex tasks are introduced, the purpose of attention training at this level can be viewed as an attempt to retrain automaticity in information processing, to move from information processing that is under effortful conscious control back to a more automatic control. While it is difficult to dissociate in practice lower and higher level attentional training, an awareness of this distinction is beneficial for the rehabilitation specialist.

Executive Functions (Level 2)

We now move to the second level postulated in Figure 10.1, that of executive functions. At this level, there is an assumption that there is a rudimentary attentional capacity and no disorder of arousal and functioning. However, frontal functions, including the capacity to organize sequences and carry out novel activities, are likely to be disrupted and must be rehabilitated. At this level, a variety of management and treatment activities might be utilized to train subfunctions of anticipation, goal articulation, and plan formulation. Since most activities have to be done within somewhat specified time frames, time management strategies should be considered. It is important to keep data on tasks presented, and to build skills in a hierarchical fashion going from more to less structured tasks and to tasks of increasing complexity.

Modulating Output Mechanisms

Functions intimately associated with the frontal lobes are essential for the effective initiation and sequencing of action programs. The facilitation of drive and the energizing of behavior will be a necessary step in rehabilitation at this level. Clinically, a disorder of drive is often manifested in apparent disinterest or inactivity. Generally, it is not the case that the patient with frontal lobe deficits cannot perform an action at all; rather, they do not independently initiate the action at a particular time or place.

Such patients may respond to external cues or prompts to initiate activity and their behavior can be modified through traditional behavior modification techniques. The following discussion uses the example of working with someone who has difficulty initiating verbal output.

Increasing Initiation of Conversation

Some individuals with frontal system impairment may demonstrate adequate knowledge of what is going on in the environment, but show little apparent interest or involvement. As part of the intervention, the patient is told that they will be practicing the initiation of conversation. They are provided with samples of how to carry out this activity. For example, the clinician might provide a list of typical phrases that are useful for initiating conversations (e.g., How is it going today? What are you going to do this weekend?) as well as sample conversational situations (e.g., sitting at a cafeteria table in the hospital or waiting for group therapy to begin). The clinician chooses a situation in which this behavior will be monitored (e.g., accompanying the patient to the cafeteria). The clinician then gathers data on a scorecard designed for this purpose. Analogous initiation activities are easily developed for other behaviors. The important steps are first to increase the patient's awareness of the initiation problem and then to provide structured opportunities to practice the initiation of the target activity. The awareness training and self-correction aspects of the task might be considered operations relevant to the third level (self-reflectiveness, metacognition), while the practice part of training would relate to the second level of the proposed model (executive functions).

In a single case study by Sohlberg, Sprunk, and Metzelaar (1988), it was shown that an individual with severe frontal lobe impairment and marked initiation problems did respond differentially with two types of cuing. During a group activity, this patient was provided with a cue at which time he was to ask himself whether or not he was initiating conversation. His verbal interactions during group clearly increased over a baseline period during and following a treatment phase in which such prompts were provided. Experimental control of the behavior was demonstrated by means of comparison to another measured behavior, response acknowledgements; these responses did not increase during the baseline or initial intervention stage but only when response acknowledgements were specifically trained and then cued by a similar prompted self-evaluation system. The opportunity for repeated practice initiating conversation would be considered part of training the executive functions. The ability to self-evaluate and modify behavior based upon cued self-reflection would correspond to the metacognitive portion of training.

Training Higher Level Attentional Skills

Many patients with frontal lobe impairments retain substantial general basic knowledge and essentially intact language processing capabilities. They are unlikely to have primary auditory, visual, or somatosensory impairments. They are very likely, however, to demonstrate problems with higher order attention. If brainstem and midbrain systems are essentially intact, it is likely that basic arousal mechanisms will be spared. However, patients with frontal lobe impairment may have difficulty with smooth and effective allocation of attentional resources on more complex tasks. Focused attention deficits may be intermittently revealed (Stuss, et al., 1989). They are also likely to have difficulty shifting attention and performing efficiently on tasks that require divided attention capabilities.

Several studies have suggested that individuals with TBI benefit from exercise and training of attentional skills. Indeed, some of the earliest work in cognitive rehabilitation demonstrating positive findings involved systematic intervention with the attentional system (Ben-Yishay, Piasetsky, and Rattok, 1987; Kewman, et al., 1985). Sohlberg and Mateer (1986) developed a package of attention training materials (Attention Process Training) which was based on 5–levels of attention including focused, sustained, selective, alternating, and divided attention. The efficacy of this training in improving attentional capacities has been supported in a series of single case designs and in group pre- and posttreatment comparisons (Mateer, 1992; Mateer, Sohlberg and Youngman, 1990; Sohlberg and Mateer, 1986). Improved attentional function has also been associated with improved memory function in individuals who received attention but not memory training (Mateer and Sohlberg, 1988; Niemann, 1989; Ruff, et al., 1989). Improved attentional control, with increased vigilance, decreased susceptibility to distraction, and improved capacity to deal with more than one task at a time positively influences problem solving, organizational and communication skills.

Compensatory Techniques: The Externalization and Internalization of Executive Functions

In this section we describe the attempt to reinstate at least some executive functions in certain patients where this is deemed possible. This rehabilitative strategy differs from the lower level compensatory approach where the focus is on environmental control and reinstitution of lower level processes. The conceptual approach is based on the teachings and research of Vygotsky (1962), Luria (1960, 1973), and Meichenbaum (Meichenbaum and Cameron, 1973; Meichenbaum and Goodman, 1971). Directive functions are externalized through various procedures and, hopefully, become internalized.

Cuing systems may be established which allow patients to plan, organize, and follow through with multiple step activities. Examples of such systems include training in the use of a watch with an alarm, a calendar system, or a card cuing system to prompt activities throughout the day. More complex computer-based or interactive systems (e.g., electronic memories) could provide greater flexibility in tasks, but also might prove more costly and difficult to manage. Such factors become important to realistic implementation of strategies as it often falls to the family, friends, or others to monitor their disposition and use. Indeed, family education and support are critical when rehabilitative efforts are targeted at this level. Clinicians themselves, while likely to introduce a variety of compensatory strategies, may not spare sufficient time in training their use. Experience in rehabilitation has shown that active and systematic training is required for effective utilization of compensatory strategies.

Stuss, Delgado, and Guzman (1987), employed verbal self-regulation to rehabilitate a deficit in sustaining motor actions (motor impersistence) in two patients with focal right hemisphere pathology. Both demonstrated spontaneously some ability to generalize the use of this technique. The case studies also suggest the possible importance of lesion localization in the success of specific rehabilitative procedures.

Sohlberg and Mateer (1989b) describe a comprehensive 3–stage behavioral approach to training use of a memory/organizational book in an individual with severe amnesia and executive function disorder. The first stage of training relates to the first level of the model as it focuses on increasing the patient's *knowledge* of how this system works. The second training phase involves practice using the system to *plan* and *execute* tasks and this relates to the executive function level of the model. The third training phase works on *generalization* and corresponds to the meta-cognitive stage.

Training Prospective Memory

Another way in which difficulties at the action program level might be manifest is in failures of what has been termed prospective memory (Sohlberg, White, Evans, and Mateer, 1991a, b). Prospective memory requires that the person carry out a particular action at a specified time in the future based on a self-initiated and internally generated plan of action. Patients may have formed an intent to do something, but at the time that the action is required, they may fail to remember to act. Prospective memory can involve such practical and useful activities as remembering to take medications, remembering to make a phone call, or remembering to bring home items when shopping. This capacity may differ sharply from performance on more traditional measures of anterograde, semantic, or episodic memory which are traditionally tested by providing a cue or prompt for recall. Performance on specific prospective memory tasks such as are included on the *Rivermead Everyday Memory Test* (Wilson, Cockburn, and Baddeley, 1985) has been shown to be more closely correlated with functional independence in the community than has performance on more traditional measures of cued recall.

The possibility of improving prospective memory functioning has been suggested (Sohlberg, et al., 1991a, b). The goal of prospective memory training is to increase the amount of time between the instruction and the carrying out of a specific action and the gradual introduction of distractors during the prospective memory interval. Using this procedure, patients initially unable to hold an instruction for even 1–2 minutes could increase their prospective memory performance to 15 minutes. It is hoped that, through improved prospective memory, patients may be better able to utilize other memory and organizational systems. As described earlier, failure to restore or improve a capacity sufficiently may necessitate a compensatory approach utilizing the knowledge of lower level processes. In such cases, prospective memory may be compensated for by environmental cues or training in task-specific routines.

Facilitating, Planning and Organizational Skills

The major disorder of executive abilities in patients with TBI are impairments in planning and organization. It is proposed that patients may benefit from structured exercises which would provide multiple opportunities for initiation, planning and carrying out of goal-directed activities. An example for training initiation was presented earlier in this section. The intended aim is that patients would improve in developing and carrying out multistep plans. Several procedures have been utilized. Although their efficacy has not yet been experimentally demonstrated, studies are underway and description of several procedures is provided here.

Therapy Planning Exercises

In most formal therapy sessions in rehabilitation settings, the actual planning and scheduling of the treatment period are under control of the therapist. The therapist usually decides what activities will be done, over what duration of time and in what order, thereby in some sense obviating the need for the patient's management of that period of time. When working with an individual with executive function compromise, the requirement for treatment session planning can be gradually turned over to the patient. The patient can be told that a certain number of tasks should probably be used and what time frame is available, but the patient decides in what sequence and for what duration each particular activity is undertaken. One could look, for example, at the capacity to plan a period of time and then look at the capability of the patient to stay within that scheduled plan. Once a patient is able to plan and maintain the time schedule, it would be useful to introduce something which would require that the patient alter or modify the plan. The therapist could indicate that certain materials need to be utilized by someone else and are not available or that the entire session needs to be shortened but that the same number of tasks must be incorporated. This would allow for observations as to whether or not the patient can modify the plan in accordance with new information or new requirements. Independent scheduling of activity on the part of the patient may be revealing with regard to their capacity for scheduling and time management in everyday life. These procedures are based on data reported by Shallice and Burgess (1991) which indicated impairment in completing a number of simple tasks in a specified time frame according to simple rules.

If possible, the clinician should move from hypothetical planning exercises to actually carrying out the planning for a real life activity. Clinicians may need to be creative in providing opportunities that meet the constraints of a particular work setting. If a clinician is working one-on-one in a private practice, he or she might suggest the patients plan to arrange for refreshments. In a group setting, the clinician may ask the patient to plan an activity for the group, e.g., a breakfast, a birthday party, or a community outing. Data collection pertaining to the ability to plan hypothetical and/or real activities can be scored using a variety of charts or checklists. Again, opportunities for modifying plans are a necessity. In real life, for example, if one were organizing refreshments, someone could be allergic to a particular food that had been planned; such contingencies should be posed to the patient to increase flexibility and divergent thinking.

Route Finding Tasks

The Executive Route Finding Task (ERFT) developed by Boyd, Sautter, Bailey, Echols, and Douglas (1987), was designed to target frontal lobe functions. These researchers gave patients open-ended instructions, indicating that they should find the location of a particular office on a hospital campus in as efficient a manner as possible. The examiner could not give them any cues, but would accompany them. Patients variously demonstrated more or less effective techniques. Some demonstrated what was called "aimless wandering," a kind of nondirected, nonsystematic walking about the facility. Some used a "trial and error" method characterized by continuous guessing and a gradual process of elimination. Use of a "step-by-step" approach suggested that patients were recognizing limitations and were systematically narrowing in on the target location by asking for information limited to the next closest location. Finally, there were patients who used a strategy approach in which they took notes, asked for a map, or performed some other higher level strategy to maximize their chances of successfully finding the target. Boyd and colleagues (1987) suggested that route finding tasks should be evaluated on the following parameters: 1) Task understanding, 2) incorporation of information seeking, 3) retaining the directions, 4) error detection, 5) error correction, and 6) on-task behavior. The second parameter directly relates to the executive function of planning. The fourth and fifth parameters require self-monitoring and use of feedback, which relate to the third level of the theoretical model. Contributory problems related to emotional, communication and/or perceptual barriers can be recorded to note any variables that might confound completion of the task.

The cuing system used in the *ERFT* is a unique system that can be applied to a variety of tasks involving executive functions. Nonspecific cues are used to remind the patient to self-monitor. An example might be "What should you do now?" Specific cues provide information relevant to how to actually execute the task. These two cue levels can provide an excellent hierarchy for training executive functions. Over the course of training, one would hope to see fewer needs for specific cues and greater dependence on nonspecific cues and eventually a reduction in the need for cues in general.

von Cramon and Matthes-von Cramon (1990) described positive results in a series of patients with frontal lobe dysfunction using a training procedure which involved enabling patients to help reduce the complexity of a multistage problem by breaking it down into more manageable proportions. Problem solving training incorporated four modules. The first involved the generation of goal-directed ideas, a kind of "brainstorming" designed to produce a variety of alternatives to a given problem. The second involved training in systematic and careful comparison of information provided to them. The third consisted of tasks where multiple information needed to be processed simultaneously, such as having the patient compare catalogues of several tourist offices in order to find the most favorable trip to England for a family of four. The fourth focused on improving the patient's abilities in drawing inferences. They utilized short detective stories and had subjects uncover discrepancies and detect hints about how crimes could have been committed. The researcher reported significant psychometric as well as functional gains in a group receiving this training as opposed to a group receiving more generic memory training.

The therapy planning exercises and route finding tasks are included under the executive function component as they all require the organization of output and the integration of complex patterns, relationships and associations. Many patients with severe frontal lobe compromise may demonstrate only partial recovery of function at this level, and may need to rely on compensatory approaches as described earlier. There is growing indication, however, that some patients may improve significantly in executive functions and may benefit from specific intervention and treatment addressing the highest level in Figure 10.1, that of self-reflectiveness and metacognition.

Self-Reflectiveness/Metacognition

Functioning at this level, with awareness and self-regulatory capacity, may, more than any other area, define the essence of frontal lobe activity. It is the experience of most clinicians that many persons with frontal lobe damage have limited insight into their problems and require explicit behavioral objectives in order to understand and progress in therapy. Treatment in this area presents a tremendous challenge for the rehabilitation professional.

Awareness training can take a variety of forms. Usually, patients are given didactic information about the nature of their injury, the way in which it affects their behavior, and the reasons why a particular behavior is not appropriate or acceptable. Although sometimes helpful and often necessary, such didactic training is usually not sufficient to bring about a durable change in behavior. Awareness training may be most effective as the first stage of a training sequence. For example, the previously described study by Sohlberg, et al. (1989b), targeted increasing initiation of conversation in a severely brain-injured individual. The first training phase involved increasing the subject's awareness of the initiation deficit. This approach builds on the didactic training. The patient is informed that he or she tends to exhibit a particular behavior, either desirable or undesirable (e.g., escalating to a loud voice, limited eye contact). The patient is then told to mark a piece of paper every time he or she exhibits the behavior during a designated time period. The clinician simultaneously keeps track of the behavior; videotapes may be made as a tertiary source of information. The patient's awareness may be increased by comparing his or her observations to those of the clinician or observed on a tape. Ylvisaker and Szekeres (1989) has proposed a 4–step program for improving self-regulatory behavior in adolescents with brain injury.

Another kind of intervention at this level involves teaching self-instructional procedures before and during the execution of a training task. Cicerone and Wood (1987) reported successful treatment of a patient who exhibited impaired planning ability and poor self-control 4 years after closed head injury using such a procedure. They used as a training task a modified version of the *Tower of London*. Training in the self-instructional technique involved 3 distinct phases involving overt verbalization, overt self-guidance, and covert internalized self-monitoring. Following this program, and to promote generalization, the client was presented with a structured interpersonal problem and asked to solve it applying principles learned in the self-instructional training. The results supported the clinical efficacy of verbal mediation training in treating executive functions. The authors noted, however, that generalization of training occurred only after direct, extended training using real life situations.

As with other areas discussed, the use of metacognitive strategies and self-instructional programs is in its infancy with regard to the adult brain-injured population. Encouraging, however, are numerous reports of success with such approaches in children and adolescents with learning disability for whom they have been used over the past decade (Lawson and Rice, 1989).

DISCUSSION

We have presented evidence that impairment of executive functions is the most significant sequela after traumatic brain injury. Based on a model of brain functioning, we then proposed a variety of approaches have been discussed with reference to the treatment of individuals with frontal lobe impairment. In general, they involve moving from simple structured activities with significant external cuing and support to more complex, multistep activities in which external support is gradually reduced and internal support or self-direction is enhanced. Although a variety of articles have suggested success in using these techniques, there are as yet a very small number of cases and a limited number of studies in which such techniques have been experimentally manipulated. Clearly more work in this area is needed. In addition to the more formal intervention procedures, some generic interventions should not be forgotten. Certainly education of the family and significant others in how to respond to a person with frontal lobe injury will be important. Often an appreciation for the organic or nonvolitional nature of the behavior is helpful in alleviating fears and misconceptions. As many different terms can be used to describe these behaviors and capacities, it is important to use consistent language and understandable terminology. Repetition will be a key factor and no matter what kind of intervention is utilized, whether it be restorative or compensatory, multiple opportunities for practice must be incorporated into the treatment program. Finally, it is vital that clinicians actively train for generalization. One should not expect generalization, but rather provide systematic opportunities during which skills and behaviors can be trained and stabilized.

Individuals with executive function impairments pose one of the greatest challenges to clinicians and to the rehabilitation system. In the last decade, we have made great strides in understanding at least some of the many functions of the frontal lobes. It is important to recognize, however, that the development of rehabilitative strategies directed to these disorders is in an embryonic state. With greater knowledge and understanding, we should be able to identify, develop, apply, and test specific interventions to mediate the effect of frontal system impairments. More than physical limitations, or even many other cognitive impairments, executive dysfunction has the potential to disrupt and limit an individual's capacity for independent, meaningful, and socially integrated functioning. Strides that we make in the understanding and treatment of these impairments will be valuable and rewarding to our patients, their families, and society.

Acknowledgements

During the preparation of this manuscript, D. Stuss was funded by the Ontario Mental Health Foundation. We are grateful for assistance in typing, library research, figure preparation, and editing provided by P. Mathews, L. Buckle, J. Pogue, and R. Hetherington.

References

Adams, J.H., Doyle, D., Graham, D.I., et al. (1985). The contusion index: A reappraisal in human and experimental nonmissile head injury. Neuropathology and Applied Neurobiology, 11:299–308.

Agid, Y., Ruberg, M., Dubois, B., and Pillon, B. (1987). Anatomoclinical and biochemical concepts of subcortical dementia. In: Stahl, S.M., Iversen, S.D., and Goodman, E.C. (eds). Cognitive neurochemistry. Oxford: Oxford University Press, 248–71.

Alexander, M.P. (1982). Traumatic brain injury. In: Benson, D.F., and Blumer, D. (eds). Psychiatric aspects of neurologic disease: Vol. 2. New York: Grune and Stratton, 219–50.

Alexander, M.P. (1987). The role of neurobehavioral syndromes in the rehabilitation and outcome of closed head injury. In: Levin, H.S., Grafman, J., and Eisenberg, H.M. (eds). Neurobehavioral recovery from head injury. New York: Oxford University Press, 191–205.

Alexander, M.P., Benson, D.F., and Stuss, D.T. (1989). Frontal lobes and language. Brain and Language, 37:656–91.

Arnot, R. (1952). A theory of frontal lobe function. Archives of Neurology and Psychiatry, 67:487–95.

Barth, J.T., Macciocchi, S.N., Giordani, B., Rimel, R., Jane, J.A., and Boll, J.T. (1983). Neuropsychological sequelae of minor head injury. Neurosurgery, 13:529–33.

Benson, D.F., and Stuss, D.T. (1982). Motor abilities after frontal leukotomy. Neurology (NY), 32:1353–57.

Ben-Yishay, Y., Piasetsky, E.B., and Rettok, J. (1987). A systematic method for ameliorating disorders in basic attention. In: Meier, M., Benton, A., and Diller, L. (eds). Neuropsychological rehabilitation. New York: Guilford Press, 163–81.

Blumer, D., and Benson, D.F. (1975). Personality changes with frontal and temporal lobe lesions. In: Benson, D.F., and Blumer, D. (eds). Psychiatric aspects of neurologic disease: Vol. 1. New York: Grune and Stratton, 151–70.

Bond, M. (1984). The psychiatry of closed head injury. In: Brooks, N. (ed). Closed head injury: Psychological, social, and family consequences. Oxford: Oxford University Press, 148–78.

Boyd, T.M., Sautter, S., Bailey, M.D., Echols, L.D., and Douglas, J.W. (1987). Reliability and validity of a measure of everyday problem solving. Paper presented at the annual meeting of the International Neuropsychological Society, Washington, DC.

Brickner, R.M. (1936). The intellectual functions of the frontal lobes. New York: Macmillan.

Carver, C.S., and Scheier, M.F. (1982). Self-awareness and the self-regulation of behaviour. In: Underwood, G. (ed). Aspects of consciousness: Vol. 3. Awareness and self-awareness. New York: Academic Press, 235–66.

Cicerone, K.D., and Wood, J.C. (1987). Planning disorder after closed head injury: A case study. Archives of Physical Medicine and Rehabilitation, 68:111–15.

Clifton, G.L., Grossman, R.G., Makela, M.E., Miner, M.E., Handel, S., and Sadhu, V. (1980). Neurological course and correlated computerized tomography findings after severe closed head injury. Journal of Neurosurgery, 52:611–24.

Courville, C.B. (1937). Pathology of the central nervous system: Part 4. Mountain View, CA: Pacific Publishers.

Craine, S.F. (1982). The retraining of frontal lobe dysfunction. In: Trexler, L.E. (ed). Cognitive rehabilitation: Conceptualization and intervention. New York: Plenum, 239–62.

Cullum, C.M., and Bigler, E.D. (1986). Ventricle size, cortical atrophy, and the relationship with neuropsychological status in closed head injury: A quantitative analysis. Journal of Clinical and Experimental Neuropsychology, 8:437–52.

DeRenzi, E., Colombo, A., Faglioni, P., and Gibertoni, M. (1982). Conjugate gaze paresis in stroke patients with unilateral damage: An unexpected instance of hemispheric asymmetry. Archives of Neurology, 39:482–86.

Eisenberg, H.M., and Weiner, R.L. (1987). Input variables: How information from the acute injury can be used to characterize groups of patients for studies of outcome. In: Levin, H.S., Grafman, J., and Eisenberg, H.M. (eds). Neurobehavioral recovery from head injury. New York: Oxford University Press, 13–29.

Eslinger, P.J., and Damasio, A.R. (1985). Severe disturbance of higher cognition following bilateral frontal lobe ablation: Patient EVR. Neurology, 35:1731–41.

Fisher, J.M. (1985). Cognitive and behavioural consequences of closed head injury. Seminars in Neurology, 5:197–204.

Freedman, P.E., Bleiberg, J., and Freedland, K. (1987). Anticipatory behaviour deficits in closed head injury. Journal of Neurology, Neurosurgery, and Psychiatry, 50:398–401.

Fuster, J.M. (1989). The prefrontal cortex. Anatomy, physiology, and neuropsychology of the frontal lobe (2nd ed). New York: Raven Press.

Fuster, J.M., and Bauer, R.H. (1974). Visual short-term memory deficit from hypothermia of frontal cortex. Brain Research, 81:393–400.

Gentry, L.R., Godersky, J.C., and Thompson, B. (1988a). MR imaging of head trauma: Review of the distribution and radiopathologic features of traumatic lesions. American Journal of Neuroradiology, 9:101–10.

Gentry, L.R., Godersky, J.C., Thompson, B., and Dunn, V.D. (1988b). Prospective comparative study of intermediate-field MR and CT in the evaluation of closed head trauma. American Journal of Roentgenology, 150:673–82.

Geyer, S. (1988). Executive functions: Model and management. Puyallup: Good Samaritan Hospital.

Glowinski, J., Tassin, J.P., and Thierry, A.M. (1984). The mesocortico-prefrontal dopaminergic neurons. Trends in NeuroScience, 7:415–18.

Goldberg, E., and Bilder, R.M., Jr. (1987). The frontal lobes and hierarchical organization of cognitive control. In: Perecman, E. (ed). The frontal lobes revisited. New York: IRBN Press, 159-87.

Goldman-Rakic, P.S. (1987). Circuitry of primate prefrontal cortex and regulation of behavior by representational memory. In: Plum, F. (ed). Handbook of physiology: The nervous system: Vol. 5. Hillsdale, NJ: Lawrence Erlbaum Associates, 373-417.

Grafman, J. (1989). Plans, actions, and mental sets: Managerial knowledge units in the frontal lobes. In: Perecman, E. (ed). Integrating theory and practice in neuropsychology. Hillsdale, NJ: Lawrence Erlbaum Associates, 93-138.

Hebb, D.O., and Penfield, W. (1940). Human behavior after extensive bilateral removal from the frontal lobes. Archives of Neurology and Psychiatry, 44:421-38.

Herscovitch, J., Stuss, D., and Broughton, R. (1980). Changes in cognitive processing following short-term cumulative partial sleep deprivation and recovery oversleeping. Journal of Clinical Neuropsychology, 2:301-19.

Holbourn, A.H.S. (1943). Mechanics of head injury. Lancet, 2:438-41.

Jane, J.A., Steward, O., and Gennarelli, T. (1985). Axonal degeneration induced by experimental noninvasive minor head injury. Journal of Neurosurgery, 62(1):96-100.

Jarvie, H.F. (1954). Frontal lobe wounds causing disinhibition: A study of six cases. Journal of Neurology, Neurosurgery, and Psychiatry, 17:14-32.

Jefferson, G. (1933). Remarks on the treatment of acute head injuries. British Medical Journal, 2:807-12.

Kaplan, E. (1983). Process and achievement revisited. In: Wapner, S., and Kaplan, B. (eds). Toward a holistic developmental psychology. Hillsdale, NJ: Lawrence Erlbaum Associates, 143-56.

Kewman, D.G., Seigerman, C., Kintner, H., Chu, S., Henson, D., and Reeder, C. (1985) Simulation and training of psychomotor skills: Teaching the brain-injured to drive. Rehabilitation Psychology, 30:11-27.

Kinsbourne, M. (1977). Cognitive decline with advancing age: An interpretation. In: Smith, W.L., and Kinsbourne, M. (eds). Aging and dementia. New York: Spectrum, 217-35.

Lambooy, N., Van der Zwan, A., and Fossen, A. (1965). End-results after long-term unconsciousness due to head-injury. Psychiatria, Neurologia, Neurochirurgia, 68:431-42.

Lawson, M.J., and Rice, D.D. (1989). Effects of training in use of executive strategies on a verbal memory problem resulting from closed head injury. Journal of Clinical and Experimental Neuropsychology, 11:842-54.

Levin, H.S., and Goldstein, F.C. (1986). Organization of verbal memory after severe closed-head injury. Journal of Clinical and Experimental Neuropsychology, 8:643-56.

Levin, H.S., High, W.M., Goethe, K.E., et al. (1987). The neurobehavioural rating scale: Assessment of the behavioral sequelae of head injury by the clinician. Journal of Neurology, Neurosurgery, and Psychiatry, 50:183-93.

Lezak, M.D. (1983). Neuropsychological assessment (2nd ed). New York: Oxford University Press.

Luria, A.R. (1960). Verbal regulation of behaviour. In: Brazier, M.A.B. (ed). The central nervous system and behavior. Third Macy Conference. Madison, NJ: Madison Printing Co., 359-423.

Luria, A.R. (1973). The working brain. An introduction to neuropsychology (Haigh, B., trans). New York: Basic Books.

Luria, A.R., and Homskaya, D. (1964). Disturbance in the regulative role of speech with frontal lobe lesions. In: Warren, J.M., and Akert, K. (eds). The frontal granular cortex and behavior. New York: McGraw-Hill, 353-71.

Mason, S.T. (1981). Noradrenaline in the brain: Progress in theories of behavioral function. Progressive Neurobiology, 16:263-303.

Mateer, C.A. (1992). Systems of care for postconcussion syndrome. In: Horn, L.J., and

Zasler, N.D. (eds). Physical medicine and rehabilitation: State of the art reviews. Philadelphia: Henley and Belfus, Inc., 143-60.

Mateer, C.A., and Sohlberg, M.M. (1988). A paradigm shift in memory rehabilitation. In: Whitaker, H.A. (ed). Neuropsychological studies of nonfocal brain injury: Dementia and closed head injury. New York: Springer-Verlag, 202-25.

Mateer, C.A., Sohlberg, M.M., and Youngman, P.K. (1990). The management of acquired attention and memory deficits. In: Wood, R.L., and Fussey, I. (eds). Cognitive rehabilitation in perspective. London: Taylor and Francis, 68-95.

McGlynn, S.M., and Schacter, D.L. (1989). Unawareness of deficits in neuropsychological syndromes. Journal of Clinical and Experimental Neuropsychology, 11(2):143-205.

Meichenbaum, D., and Cameron, R. (1973). Training schizophrenics to talk to themselves: A means of developing attentional controls. Behaviour Therapy, 4:515-34.

Meichenbaum, D., and Goodman, J. (1971). Training impulsive children to talk to themselves: A means of developing self-control. Journal of Abnormal Psychology, 77:115-26.

Mesulam, M.M. (1981). A cortical network for directed attention and unilateral neglect. Annals of Neurology, 10:309-25.

Miller, G.A., Galanter, E.H., and Pribram, K.H. (1960). Plans and the structure of behavior. New York: Holt, Rinehart, and Winston.

Minderhoud, J.M., van Woerkom, T.C.A.M., and van Weerden, T.W. (1976). On the nature of brainstem disorders in severe head injured patients: II. A study on caloric vestibular reactions and neurotransmitter treatment. Acta Neurochir, Urgica (Wien) 34:23-35.

Nauta, W.J.H. (1971). The problem of the frontal lobe: A reinterpretation. Journal of Psychiatric Research, 8:167-87.

Nevin, N.C. (1967). Neuropathological changes in the white matter following head injury. Journal of Neuropathology and Experimental Neurology, 26:77-84.

Newcombe, F. (1982). The psychological consequences of closed head injury: Assessment and rehabilitation. Injury, 14:111-36.

Niemann, H. (1989). Retraining of attention in head injured individuals. Unpublished doctoral dissertation, University of Victoria, British Columbia.

Norman, D.A., and Shallice, T. (1986). Attention to action. Willed and automatic control of behaviour. In: Davidson, R.J., Schwartz, G.E., and Shapiro, D. (eds). Consciousness and self-regulation. Advances in research and theory: Vol. 4. New York: Plenum, 1-18.

Ommaya, A.K., and Gennarelli, T.A. (1974). Cerebral concussion and traumatic unconsciousness: Correlation of experimental and clinical observations on blunt head injuries. Brain, 97:633-54.

Ommaya, A., Grubb, R., and Naumann, R. (1971). Coup and contre-coup injury. Observations on the mechanics of visible brain injuries in the rhesus monkey. Journal of Neurosurgery, 35:503-16.

Pandya, D.N., and Barnes, C.L. (1987). Architecture and connections of the frontal lobe. In: Perecman, E. (ed). The frontal lobes revisited. New York: IRBN Press, 41-72.

Papo, I., Caruselli, G., Scarpelli, M., and Luongo, A. (1982). Mass lesions of the frontal lobes in acute head injuries: A comparison with temporal lesions. Acta Neurochirurgica (Wien), 62:47-72.

Perret, E. (1974). The left frontal lobe of man and the suppression of habitual responses in verbal categorical behaviour. Neuropsychologia, 12:323-30.

Petrides, M. (1987). Conditional learning and the primate frontal cortex. In: Perecman, E. (ed). The frontal lobes revisited. New York: IRBN Press, 91-108.

Pisa, M., and Fibiger, H.C. (1983). Evidence against a role of the rat's dorsal noradrenergic bundle in selective attention and place memory. Brain Research, 272:319-29.

Povlishock, J.T., Becker, D.P., Cheng, C.L.Y., and Vaughan, G.W. (1983). Axonal changes in minor head injury. Journal of Neuropathology and Experimental Neurology, 42:225-42.

Powers, W.T. (1973). Behavior: The control of perception. Chicago: Aldine.

Pribram, K.H. (1971). Languages of the brain: Experimental paradoxes and principles in neuropsychology. Englewood Cliffs, NJ: Prentice Hall.

Prigatano, G.P. (1987). Psychiatric aspects of head injury: Problem areas and suggested guidelines for research. In: Levin, H.S., Grafman, J., and Eisenberg, H.M. (eds). Neurobehavioral recovery from head injury. New York: Oxford University Press, 215-31.

Rizzo, P.A., Amabile, G., Caporali, M., et al. (1978). A CNV study in a group of patients with traumatic head injuries. Electroencephalography and Clinical Neurophysiology, 45:281-85.

Robinson, M.F., and Freeman, W. (1954). Psychosurgery and the self. New York: Grune and Stratton.

Ruff, R.M., Baser, C.A., Johnson, J.W., et al. (1989). Neuropsychological rehabilitation: An experimental study with head injured patients. Journal of Head Trauma Rehabilitation, 4:20-36.

Sekino, H., Nakamura, N., Yuki, K., Satoh, J., Kikuchi, K., and Sanada, S. (1981). Brain lesions detected by CT scans in cases of minor head injuries. Neurologica Medico-Chirurgica, 21:677-83.

Shallice, T. (1988). From neuropsychology to mental structure. Cambridge: Cambridge University Press.

Shallice, T., and Burgess, P.W. (1991). Higher-order cognitive impairments and frontal-lobe lesions in man. In: Levin, H., Eisenberg, H.M., and Benton, A.L. (eds). Frontal lobe function and injury. Oxford: Oxford University Press.

Shiffrin, R.M., and Schneider, W. (1977). Controlled and automatic human information processing, II. Perceptual learning, automatic attending, and a general theory. Psychological Review, 84:127-90.

Simon, H. (1981). Neurones dopaminergiques A10 et systeme frontal. Journal of Physiology (Paris), 77:81-95.

Slater, E., and Roth, M. (1969). Clinical psychiatry (3rd ed). Baltimore: Williams and Wilkins.

Sohlberg, M.M., White, O., Evans, E., and Mateer, C.A. (1991a). Background and initial case studies into the effects of prospective memory training. Brain Injury, 5:129-38.

Sohlberg, M.M., White, O., Evans, E., and Mateer, C.A. (1991b). An investigation of the effects of prospective memory training. Brain Injury, 5:139-54.

Sohlberg, M.M., and Geyer, S. (1986). Executive Function Behavioral Rating Scale. Paper presented at Whittier College Conference Series, Whittier, CA.

Sohlberg, M.M., and Mateer, C.A. (1989b). Training use of compensatory memory books: A three stage behavioral approach. Journal of Clinical and Experimental Neuropsychology, 11:871-91.

Sohlberg, M.M., and Mateer, C.A. (1989a). Introduction to cognitive rehabilitation: Theory and practice. New York: Guilford Press, 232-63.

Sohlberg, M.M., Sprunk, H., and Metzelaar, K. (1988). Efficacy of an external cuing system in an individual with severe frontal lobe damage. Cognitive Rehabilitation, 6:36-41.

Stuss, D.T. (1987). Contribution of frontal lobe injury to cognitive impairment after closed head injury: Methods of assessment and recent findings. In: Levin, H.S., Grafman, J., and Eisenberg, H.M. (eds). Neurobehavioral recovery from head injury. New York: Oxford University Press, 166-77.

Stuss, D.T. (1991a). Disturbance of self-awareness after frontal system damage. In: Prigatano, G., and Schacter, D. (eds). Awareness of deficit after brain injury. New York: Oxford University Press, 63-83.

Stuss, D.T. (1991b). Self, awareness and the frontal lobes: A neuropsychological perspective. In: Goethals, G.R., and Strauss, J. (eds). The self: An interdisciplinary approach. New York: Springer-Verlag.

Stuss, D.T. (1992). Biological and psychological development of "frontal" executive functions. Brain and Cognition, 20:8–23.

Stuss, D.T., and Benson, D.F. (1986). The frontal lobes. Raven Press: New York.

Stuss, D.T., Benson, D.F., Kaplan, E.F., Weir, W.S., and Della Malva, C. (1981). Leukotomized and nonleukotomized schizophrenics: Comparison on tests of attention. Biological Psychiatry, 16:1085–1100.

Stuss, D.T., Delgado, M., and Guzman, D.A. (1987). Verbal regulation in the control of motor impersistence: A proposed rehabilitation procedure. Journal of Neurologic Rehabilitation, 1:1–6.

Stuss, D.T., Ely, P., Hugenholtz, H., et al. (1985). Subtle neuropsychological deficits in patients with good recovery after closed head injury. Neurosurgery, 17:41–47.

Stuss, D.T., and Gow, C.A. (1992). Frontal dysfunction after traumatic brain injury. Neuropsychiatry, Neuropsychology, and Behavioural Neurology, 5(4):272–82.

Stuss, D.T., Stethem, L.L., Hugenholtz, H., Picton, T., Pivik, J., and Richard, M.T. (1989). Reaction time after head injury: Fatigue, divided and focused attention, and consistency of performance. Journal of Neurology, Neurosurgery, and Psychiatry, 52:742–48.

Tanaka, D. (1974). Sparing of an escape response following serial prefrontal decortication in the monkey. Brain Research 54:195–201.

Tanaka, D. (1973). Effects of selective prefrontal decortication on escape behavior in the monkey. Brain Research, 53:161–73.

Tecce, J. (1977). Electrical brain activity (Contingent Negative Variation) and related neuropsychological functions. In: Appendix Psychosurgery. The National Commission for the Protection of Human Subjects of Biomedical and Behavioral Research. Washington, DC: DHEW Publication No. (OS) 77-0002, II-44–II-64.

Teuber, H.L. (1964). The riddle of frontal lobe function in man. In: Warren, J.M., and Akert, K. (eds). The frontal granular cortex and behavior. New York: McGraw-Hill, 410–44.

von Cramon, D.Y., and Matthes-von Cramon, G. (1990). Frontal lobe dysfunction in patients—Theoretical approaches. In: Wood, R.L., and Fussey, I. (eds). Cognitive rehabilitation in perspective. London: Taylor and Francis.

Vygotsky, L.S. (1962). Thought and language (Hanfmann, E., and Vakar, G. eds and transl). Cambridge, MA: MIT Press.

Walsh, K. (1987). Neuropsychology. A clinical approach (2nd ed). Edinburgh: Churchill Livingstone.

Walter, W.G. (1973). Human frontal lobe function in sensory-motor association. In: Pribram, K.H., and Luria, A.R. (eds). Psychophysiology of the frontal lobes. New York: Academic Press, 109–22.

Wilson, B., Cockburn, J., and Baddeley, A. (1985). The Rivermead behavioral memory test. Reading, England: Thames Valley Test Company.

Ylvisaker, M., and Szekeres, S.F. (1989). Metacognitive and executive impairments in head-injured children and adults. Topics in Language Disorders, 9:34–49.

Zatorre, R.J., and McEntee, W.J. (1983). Semantic encoding in a case of traumatic amnesia. Brain and Cognition, 2:331–45.

11

Information Technology and Brain Injury Rehabilitation

KENNETH W. DUNN

In the past decade we have witnessed an unprecedented technological revolution. In particular, technology involving "the mechanical processing of information" (Soede, 1989, p. 5) has become an integral part of modern life. The best example of this new information technology is the microcomputer. With its technological sophistication and availability to the point where it is a common and accepted appliance at both work and home.

There are many advantages in the use of microcomputers. There is also a tendency for society to view technology as a cure. Consequently, the potential of microcomputers has been overestimated and their application oversimplified (Vanderheiden, 1983). This is particularly evident in the field of rehabilitation where this technology has become increasingly employed in both physical and cognitive assessment and treatment, communication, education, vocational training, and environmental control (Burkehead, Sampson, and McMahon, 1986; Links and Frydenberg, 1989; Soede, 1989).

There is a general belief that the use of microcomputers has increased the quality of life of handicapped people especially in terms of independence (Soede, 1989). However, as with many new realms of endeavor, there are few models to guide systematic application of this technology and little empirical evidence to support its effectiveness. Although microcomputers may be a helpful adjunct to the rehabilitation process (Links and Frydenberg, 1989), there is a need for both theoretical models capable of guiding the use of technology in rehabilitation, and a systematic empirical research program capable of evaluating those efforts.

REHABILITATION AND TECHNOLOGY

Rehabilitation involves the alleviation of impairment, disability, and/or handicap (World Health Organization, 1980). Impairment refers to underlying physical or psychologic deficits; disability describes the behavioral effect of impairment; and handicap refers to the subsequent impact on role performance (World Health Organization, 1980). Effective rehabilitation requires an understanding of the relationship among impairment, disability, and handicap. One model which can assist in this regard involves the concept of person-environment fit (Coulton, 1984). In terms of this concept, the goal of rehabilitation is to maximize congruence between the individual's needs, abilities, and aspirations, and the demands, resources, and opportunities of the environment (Coulton, 1984, p. 120).

As such, impairment and disability will result in handicap only when environmental demands exceed the individual's capacity to cope with such demands (Coulton, 1984). Taken to the extreme, it has been argued that handicap is nothing more than environmental artifact (Goldenberg, 1979). Although this position overstates the case by minimizing the role of impairment and disability, it serves to highlight the importance of matching the environment to the needs of the person in the process of rehabilitation.

Human-machine systems (Chapanis, 1965) describe a specific application of the person-environment fit approach to rehabilitation whereby technology is conceptualized as a highly complex, mechanized aspect of the environment. Interactions between the person and technology can be conceptualized, like in any other system, as a process of input, processing, output, and feedback (Boulding, 1968).

There are two important practical implications of the human-machine systems model. First, a distinction must be drawn between machine-assisted and machine-dependent approaches to the use of technology in rehabilitation (Dunn, 1988a, b). The machine-assisted approach involves the temporary use of technology to reduce the impairments which can lead to disability and handicap. On the other hand, the machine-dependent approach involves a relatively permanent application of technology to accommodate impairment.

One example of a machine-assisted approach is cognitive rehabilitation of attentional deficits. The goal here is to develop machine-independent attentional skills which will generalize to activities of daily living. One would question whether attention had truly improved if such skills were manifest only during microcomputer use. On the other hand, use of a digital speech synthesizer with a nonvocal person illustrates a machine-dependent approach. There is no expectation that independent speech will be restored through use of the technology. Rather, it is assumed that any speech produced will depend on the technology in use.

Secondly, a machine-dependent approach may or may not address the issues of disability and handicap as effectively as a machine-assisted approach since the underlying impairment will not have been dealt with in the former. The success with which a machine-dependent approach deals with disability and handicap also depends on the social acceptance of technological dependency in the fulfillment of a person's adaptive behavioral and role expectations. Although attitudes toward the handicapped have improved markedly, there is still some perception of technological dependence as abnormal. This is evident when one considers the reaction a person using an electronic voice may encounter.

For the reasons outlined above, it makes clinical sense to attempt a machine-assisted approach prior to implementation of a machine-dependent one. This would ensure that human capabilities develop as fully and independently as possible, increasing the chance of impairment reduction, and minimizing unnecessary technological dependence (Burkehead, et al., 1986; Dunn, 1988a, b). On the other hand, there are situations in which technological dependence is unavoidable. Therefore, efforts should be maintained to enhance the social acceptance of technological dependence as a strategy for the reduction of disability and handicap.

APPLICATIONS TO BRAIN INJURY REHABILITATION
Physical Rehabilitation

In general, the application of information technologies is more established in physical rehabilitation than it is in other areas, for example, the field of biofeedback. Biofeedback therapy has been helpful in the treatment of paralysis due to head injury and stroke (Brucker, 1984). The application of microcomputers in biofeedback has been extensive. The interested reader is referred to treatments of the subject by Brucker (1984) and Ince (1988). However, the advantages of incorporating technology in this area have been described as the provision of more sophisticated auditory and visual feedback, more accurate data collection and analysis, as well as an increased ability to tailor treatment programs to individual patient needs (Ince, 1988). In other words, the use of microcomputers in biofeedback has facilitated the process of person-environment fit in rehabilitation.

Microcomputers have also been used in the assessment and treatment of hemiplegic gait (Bogataj, 1989; Wall and Turnbull, 1986). Bogataj (1989) utilized a microcomputer-based multichannel functional electrical stimulator to improve gait in 20 patients with severe hemiplegia secondary to either stroke or head injury. Although further study is required in order to compare this approach with traditional physical therapy, the author suggests that one advantage of microcomputer-based systems is the capability for complex multichannel signal processing (Bogataj, 1989).

Another area where microcomputers are beginning to be utilized is in neurodiagnosis. Recent technological advances have allowed the clinician greater access to evoked potential and electroencephalographic (EEG) data. In addition, it has been suggested that computerized quantification and mapping techniques for EEG may allow more accurate neurologic diagnoses in brain injury (MacCrimmon, Finlayson, Mosher, and Garner, 1991; Randolph and Miller, 1988; Thatch, Gerson, and Geisler, 1989).

Visual Neglect

Disturbances of perception are often encountered in brain injury (Bond, 1986; Rosenthal, et al., 1990). One common perceptual impairment is unilateral visual neglect. Microcomputer-based assessment and rehabilitation of this impairment has now been evaluated in a number of empirical studies. Dick, Wood, Bradshaw, and Bradshaw (1987), studied the effectiveness of a computerized display unit in the treatment of unilateral visual neglect. Although no conclusive data were presented, the authors suggest that such an approach might be helpful.

Using an uncontrolled single-case design, Halligan and Marshall (1989) compared computerized and noncomputerized horizontal line bisection task performance as assessment methods for left visual neglect in a 49-year-old woman who had sustained a right hemisphere aneurysm. The subject's performance was more accurate on the computer task. The authors suggest this greater accuracy is due to the computer's ability to introduce visual cues linked to the nature of the task performance (i.e., the cursor). They further suggest that use of the computer in this manner may be helpful in the rehabilitation of neglect although no data are presented.

Robertson, Gray, Pentland, and Waite (1990), compared the effectiveness of computerized versus noncomputerized applications of Weinberg's approach to visual neglect rehabilitation (Weinberg, Diller, and Gordon, 1977). The subjects were 36 patients with brain injury, mainly due to stroke and head injury. Improvements were found in both treatment groups; however, there were no significant differences between computerized and noncomputerized approaches immediately after treatment or at a 6-month follow-up. Although the authors acknowledge that several patient, therapist, and therapy variables require further investigations in this area, they conclude that there is no evidence for the superiority of the computerized approach.

Therefore, although there have been suggestions that the use of microcomputers can assist in the rehabilitation of unilateral visual neglect (Dick, et al., 1987; Halligan and Marshall, 1989), there is no conclusive evidence that computerized therapy is superior to noncomputerized approaches.

Communication

Communication disorders involving motor, speech, and cognitive impairments often result from brain injury (Soede, 1989; Ylvisaker, this volume). Due to the importance of communication abilities in social interaction and acceptance, rehabilitation in this area must be considered a high priority in brain injury. Information technologies such as the microcomputer offer two distinct advantages in the rehabilitation of communication-speed and flexibility. Information can be rapidly translated from one sensory modality to another and flexible user-specific symbol systems can be quickly developed (Fairhurst and Stephanidis, 1989). In other words, computer technology capitalizes on the interaction between information processing capabilities and symbol form, facilitating the process of person-symbol matching, a specific example of person-environment fit.

The development and use of digital speech synthesizers has had a significant impact on the communication possibilities available to individuals with speech impairments (Soede, 1989). However, despite the fact that inexpensive and functional digital speech synthesizers are readily available for microcomputers (Romanczyk, 1986), the rate of speech production remains unacceptably low, a problem which has prompted the observation that devices capable of approximating normal speech production are yet to be developed (Desch, 1986; Soede, 1989). The problem is primarily one of slow input speed due to motor impairments. Communication rates of 3 words per minute are not uncommon (Soede, van Balkom, Deroost, van Knippenberg, and Kamphuis, 1989).

Several methods of input interface modification have been employed to deal with this problem. Soede, et al. (1989), describe the development of a combined hardware-software system capable of "reducing linguistic redundancy" (Soede, 1989, p. 5) by predicting subsequent characters, words, and phrases from existing input. In this way, speed of communication has been increased by 50% (Soede, et al., 1989). Apart from the advantages of increased rate of communication, the authors suggest that this approach can reduce the conscious effort required for motor performance, an effort which may interfere with cognitive processes (Soede, et al., 1989).

The use of artificial intelligence software in the design of communication systems may also hold promise in increasing the rate of symbol production. Predictive natural language processing software may be capable of translating minimal cues into complex communicative structures (Soede, 1989). This is a potential and speculative future application. Even so, microcomputers with speech output have already been found effective in language learning (Rosegrant, 1985).

Another promising application of technology in the area of communication is that of voice recognition (Bowe, 1984). Even persons capable of producing the most primitive speech sounds could utilize user-dependent voice recognition systems to communicate and control various aspects of their environment. In contrast to user-independent systems, the former are capable of "learning" and responding to the specific voice patterns of their users.

Although microcomputer-based communication aids have been used extensively in the past several years, there is little research in the area. Colquhoun, McNaughton, Wilson, and Izzard (1981), compared the effectiveness of microcomputers with that of more traditional dedicated communication aids and obtained support for the superiority of microcomputers due to their increased flexibility. However, the relative lack of portability has remained a problem limiting the use of microcomputers as communication aids. Furthermore, software capable of utilizing both digitized speech output and voice recognition systems to assess and remediate language production and formulation is only now in the process of development (Johnson and Stonell-Thomas, 1989).

Communication disorders in brain injury can also be due to cognitive as opposed to strictly speech or motoric impairments (Story and Sbordone, 1988). Aphasias for example comprise a family of disorders involving impaired expressive and/or receptive communication due to damage in areas associated with cognition and language. In addition, problems with communication may also be due primarily to underlying cognitive impairments in attention, memory, and executive functions (Story and Sbordone, 1988).

The complexity of cognitive-communication assessment and analysis systems in brain injury rehabilitation has often limited their clinical feasibility. However, the development of computerized communication systems has allowed for the cost effective analysis of communication patterns in aphasia and a method of assessing treatment effects (Merbitz, Grip, Harper, Mogil, Cherney, and Bellaire, 1989). These authors describe a computerized system which can analyze the pragmatics of speech in brain injury, resulting in "cost effective clinical decision making and effective application of appropriate treatment techniques" (Merbitz, et al., 1989, p. 120).

Using a series of 5 single-case experimental designs, Steele, Seinrich, Wertz, Kleczewska, and Carlson (1989), evaluated the ability of patients with aphasia, due to head injury or stroke, to use an icon-based computerized communication system. They compared performance on the computerized system with a similar noncomputerized paper and pencil system (Gardner, Zurif, Berry, and Baker, 1976). Response times were faster and there was less variability of performance on the computer as compared with the traditional approach. There were also less errors, a wider variety of communicative behaviors, and more creative use of communication strategies using the computer. Finally, more independence in communication was facilitated by the computerized approach since subjects did not require as much therapist assistance and could take their computers home (Steele, et al., 1989). The authors conclude that patients with severe chronic aphasia can quickly learn to master use of an icon-based computer interface.

There is some preliminary evidence to suggest that microcomputer-based technology may be beneficial in the assessment and rehabilitation of communication disorders in brain injury, although there is clearly a need for more research in this area.

Neuropsychologic Assessment and Diagnosis

The use of microcomputer-based technology in neuropsychologic assessment and diagnosis has become commonplace in the past few years. Three major areas of application can be identified: 1) Scoring, data analysis, and test interpretation; 2) development of computer-based test formats; and 3) expert systems.

Scoring, Data Analysis, and Test Interpretation

Although the least complex from a technological perspective, the use of microcomputers in the scoring and preliminary analysis of psychologic test data is the most common, and perhaps most promising (Adams and Brown, 1986), application of technology in psychologic assessment. The use of computers can increase both the reliability and rapidity of repetitive task performance since computers are, by design, fast and precise (Adams and Brown, 1986; Meehl, 1973).

Such repetitive tasks include scoring, calculation of indices and quotients, flagging of critical item responses, and statistical calculations. On the other hand, computerized test interpretation requires a more cautious approach (American Psychological Association, 1986). Although several software programs available can produce preliminary interpretive reports (Adams, 1975; Adams and Heaton, 1985), in the final analysis, the process must always be guided by the clinician.

Computer-Based Assessment Formats

Clinicians have become increasingly concerned about the appropriateness of using psychologic tests with persons having severe physical disabilities. Because most conventional tests require intact speech and motor skills, the danger is that of "confounding motor and cognitive impairments" (Wilson and McMillan, 1986, p. 1445). The perils of such confounding are underscored by consideration of the following patient perspective:

I rusted away in St. Nicholas until Rosemary showed me that some people did know our helpless bodies could contain a mind, even if she did not realize we would be normal. However, just being thought of as an animal, not a vegetable, was reason for hope (Crossley and McDonald, 1982, p. 37).

Microcomputers provide one possible method of overcoming these problems, especially through the use of speech synthesizers and input interfaces which require minimal motor capabilities. For example, Wilson and McMillan (1986) have developed a computerized neuropsychologic test battery which they claim has been used successfully with over 150 patients who would otherwise have been untestable.

In addition, the precision and control with which test stimuli can be presented has spawned a great deal of interest in the development of computer-based neuropsychologic test formats (Baker, Letz, and Fidler, 1985; Fowler, 1985; Hofer and Green, 1985; Laursen, 1990; Wilson and McMillan, 1986). This has primarily involved the adaptation of existing paper and pencil measures to a computer-based format or the development of new tests designed specifically for the computer environment.

The adaptation of existing psychologic tests to a computer-based format presents a number of problems. Computer versions of existing paper and pencil measures do not automatically conform to accepted technical and psychometric standards (American Psychological Association, 1986). A number of factors may alter the reliability and validity of computerized tests including differences in item presentation mode and timing, task and recording requirements, ability to skip items, and typing or computer skills (Adams and Brown, 1986; Jackson, 1985; Moreland, 1985).

Given the potential for differences between traditional and computer-based assessment methods, it is somewhat surprising to find the results of preliminary studies providing support for equivalence of forms in a wide variety of psychologic tests including the MMPI (Biskin and Kolotkin, 1977; Harrell, Honaker, Hetu, and Oberwager, 1987; Hofer and Green, 1985; Lambert, Andrews, Rylee, and Skinner, 1987; Russell, Peace, and Mellsop, 1986; White, Clements, and Fowler, 1985). More process-oriented assessment methods such as those involved in neuropsychology, however, may be more sensitive to changes as a function of format translation to the microcomputer environment.

Another interesting finding in relation to computer-based assessments is a more positive patient perception of the process (Adams and Brown, 1986; Lambert, et al., 1987; Laursen, 1990). This reported acceptance of computer-based testing formats by those being tested is in contrast to the hypothesis that computers are perceived as cold and dehumanizing (Weizenbaum, 1976). One possible explanation may be that as our societies have moved into the information age, technophobia is gradually being replaced by trust in the reliability and power of computers. Along these lines, Laursen (1990) suggests that the use of computers in neuropsychologic assessment may enhance the public perception of such an endeavor as important and scientific.

Other potential advantages of computer-based neuropsychologic assessment are the enhanced freedom of the psychologist to observe process-oriented variables during the assessment and the increased potential for standardized administration. However, the ethics of computer-based psychologic assessment must be carefully examined, as with the introduction of any new technology. The guidelines published by the American Psychological Association (1986) seek to ensure that the standards relevant to traditional tests will also apply to computer-based formats.

Expert Systems

One of the most promising and controversial applications of information technology in neuropsychologic diagnosis and assessment may be the expert system. Such systems, which have emerged from the field of artificial intelligence, seek to replicate the results of clinical decision making. At present, this type of software is quite limited in its utility. As such, its use presents another challenge for the clinician to maintain ultimate responsibility and decision making when interpreting results generated by expert systems.

In general, three approaches to the use of expert systems in neuropsychologic diagnosis have been identified (Adams and Brown, 1986). The taxonomic approach places the patient within some existing classification scheme using known diagnostic criteria. One example of this approach is the early system designed by Russell, Neuringer, and Goldstein (1970), which demonstrated good agreement with human experts.

A second method is primarily statistical in nature. This involves matching patient data with models of brain function. Diagnosis or assessment is accomplished statistically using goodness-of-fit criteria. Unfortunately, the complex mathematic models used often exhibit limited practical utility from a clinical perspective (Adams and Brown, 1986).

Finally, some expert systems seek to model the cognitive activity of the clinician. Some early attempts were the BRAIN 1 program by Finklestein (1976), and Adams' Revised Program (Adams, 1975). In general, these expert systems were inadequate. Although cerebral dysfunction could be identified, specifics regarding lateralization, localization, and severity could not be identified. Although recent attempts (e.g., Plugge, Verhey, and Jolles, 1990) have continued to improve the differential diagnostic capabilities of expert systems, this area requires much more development before it will find a place in everyday clinical practice.

Cognitive Rehabilitation

The extent to which the brain-injured individual can recover from or compensate for cognitive impairments remains an open question (Prigatano, 1986; Zangwill, 1947; Fordyce, this volume). The term spontaneous recovery usually refers to improved brain function as a result of neurologic factors. On the other hand, cognitive rehabilitation describes environmental strategies designed to facilitate such improvement (Sohlberg and Mateer, 1989).

The use of microcomputers in cognitive rehabilitation has become established practice in the United States, Canada, Great Britain, Australia, and other developed countries. In fact, the large majority of clinical centers providing cognitive rehabilitation to the brain-injured employ microcomputers (Bracy, 1986).

Historically, commercially available computer games were among the first software programs to be used in computerized cognitive rehabilitation (Wilson and McMillan, 1986; Wood, 1984). Although game mastery involves many of the cognitive skills which are likely to require rehabilitation following brain injury (Finlayson, et al., 1987), an increasing selection of programs developed specifically for the purpose of cognitive rehabilitation are now available (Bracy, 1984, 1990; Sandford and Browne, 1986; Skilbeck, 1984; Smith, 1984). A comprehensive list, with supplier addresses can be found in Sohlberg and Mateer (1989).

Rehabilitation professionals have clearly embraced the application of technology in this area of clinical practice. Such overwhelming acceptance begs the question—What evidence exists for the efficacy of computerized cognitive rehabilitation? In this regard, a number of studies have evaluated the effect of this treatment on a variety of diverse cognitive functions.

Using Reitan's REHABIT model (Reitan Evaluation of Hemispheric Ability and Brain Improvement Training; Reitan, 1979) as a guide, Finlayson, et al. (1987), evaluated the effectiveness of computerized cognitive rehabilitation employing a single case study. Their results were encouraging in that neuropsychologic test performance improved as a result of training a number of cognitive skill areas. Similar results were found by Ethier, Braun, and Baribeau (1989a, b) using a controlled group design. Batchelor and colleagues (Batchelor, et al., 1988), at Westmead Hospital in Australia, also utilized a controlled group design to compare both computerized and noncomputerized cognitive rehabilitation. The effect on a number of cognitive skills including attention, memory, and problem solving was examined. Although both groups improved as a function of training, there was no significant difference found between computerized and noncomputerized cognitive rehabilitation.

In addition to the more general studies mentioned above, a number of investigators have chosen to focus on specific cognitive functions. In particular, the efficacy of computer-based cognitive rehabilitation has been examined in relation to attentional skills and memory.

Attentional Skills

Deficits in attention are common following brain injury (Ponsford and Kinsella, 1988; Van Zomeren, 1981). Therefore, it is not surprising to find that a number of studies have focused their efforts at computerized cognitive rehabilitation specifically in this area. Furthermore, the importance of attentional skills in cognition is understood if a hierarchical model is adopted. Such models view attention as a foundation skill, one that other skills, such as memory and problem solving, are based upon (Ponsford and Kinsella, 1988; Sohlberg and Mateer, 1989).

Ponsford and Kinsella (1988) compared computerized attentional training with and without therapist feedback and reinforcement in 15 closed-head injured patients in the spontaneous recovery phase. Controlled single-case experimental designs were utilized. Although subjects' attentional skills improved in both conditions, spontaneous recovery could not be ruled out as an explanatory factor. Based on the results of their study, the authors concluded that there was little evidence to suggest that attentional skills improved as a function of either computerized treatment. Malec, Jones, Rao, and Stubbs (1984), have also reported negative results in this area.

On the other hand, positive results have been found by a number of investigators (Baribeau, Ethier, and Braun, 1989; Gray and Robertson, 1988; Skinner and Trachtman, 1985; Sohlberg and Mateer, 1989). Skinner and Trachtman (1985) found improvements in attentional skills in a subject with acquired brain injury, utilizing an uncontrolled single-case research design. Sohlberg and Mateer (1989) found similar results using a series of controlled single-case designs.

Using a group experimental design, Gray and Robertson (1988) found evidence for the superiority of a microcomputer-based approach to the rehabilitation of attentional skills in brain injury. Also using a group experimental design, Baribeau, et al. (1989), examined the effects of computerized cognitive rehabilitation on selective attention in closed-head injury patients using auditory event related potentials (ERP) as a dependent variable. Improvements on ERP measures as a function of computerized cognitive rehabilitation were attributed to "improved motivation, more effort, and better capacity to follow experimental instructions" (Baribeau, et al., p. 91), as opposed to improvement in selective attentional mechanisms. Skinner and Trachtman (1985) also found improvements in motivation which could, in part, explain the increases in attention found.

The equivocal results in this area of computerized cognitive rehabilitation have been attributed to differences in the definition and measurement of attentional skills, as well as various treatment and patient parameters (Ponsford and Kinsella, 1988). Although more research is required in order to clarify the mechanisms involved, the research to date suggests that the remediation of attentional skills may be one of the more promising areas of computerized cognitive rehabilitation.

Memory

Memory impairments are one of the most common and devastating consequences of brain injury (Glisky, Schacter, and Tulving, 1986). Although a few studies have reported positive results in this area (see review by Lynch, 1988), direct rehabilitation of memory or mnemonic function itself has generally been considered untenable (Glisky, et al., 1986; Miller, 1978; Sohlberg and Mateer, 1989). Instead, it has been suggested that microcomputers may be helpful as a technological memory prosthesis for individuals with memory impairments (Glisky, et al., 1986; Harris, 1984; Skilbeck, 1984). In this regard, spared cognitive abilities might be utilized in teaching domain-specific knowledge, for example, how to use a microcomputer. Use of the computer, in turn, may assist the memory-impaired individual in the storage and retrieval of information pertinent to daily living (Glisky, et al., 1986).

Using the method of vanishing cues, where the letters of instructional words are gradually faded, Glisky, et al. (1986), found that individuals with memory impairments could successfully retain computer-related vocabulary and learn to use microcomputers. The question remains, however, as to the extent microcomputer usage was helpful in itself.

Giles and Shore (1989) examined the effectiveness of a microcomputer-based memory prosthesis with a brain-injured adult with normal intelligence and a severe memory impairment. Eighteen months postinjury, a single-case experimental design was utilized to compare the effectiveness of a pocket diary with that of an electronic organizer on functional task performance. The electronic organizer was found to be superior in that a greater number of functional tasks were performed when it was used. This effect was attributed primarily to an alarm feature on this device. The authors suggest that microcomputerized organizers may be helpful in compensating for memory impairments by increasing functional task performance in brain-injured adults with average intelligence, executive skills, and motivation (Giles and Shore, 1989).

Methodological Consideration

The results obtained thus far are inconclusive with respect to the efficacy of computer-based cognitive rehabilitation. This is likely due to a number of variables. First, it would appear that the effectiveness of such treatment may be process-specific. That is, certain cognitive processes such as attentional skills may respond more than others such as mnemonic function. In addition, a number of other patient and therapeutic variables may have an impact on computer-based cognitive rehabilitation. For example, it may be that certain patient variables are more amenable to change than others. Post-onset time, location, and extent of brain damage, and length of time in coma have all been suggested as patient variables which could influence the outcome of computerized cognitive rehabilitation (Ethier, et al., 1989a, b).

In addition, a number of therapeutic variables require consideration (Ethier, et al., 1989; Prigatano, Fordyce, Zeiker, Roueche, Pepping, and Case-Wood, 1984). The vast array of software being utilized underscores the need for an integrative conceptual framework to guide computerized cognitive rehabilitation efforts and allow for the categorization of software in terms of specific cognitive functions. Several practical models of brain function have been proposed for this purpose (Armstrong, 1989; Bracy, 1986; Finlayson, et al., 1987; Sohlberg and Mateer, 1989). Furthermore, it is important that software be matched to individual patient needs. In this regard, Shaw and McKenna (1989) have developed a simple framework which allows for the evaluation of software in terms of the cognitive skills required by the patient.

Not only is the content of therapy important but the process by which it is delivered requires consideration as well. Little is known about the frequency, duration, and timing variables which might contribute to the effectiveness of computerized cognitive rehabilitation (Ethier, et al., 1989a, b). The context within which therapy is provided also requires further investigation. Effective therapy necessitates that the therapist do more than just sit the patient down in front of the computer (Sohlberg and Mateer, 1989). Instead, the microcomputer should be viewed as a tool which augments, but does not replace traditional forms of therapy (Finlayson, et al., 1987). The use of this technology in rehabilitation must be viewed within the context of good clinical practice. As such, the therapeutic relationship is very important, and the practice of computerized cognitive rehabilitation should involve appreciation for a comprehensive systems or biopsychosocial approach.

This systematic examination of patient and therapeutic variables must be conducted within the context of adequate research designs. Much of the research on computerized cognitive rehabilitation to date has lacked adequate control, whether single-case or group designs were used. As a result, alternative explanations for patient change, such as spontaneous recovery or therapist attention cannot always be ruled out. In addition, more studies are required to compare computerized and noncomputerized cognitive rehabilitation to investigate what, if any, specific advantages might be found with computers. These goals can be best achieved through a coordinated, multicenter effort, due to the inherent complexity of brain injury and the subsequent need to study large groups of subjects.

Despite the promise of impairment reduction, the research to date would suggest that microcomputers are more effective as cognitive prostheses (Lynch, 1990; Matthews, Harley and Malec, 1990). This prosthetic application of technology can be conceptualized within the context of a machine-dependent approach (Dunn, 1988a, b), whereby the permanent application of technology seeking to accommodate impairment may have more utility in the reduction of disability and handicap as opposed to the alleviation of impairment per se. This is the thrust behind the current movement to train compensatory skills in cognitive rehabilitation. Nonetheless, the search for ways to reduce impairment must be continued. In this regard, the most promising area to date would appear to involve the remediation of attentional skills.

Finally, in evaluating the outcome of cognitive rehabilitation, it is important to consider not only the effect on cognitive skills, but also generalization to activities of daily living, and maintenance over time (Ben-Yishay, 1983; Ethier, et al., 1989a, b; Finlayson, et al., 1987; Prigatano, et al., 1984; Scherzer, 1986).

Microcomputers and Living Skills

In addition to specific therapeutic uses such as cognitive rehabilitation, microcomputers and related technology may facilitate the brain-injured individual's ability to accomplish many of the same daily living activities as they did prior to their injury. This technology may also provide an opportunity to develop new life skills. For example, learning to use a microcomputer is in itself becoming an increasingly important life skill. Therefore, it is not surprising to find that rehabilitation programs are focusing on teaching computer literacy, word processing, data entry, spreadsheet, and programming skills to their clients (Links and Frydenberg, 1989; Soede, 1989).

Microcomputers may also assist brain-injured individuals in the acquisition of academic skills. A common application in this regard is use of the computer as a writing aid (Soede, 1989). One potential benefit is increased employment opportunities (Glisky, et al., 1986) since computers have become a fixture in the office environment (Soede, 1989).

Links and Frydenberg (1989) examined the effects of teaching microcomputer skills on vocational activity in a single individual who sustained a severe brain injury. Although the subject's ability to perform avocational activities using the microcomputer improved, no change in vocational activity was found. The authors conclude that although competitive employment may not be a realistic goal for those with severe impairments, the "quality of life during extended hospitalization is enhanced" (Links and Frydenberg, 1989, p. 139) by using microcomputers. It should be kept in mind that this is one study involving only one subject, utilizing an uncontrolled design.

Information technology may also be used by the brain-injured individual to directly control various aspects of the physical environment, thus increasing the possibility of more independent living (Desch, 1986; Soede, 1989). For example, environmental control systems capable of operating any household appliance including televisions, radios, telephones, doors, windows, and security systems (Romanczyk, 1980; Soede, 1989) have been widely used by quadriplegics for several years. Such technology may allow more independent living for brain-injured individuals whose residual impairments are primarily physical in nature.

Microprocessor controlled robotics may also be helpful in environmental control in some cases (Soede, 1989). Robotics may play an especially important role in the cognitive development of brain-injured children. To the extent that action is important in cognitive development (Inhelder, 1980; Piaget, 1970), a reduced ability to interact with 3-dimensional objects may further impede the brain-injured child's ability for continued cognitive development. Interaction with microcomputers may be helpful, but the computer screen is limited in the information it can convey since it is only 2-dimensional in nature. Recent work on the development of an "intelligent end-effector" (Gosine, Harwin, Furby, and Jackson, 1989, p. 37) robot holds promise in terms of providing brain-injured children with 3-dimensional feedback about their environments. The robot incorporates a design which allows the provision of complex sensory feedback to the operator.

The telecommunications capabilities of microcomputers, as exemplified by modems and networks, can be utilized for the purposes of telebanking, shopping, and social interaction. It is possible that this type of "telecommunication enhances the desire to make contact and, therefore, enhances mobility" (Soede, 1989, p. 6). Also, in relation to mobility, microcomputerized systems for the assessment of wheelchair and automobile driving skills have been developed (Ranu, 1986). In addition, microprocessors are increasingly being used in wheelchairs (Soede, 1989). The advent of smart wheelchairs capable of being programmed to accommodate to the motor impairments of their drivers may be a viable future application. This could result in increased accuracy and safety, greater mobility, and thus increased independence.

In summary, there are many microcomputer applications which have the potential for increasing the independence and social integration of the brain-injured individual. However, there remains a paucity of research on the efficacy of such applications.

Administration and Program Evaluation

In addition to direct patient care applications, microcomputers are being increasingly utilized in the administration and evaluation of rehabilitation programs. An integrated microcomputerized database system for monitoring the effectiveness of patient care in rehabilitation has been developed by Sulton, Hardisty, Bisterfeldt, and Harvey (1987). In this regard, a common database is used in program evaluation, utilization review, and quality assurance, in order to document patient potential, status, progress, and outcome in an integrated fashion. Microcomputers have been used effectively for practice management as well including patient scheduling, billing, and word processing (Adams and Brown, 1986).

It is important that several nontechnical factors be taken into consideration in the development of a rehabilitation database, including the application of appropriate decision making for the selection and operationalization of variables to be included in the database. Failure to consider such factors has resulted in serious database utilization problems (Renwick, 1989).

FUTURE DIRECTIONS

Research

Since assessment and treatment protocols in brain injury rehabilitation must often be individually tailored, single-case experimental designs can be a valuable clinical research tool (Daniel, Webster, and Scott, 1986; Wilson, 1987). However, there is also a need for more controlled group experimental studies in the evaluation of microcomputers and technology in brain injury rehabilitation (Batchelor, et al., 1988; Finlayson, et al., 1987).

Due to the complexity and variability in head injury, advances in clinical research will increasingly rely on sophisticated statistical analyses which will, in themselves, require a computerized approach (Kaufman, Bretaudierre, Towlands, Stein, Bernstein, Wagner, and Gildenberg, 1989). The complexity of these variables also necessitates that a coordinated, multicenter effort is required in order to more specifically delineate the therapeutic and patient variables influencing the outcome of computerized brain injury rehabilitation (Ethier, et al., 1989b; Prigatano, et al., 1984).

Problems and Potentials

Independent of their ability in the rehabilitation process, per se, access to technology and microcomputers is becoming increasingly important for brain-injured individuals since the role of such technology is expanding in society at large (Vanderheiden, 1983). Even if microcomputers do not facilitate the process of rehabilitation, their accessibility to the brain-injured is important since society has embraced this new technology wholeheartedly. In a sense, mastery of at least some microcomputer skills has become an important adaptive behavior. Furthermore, as Olson (1976) contended, in any given culture, that which is considered intelligent behavior is dependent on the technology in use. This phenomenon was apparent during a recent open house inviting the community to visit the computerized rehabilitation program at our hospital. The sight of severely brain-injured individuals actually producing something valuable on microcomputers prompted several surprised comments about the intelligence of our patients.

Accessibility to the environment by handicapped people has been one of the major issues of the past several years. Advances have been made both architecturally, and in terms of transportation. Burkehead, et al. (1986), suggest that access to technological environments will be the next major challenge for those with handicaps. Given the increasing importance of microcomputers in our culture, it is possible to infer that integration of brain-injured persons in society will by necessity require access to technology. However, such access is hampered by a number of technological and human issues.

Technological Issues

Restricted access to technology can be an engineering problem. Microcomputers are designed for use with able minds and bodies. The physical and cognitive limitations resulting from brain injury often require modification of existing technology. Such modification is inevitably expensive and time consuming. Nonetheless, there are a wide variety of adaptive or assistive devices which have been developed and are currently in use. These can be divided into software and hardware approaches. Adapting software so that a handicapped user can use existing technology has proven to be largely unfeasible due to the great expense and effort required in order to individually tailor software to each unique user (Burkehead, et al., 1986; Vanderheiden, 1983). However, advances in the flexibility of software have allowed for the reevaluation of such an approach. Modifications involving speed of program execution, screen attributes, and the user interface can be made by the user without knowledge of computer programming. For example, it is possible to insert visual and auditory cues, change the complexity and location of pull down menus and reconfigure keyboard layouts to meet the user's special needs (Lynch, 1990).

Hardware modification has also proven to be an effective approach to the access problem. In general, this involves attempts to create hardware interfaces which are software transparent (Burkehead, et al., 1986; Vanderheiden, 1983). That is, hardware capable of running existing software programs. Some examples of this approach are touch sensitive tablets, voice recognition systems, head control sensors, eye position sensors, single switches and adapted keyboards (Soede, 1989). Development in this area has progressed to the point where it can now be said there is no lack of assistive devices, only a lack of research on their cost effectiveness (Burkehead, et al., 1986). The same authors suggest that greater consumer participation by individuals with handicaps in the development of such devices would enhance their cost effectiveness.

Rossler (1986) contends that the problem of technological access can only be solved through the development of "the universal product" (p. 171). Such a product would allow for a wide variety of inputs and outputs in the operation of the computer. In this way, almost any human impairment could be accommodated. The development of such a dedicated device would clearly provide an unprecedented level of functionality for any handicapped user. Unfortunately, such technology has proven prohibitively expensive (Soede, 1989). As a result, adaptation of existing technology has been, thus far, more economically feasible (Soede, 1989).

Obsolescence is also a problem, since developments in microcomputer technology are occurring so quickly (Roessler, 1986). This has the potential for increasing costs well beyond the savings in therapist time attributed to the use of microcomputer technology. One potential solution is distinguishing between technological and functional obsolescence. Although technology may be obsolete in the sense that newer and better systems are available, it may nonetheless serve a very useful purpose. In our clinic, patients effectively utilize vintage Apple II systems, as well as more advanced technology.

The rapid pace of technological change has a positive side as well. Decreased cost and increased portability will enhance access to microcomputers. In addition, new technologies, such as interactive videodiscs, hypercards, and CD-ROMs, have greatly increased the power of microcomputer systems.

A final technological issue involves the fact that classification systems for adaptive technology have been based on the characteristics of the technology as opposed to the client (Burkehead, et al., 1986; Szeto, Tingle, and Cronk, 1981). As a result, the implications of adaptive hardware for the brain-injured patient are not well understood by the rehabilitation professional. A classification system is needed based on the physical, cognitive, and functional capabilities of the patient (Soede, 1989). In other words, there is a need to approach the problem of human-machine interaction from the human perspective, matching hardware and software to human needs as opposed to the other way around (Burkehead, et al., 1986; Lynch, 1990). If a brain-injured individual cannot use a computer, this should be conceptualized as a design failure, as opposed to a user failure (Lynch, 1990).

Human Issues

Access to, and appropriate utilization of, rehabilitation technology requires more than just a technological approach. An equal focus must be given to development of adequate human resources as well (Bowe, 1984). As mentioned previously, the appropriate use of technology requires more than simply placing the client in front of a computer. It is also necessary to develop an adequate human infrastructure capable of supporting the use of such technology (Cohen, 1989; Dudek and Marcy, 1984). In other words, the effective utilization of rehabilitation technology requires consideration of not only hardware and software, but "orgware" as well.

Orgware has been defined as the organization within which a technological application is embedded (Soede, 1989). It refers to the human systems required for appropriate utilization of technology, and once again underscores the importance of person-environment fit in rehabilitation. The development of appropriate orgware involves adaptation of the brain-injured individual's social environment and is directly involved in the reduction of handicap. For example, service delivery systems must be developed for not only product support and maintenance (Roessler, 1986; Vanderheiden, 1983), but also human resource development. Rehabilitation workers require better training in relation to the potential and limitations of technology so that this information can be utilized effectively in the rehabilitation process (Legrand, 1989; Roessler, 1986). Furthermore, the appropriate use of technology in rehabilitation requires an interdisciplinary approach with information sharing across disciplines (Ranu, 1986). Several regional, national, and international databases have been developed for this purpose.

Information regarding technology must not only be made available to the rehabilitation professional but to the brain-injured individual and his or her family as well. In addition, the process of technological development must involve more consumer participation. In other words, technology for individuals with brain injury should be a consumer-driven process. Such approaches, in general, have been found to enhance the acceptability of the technology being developed (Roessler, 1986). This is an important consideration given that technophobia is a problem encountered in both therapists and patients (Burkehead, et al., 1986).

Another human problem impeding access to technology by individuals with brain injury is the vestigial perception of microcomputer as a toy.

Funding agencies are often reluctant to provide computers for recreational purposes, even though an argument in favor of therapeutic recreation could easily be made. In our own clinic, early attempts to obtain appropriate technology for the purpose of cognitive rehabilitation were met with bemused comments about the therapists wanting to play Pacman. Although the analogy is a simple one, it was not until computerized cognitive rehabilitation was likened to "physiotherapy of the mind" that we were successful in securing a source of funding.

The funding problem, however, is much wider in its scope. Those with brain injuries and their families often cannot afford microcomputers. Government reimbursement policies focus on medical, as opposed to independent living, considerations (Roessler, 1986), and as such must be reexamined. Incentives to employers to implement technological modifications in the workplace are also required if greater employment opportunities are to be made available to the brain-injured (Roessler, 1986).

Although more funding is required for research and development into new technologies (Roessler, 1986), some government and private sector cooperation has already been effective in the development of new rehabilitation technologies. For example, in Canada, Technological Aids and Systems for the Handicapped, Inc. (TASH), has received international recognition for its ability to work effectively with government in the development of new technologies (Office of Technology Assessment, 1983).

Finally, there is always danger that technology will be overutilized, a situation which could result in isolation, depersonalization, and a lack of social contact (Brown, 1984). Computers are no substitute for human interaction, and technological advances must not be allowed to decrease the commitment of society to the integration of the brain-injured. There is a need for standards with respect to the development and utilization of technology in rehabilitation. Recent efforts in this direction have resulted in the development of technological standards in specific areas such as cognitive rehabilitation (Matthews, Harley, and Malec, 1990) and psychologic assessment (American Psychological Association, 1986). More generally, the World Health Organization (WHO) has established guidelines for the appropriate use of technology in primary health care. These guidelines require that new technologies conform to the principle of developing self-reliance by being scientifically sound, practical, and socially acceptable (Cohen, 1989).

If information technologies are to assist in the process of developing self-reliance in brain-injured individuals, then these goals must be achieved. Scientific soundness requires effective research strategies, practicality involves overcoming the technological barriers discussed, and, finally, social acceptability requires that the human issues presented in this chapter be resolved.

References

Adams, K.M. (1975). Automated clinical interpretation of the neuropsychological battery: An ability based approach. Dissertation Abstracts Internations, 35(12-B):6085.

Adams, K.M., and Heaton, R.K. (1985). Automated interpretation of neuropsychological test data. Journal of Consulting and Clinical Psychology, 53:790–802.

Adams, K.M., and Brown, G.G. (1986). The role of the computer in neuropsychological assessment. In: Grant, I., and Adams, K.M. (eds). Neuropsychological assessment of neuropsychiatric disorders. Oxford: Oxford University Press.

American Psychological Association (1986). Guidelines for computer-based tests and interpretations. Washington, DC: Author.

Armstrong, C. (1989). Luria's theory of brain function recovery with applications to the use of computers in cognitive retraining. Cognitive Rehabilitation, 7:10–15.

Baker, E.L., Letz, R., Fidler, A. (1985). A computer-administered neurobehavioral evaluation system for occupational and environmental epidemiology. Journal of Occupational Medicine, 27:206–12.

Baribeau, J., Ethier, M., and Braun, C. (1989). A neuropsychological assessment of selective attention before and after cognitive remediation in patients with severe closed head injury. Journal of Neurologic Rehabilitation, 3:71–92.

Batchelor, J., Shores, E.A., Marosszeky, J.E., Sandanam, J., and Lovarini, M. (1988). Cognitive rehabilitation of severely closed-head-injured patients using computer-assisted, and noncomputerized treatment techniques. Journal of Head Trauma Rehabilitation, 3(3):78–85.

Ben-Yishay, Y. (1983). Cognitive remediation viewed from the perspective of a systematic clinical research program in rehabilitation. Cognitive Rehabilitation, 1:4–6.

Biskin, B.H., and Kolotkin, R.L. (1977). Effects of computerized administration on scores on the MMPI. Applied Psychological Measurement, 1:543–49.

Bogataj, U. (1989). Restoration of gait using multichannel electrical stimulation. Physical Therapy, 69(5):319–27.

Bond, M.R., (1986). Neurobehavioral sequelae of closed head injury. In: Grant, I., and Adams, K.M. (eds). Neuropsychological assessment of neuropsychiatric disorders. Oxford: Oxford University Press.

Boulding, K.E. (1968). General systems theory: The skeleton of science. In: Buckley, W. (ed). Modern systems research for the behavioral scientist: A sourcebook. Chicago: Aldine.

Bowe, F.G. (1984). Personal computers and special needs. Berkely, CA: Sybex.

Bracy, O.L. (1990). Computer Software for Cognitive Rehabilitation. Indianapolis: Psychological Software Services, Inc.

Bracy, O.L. (1986). Cognitive rehabilitation: A process approach. Cognitive Rehabilitation, 4:10–17.

Bracy, O.L. (1984). Using computers in neuropsychology. In: Schwartz, M.D. (ed). Using Computers in Clinical Practice. New York: Haworth Press, 257–64.

Brooks, D.N. (1984). Closed head injury: Psychological, social, and family consequences. Oxford: Oxford University Press.

Brown, D. (1984). Computer-assisted isolation. Disabled USA, 4:23–24.

Brucker, B.S. (1984). Biofeedback in rehabilitation. In: Golden, C.J. (ed). Current Topics in Rehabilitation Psychology. New York: Grune and Stratton, 173–99.

Burkehead, E.G., Sampson, J.P., and McMahon, B.T. (1986). The liberation of disabled persons in a technological society: Access to computer technology. Rehabilitation Literature, 47:162–68.

Chapanis, A. (1965). Man-machine engineering. Belmont, CA: Wadsworth.

Cohen, J. (1989). Appropriate technology in primary health care: Evolution and meaning of WHO's concept. International Journal of Technology Assessment in Health Care, 5:103–09.

Colquhoun, A., McNaughton, S., Wilson, B., and Izzard, M. (1981). Microcomputers and communication for the handicapped. Proceedings of the 4th Conference on Rehabilitation Engineering: Washington, DC, 188–90.

Coulton, C.J. (1984). Person-environment fit and rehabilitation. In: Krueger, D.W. (ed). Rehabilitation Psychology. Rockville, MD: Aspen Systems.

Crossley, R., and McDonald, M. (1982). Annie's coming out. Harmondsworth, UK: Pelican Books.

Daniel, M., Webster, J.S., and Scott, R.R. (1986). Single-case analysis of the brain-injured patient. The Behaviour Therapist, 4:71–75.

Desch, L.W. (1986). High technology for handicapped children: A pediatrician's viewpoint. Pediatrics, 77:71–87.

Dick, R.J., Wood, R.G., Bradshaw, J.L., and Bradshaw, J.A. (1987). Programmable visual display for diagnosing, assessing, and rehabilitating unilateral neglect. Medical and Biological Engineering and Computing, 10:21–23.

Dudek, R.A., and Marcy, W.M. (1984). Technology assessment for disablement. In: Granger, C.V., and Gresham, G.E. (eds). Functional assessment in rehabilitation medicine. London: Williams and Wilkins, 378–94).

Dunn, K.W. (1988a). A model for the application of technology in rehabilitation. Canadian Journal of Rehabilitation, 1:28–29.

Dunn, K.W. (1988b). Machine assistance versus machine dependence in rehabilitation. Canadian Psychology, 29.

Dunn, K.W., Chilly, C., Davis, J.R., and Chabria, S. (in progress). Computer-based rehabilitation of acquired brain injury in a long-term care setting.

Ethier, M., Braun, C., and Baribeau, J. (1989a). Computer-dispensed cognitive-perceptual training of closed head injury patients after spontaneous recovery. Study 1: Speeded tasks. Canadian Journal of Rehabilitation, 2(4):223–33.

Ethier, M., Braun, C., and Baribeau, J., (1989b). Computer-dispensed cognitive-perceptual training of closed head injury patients after spontaneous recovery. Study 2: Non-speeded tasks. Canadian Journal of Rehabilitation, 3(1):7–16.

Fairhurst, M.C., and Stephanidis, C. (1989). A model-based approach to the specification of computer-based communication aids. Journal of Medical Engineering and Technology, 13(1/2):13–17.

Finkelstein, J.N. (1976). Brain: A computer program for interpretation of the Halstead-Reitan neuropsychological test battery. Dissertation Abstracts Internations, 37:5349B (University Microfilms, No. 77–78).

Finlayson, M.A.J., Alfano, D., and Sullivan, J. (1987). A neuropsychological approach to cognitive remediation: Microcomputer applications. Canadian Psychology, 28:180–90.

Fowler, R.D. (1985). Landmarks in the computer-assisted psychological assessment. Journal of Consulting and Clinical Psychology, 53:748–59.

Gardner, H., Zurif, E., Berry, T., and Baker, E. (1976). Visual communication in aphasia. Neuropsychologia, 14:275–92.

Gianutsos, R., and Klitzner, C. (1982). Computer programs for rehabilitation: Personal computing for brain-injured persons. Johns Hopkins APL Digest, 3:253–54.

Giles, G., and Shore, M. (1989). The effectiveness of an electronic memory aid for a memory-impaired adult of normal intelligence. American Journal of Occupational Therapy, 43(6):409–11.

Glisky, E., Schacter, D., and Tulving, E. (1986). Learning and retention of computer-related vocabulary in memory-impaired patients: Method of vanishing cues. Journal of Clinical and Experimental Neuropsychology, 8:292–312.

Goldenberg, E.P. (1979). Special technology for special children. Baltimore: University Park Press.

Gosine, R.G., Harwin, W.S., Furby, L.J., and Jackson, R.D. (1989). An intelligent end-effector for a rehabilitation robot. Journal of Medical Engineering and Technology, 13(1/2):37–43.

Gray, J., and Robertson, I. (1988). Microcomputer-based attentional retraining after brain injury: A randomised group controlled trial. Journal of Clinical and Experimental Neuropsychology, 10:332.

Halligan, P.W., and Marshall, J.C. (1989). Two techniques for the assessment of line bisection in visuo-spatial neglect: A single case study. Journal of Neurology, Neurosurgery, and Psychiatry, 52:1300–02.

Harrell, T.H., Honaker, L.M., Hetu, M., and Oberwager, J. (1987). Computerized versus traditional administration of the multidimensional aptitude battery-verbal scale: An examination of reliability and validity. Computers in Human Behavior, 3:129–37.

Harris, J., (1984). Methods of improving memory. In: Wilson, B.A., and Moffat, N. (eds). Clinical management of memory problems. Rockville, MD: Aspen Systems, 46–62.

Hofer, P.J., and Green, B.F. (1985). The challenge of competence and creativity in computerized psychological testing. Journal of Consulting and Clinical Psychology, 53:826–38.

Ince, L.P. (1988). An operant conditioning computer program for biofeedback. In: Eisenberg, M.G., and Grzesiak, R.C. (eds). Advances in clinical rehabilitation, Vol. 2. New York: Springer.

Inhelder, B. (1980). Commentary. In: Piattelli-Palmarini, M. (ed). Language and learning: The debate between Jean Piaget and Noam Chomsky. Cambridge, MA: Harvard University Press.

Jackson, D.N. (1985). Computer-based personality testing. Computers in Human Behavior, 1:255–64.

Jennett, B., and MacMillan, R. (1981). Epidemiology of head injury. British Medical Journal, 282:101–03.

Johnson, P.C., and Stonell-Thomas, N. (1989). An interactive computer program to assess and facilitate cognitive functioning in head injured young people. Proceedings of the 3rd Annual Conference of Cognitive Rehabilitation, Clearwater, FL, 454.

Kaufman, H.H., Bretaudierre, J.P., Rowlands, B.J., Stein, D.K., Bernstein, D.P., Wagner, K.A., and Gildenberg, P.L. (1989). Head injury: Variability of course and presence of confounding factors. International Journal of Technology Assessment in Health Care, 5:631–38.

Lamber, M.E., Andrews, R.H., Rylee, K., and Skinner, J.R. (1987). Equivalence of computerized and traditional MMPI administration with substance abusers. Computers in Human Behavior, 3:139–43.

Laursen, P. (1990). A computer-aided technique for testing cognitive functions. Acta Neurologica Scandinavica (Suppl), 82:1–108.

Lawrence, G.H. (1986). Using computers for the treatment of psychological problems. Computers in Human Behavior, 2:43–62.

Legrand, C. (1989). Prerequisites for computer-aided cognitive rehabilitation. International Journal of Rehabilitation Research, 12(3):323–26.

Links, C., and Frydenberg, H. (1989). Microcomputer skills training program for the physically disabled in long-term rehabilitation. Physical and Occupational Therapy in Geriatrics, 6(3/4):133–40.

Lynch, W.J. (1988). Microcomputer technology in the rehabilitation of brain disorders. In: Eisenberg, M.G., and Grzesiak, R.C. (eds). Advances in clinical rehabilitation, Vol. 2. New York: Springer, 41–58.

Lynch, W.J. (1990). Cognitive prostheses for the brain injured. Journal of Head Trauma Rehabilitation, 5(3):78–80.

MacCrimmon, D., Finlayson, M.A.J., Mosher, M., and Garner, S.H., (1991). QEEG in psychiatry: The Ontario normative study. Psychiatry Department Rounds, McMaster University, Hamilton, Canada.

Malec, J., Jones, R., Rao, N., and Stubbs, K. (1984). Video-game practice effects on sustained attention in patients with craniocerebral trauma. Cognitive Rehabilitation, 2:18-23.

Malone, T.W. (1982). Heuristics for designing enjoyable user interfaces: Lessons from computer games. Proceedings of the Conference on Human Factors in Computer Science, 15-17.

Matthews, C., Harley, J.P., and Malec, J. (1990). Guidelines for computer-assisted neuropsychological rehabilitation and cognitive remediation. Madison, WI: American Psychological Association Division 40 (Clinical Neuropsychology).

Merbitz, C.T., Grip, J.C., Halper, A., Mogil, S., Cherney, L.R., and Bellaire, K. (1989). The communication analysis system. Archives of Physical Medicine and Rehabilitation, 70(2):118-23.

Miller, E. (1978). Is amnesia remediable? In: Gruneberg, M.M., Morris, P.E., and Sykes, R.N. (eds). Practical aspects of memory. New York: Academic Press.

Miller, R.A. (1990) (ed). Proceedings of the 14th annual symposium on computer applications in medical care. New York: IEEE Computer Society Press.

Moreland, K.L. (1985). Computer-assisted psychological assessment in 1986: A practical guide. Computers in Human Behavior, 1:221-33.

Office of Technology Assessment (1983). Technology and handicapped people. New York: Springer Publishing Company.

Olson, D.R. (1976). Culture, technology, and intellect. In: Resnick, L.B. (ed). The nature of intelligence. Hillsdale, NJ: Lawrence Erlbaum Associates.

Piaget, J. (1970). Piaget's theory. In: Musson, P.H. (ed). Carmichael's handbook of child psychology. New York: Wiley.

Plugge, L.A., Verhey, F.R.J., and Jolles, J. (1990). A desktop expert system for the differential diagnosis of dementia. International Journal of Technology Assessment in Health Care, 6:147-56.

Ponsford, J.L., and Kinsella, G. (1988). Evaluation of a remedial program for attentional deficits following closed-head injury, Journal of Clinical and Experimental Neuropsychology, 10:51-52.

Prigatano, G.P. (1986). Neuropsychological rehabilitation after brain injury. London: Johns Hopkins University Press.

Prigatano, G.P., Fordyce, D.J., Zeiker, H.K., Roueche, J.R., Pepping, M., and Case-Wood, B. (1984). Neuropsychological rehabilitation after closed head injury in young adults. Journal of Neurology, Neurosurgery, and Psychiatry, 47:505-13.

Randolph, C., and Miller, M. (1988). EEG and cognitive performance following closed head injury, Neuropsychology, 20:43-50.

Ranu, H.S. (1986). Engineering aspects of rehabilitation for the handicapped. Journal of Medical Engineering Technology, 10(1):16-20.

Renwick, R.M. (1989). Developing a computerized rehabilitation database: Nontechnical considerations. Canadian Journal of Rehabilitation, 3:29-36.

Reitan, R.M. (1979). Neuropsychology and rehabilitation. Privately published manuscript. Tucson: Author.

Robertson, I.H., Gray, J.M., Pentland, B., and Waite, L.J. (1990). Microcomputer-based rehabilitation for unilateral left visual neglect: A randomized controlled trial. Archives of Physical Medicine and Rehabilitation, 71(9):663-68.

Romanczyk, R.G. (1986). Clinical utilization of microcomputer technology. Toronto: Pergamon.

Rosenthal, M., Griffith, E.R., Bond, M.R., and Miller, J.D. (1990). Rehabilitation of the adult and child with traumatic brain injury. Philadelphia: F.A. Davis and Company.

Rosegrant, T. (1985). Using a microcomputer to assist children in their efforts to acquire beginning literacy. Paper presented at the meeting of The American Educational Research Association, Chicago.

Russell, E.W., Neuringer, C., and Goldstein, G. (1970). Assessment of brain damage: A neuropsychological key approach, New York: Wiley-Interscience.

Russell, G.K.G., Peace, K.A., and Mellsop, G.W. (1986). The reliability of a micro-computer administration of the MMPI. Journal of Clinical Psychology, 42:120-22.

Sandford, M.S., and Browne, R.J. (1986). Captain's log cognitive training system. Richmond, VA: Network Services.

Scherzer, B.P. (1986). Rehabilitation following severe head trauma: Results of a three-year program. Archives of Physical Medicine and Rehabilitation, 67:366-73.

Shaw, C., and McKenna, K. (1989). Microcomputer activities for attention training. Cognitive Rehabilitation, 7:18-21.

Skilbeck, C. (1984). Computer assistance in the management of memory and cognitive impairment. In: Wilson, B.A., and Moffat, N. (eds). Clinical management of memory problems. Beckenham, UK: Croom Helm, 148-70.

Skinner, A.D., and Trachtman, L.H. (1985). Use of a computer program (PC coloring book) in cognitive rehabilitation. American Journal of Occupational Therapy, 39:470-72.

Smith, J. (1984). Cognitive Rehabilitation Computer Programs. Dimondale, MI: Hartley Courseware, Inc.

Soede, M. (1989). The use of information technology in rehabilitation: An overview of possibilities and new directions in applications. Journal of Medical Engineering and Technology, 13(1/2):5-9.

Soede, M., van Balkom, H.L.M., Deroost, G., van Knippenberg, H.M., and Kamphuis, H. (1989). New possibilities for enhanced keyboard input for the handicapped. Journal of Medical Engineering and Technology, 13(1/2):34-36.

Sohlberg, M.M., and Mateer, C. (1987). Effectiveness of an attention-training program. Journal of Clinical and Experimental Neuropsychology, 9:117-30.

Sohlberg, M.M., and Mateer, C. (1989). Introduction to cognitive rehabilitation: Theory and practice. New York: Guilford Press.

Steele, R.D., Weinrich, M., Wertz, R.T., Kleczewska, M.K., and Carlson, G.S. (1989). Computer-based visual communication in aphasia. Neuropsychologia, 27(4):409-26.

Story, T.B., and Sbordone, R.J. (1988). The use of microcomputers in the treatment of cognitive-communicative impairments. Journal of Head Trauma Rehabilitation, 3(2):45-54.

Sulton, L.D., Hardisty, B., Bisterfeldt, J., and Harvey, R.F. (1987). Computerized data-bases: An integrated approach to monitoring quality of patient care. Archives of Physical Medicine and Rehabilitation, 68:850-53.

Szeto, A.Y., Tingle, L.A., and Cronk, S.R. (1981). Automated retrieval of information on assisted devices. Bulletin of Prosthetics Research, 10:27-34.

Thatcher, R.W., Walker, R.A., Gerson, I., and Geisler, F.H. (1989). EEG discriminant function analyses of mild head trauma. Electroencephalography and Clinical Neurophysiology, 73:94-100.

Van Zomeren, A.H. (1981). Reaction time and attention after closed head injury. Lisse: Swets Publishing Service.

Vanderheiden, G.C. (1983). The practical use of microcomputers in rehabilitation. Rehabilitation Literature, 44(3/4):66-70.

Wall, J.C., and Turnbull, G.I. (1986). Gait asymmetries in residual hemiplegia. Archives of Physical Medicine and Rehabilitation, 67:550-53.

Weinberg, J., Diller, L., and Gordon, W.A. (1977). Visual scanning effect on reading-related tasks in acquired right brain damage. Archives of Physical Medicine and Rehabilitation, 58:479-86.

Weizenbaum, J. (1976). Computer power and human reason. San Francisco: W.H. Freeman.

White, D.M., Clements, C.B., and Fowler, R.D. (1985). A comparison of computer administration with standard administration of the MMPI. Computers in Human Behavior, 1:153-62.

Wilson, B. (1987). Single-case experimental designs in neuropsychological rehabilitation. Journal of Clinical and Experimental Neuropsychology, 9(5):527-44.

Wilson, S.L., and McMillan, T.M. (1986). Finding able minds in disabled bodies. Lancet, 2:1444-46.

Wood, R.L. (1984). Management of attention disorders following head injury. In: Wilson, B.A., and Moffat, N. (eds). Clinical management of memory problems. Beckenham, UK: Croom Helm, 148-70.

World Health Organization (1980). International classification of impairment, disabilities, and handicaps: A manual of classification relating to the consequences of disease. Geneva: WHO

Zangwill, O.L. (1947). Psychological aspects of rehabilitation in cases of brain injury. British Journal of Psychology, 37:60-69.

12

Pharmacologic Interventions for Cognitive and Behavioral Impairments

C. THOMAS GUALTIERI

It is only in the past few years that the extraordinary technology of neuropharmacology has been turned, in a systematic way, to the debilitating effects of traumatic brain injury (TBI). It is an old ambition that is finally achieving fruition, since Luria wrote, in the 1940's, of the promise of cholinergic treatment (Luria, Naydin, and Tsvetkova, 1968). But only in the past year have attempts been made to set the actual practice of neuropharmacology into a modern theoretical framework, presented in a comprehensive format for clinicians who work with TBI patients (Gualtieri, 1990).

Neuropharmacology for TBI patients is oriented to correct or alleviate *specific impairments*. There are four appropriate goals:

1. To treat specific neuropsychiatric disorders that arise following TBI, like depression or psychosis; or to suppress untoward behaviors, like aggression or agitation.
2. To correct specific neuropsychologic impairments, especially inattention and memory impairment.
3. To encourage or enhance the course of cortical recovery.
4. To prevent *secondary deterioration*, the delayed neurobehavioral sequelae of TBI (Gualtieri and Cox, 1991).

The prevailing view of neuropsychopharmacology, especially among physicians, is that drug treatments are intuitive-nosologic in nature; that is, they are oriented around the treatment of specific psychiatric for neurologic disorders. Thus, the classes of drugs known as antidepressants are specifically for the treatment of depression, antipsychotics are for schizophrenia, thymoleptics are for bipolar disorder (manic-depression), and so on. This is how drugs are developed, from the animal models of a specific syndrome, to clinical trials of relatively homogeneous clinical populations, and ultimately to the marketing strategies of the pharmaceutical manufacturers. This argument has played such a compelling role in modern psychiatry, that theories have developed about the disorders themselves, based on no more evidence than the known mechanism of action of the psychotropic drugs; e.g., the "dopamine hypothesis" of schizophrenia, the "catecholamine hypothesis" of depression. The psychotropic drugs are understood in terms of their effect on neurotransmitter systems, and the disorders are understood in terms of the neurotransmitter effects of their specific drugs.

The reader recognizes the circular fallacy. The theory fails even in conventional psychiatry, since the various drugs are known to treat a wide variety of disorders (Gualtieri, 1977). It is rare to find a psychotropic that effects only one neurotransmitter system, and most of the psychiatric disorders are effectively treated by more than one drug. The conventional approach to psychopharmacology is even less successful in studies of special populations, like children, the demented elderly, the developmentally handicapped, and patients with TBI. In these groups, drug treatment is *almost purely empirical,* and the traditional psychiatric nosology has little or no relevance. In these groups, the theoretical constructions around which psychopharmacologic treatments are developed are quite different. In pediatric psychopharmacology, age and IQ are essential to the prediction of drug response (Gualtieri, 1990; Chandler, Barnhill, and Gualtieri, 1991). In mental retardation, etiology may be predictive (Gualtieri, 1990). And in TBI, the principles of psychopharmacology *may* be determined by a number of factors like the neuroanatomic locus of injury, the global severity of the patient's impairment, the specific neurochemical deficiency, or other variables which are yet to be determined. A psychiatric diagnosis like "organic personality disorder" does nothing to guide the choice of a psychotropic drug.

The psychopharmacology of special populations has suffered from inattention, probably because it has failed to conform to the prevailing wisdom of the field. The reader will note that the clinical information in this chapter is rarely supported by data from controlled clinical trials. But that is not because the empirical method is an inferior approach to psychopharmacology. It is, in fact, a rational, physiologic approach and can be "databased" through the use of behavioral methodology (N of 1 studies). This approach may be more useful than a nosologic approach that guides conventional psychiatry. It is better for treating patients.

Psychopharmacology for TBI patients may be based on principles of functional neuroanatomy. The three examples we have written about are the dopamine agonists for frontal lobe syndromes, the serotonin agonists for thalamic syndromes, and the psychotropic anticonvulsants and lithium for the temporal lobe syndromes (Gualtieri, 1990).

Psychopharmacology may also be based on the severity of the patient's impairment. An example is the use of direct acting dopamine agonists for patients who have sustained brainstem injury and indirect agonists for patients whose lesions are primarily cortical, and the presynaptic dopaminergic neuron is intact (Ross and Rush, 1981).

Psychopharmacology may also be oriented along hypothetical lines, based on the putative functions of specific neurotransmitter systems. So, one proposes to treat disorders of arousal by manipulating the dopamine system. Aggression and disorders of emotional control may be controlled by manipulating the serotonin system. Disorders of memory may be addressed by manipulating the cholinergic system (Gualtieri, 1990).

Hypothetical treatments may evolve, and become established as "rational" treatments, when the mechanism of drug action is well understood and when the physiology of the disorder is clearly mediated by its known effect on the system that is deranged. The dopamine agonists are the only treatment, thus far, that has achieved the status of a "rational" treatment in TBI (Gualtieri and Evans, 1988; Gualtieri, Chandler, Coons, and Brown, 1990).

This chapter will address the specific neurobehavioral syndromes of TBI and their appropriate treatment with psychotherapeutic drugs. The information is presented in terms of practical clinical guidelines, rather than as a literature review, as, to date, there are no controlled clinical trials to guide pharmacologic interventions.

This chapter shall present an approach to guide the use of psychopharmacologic agents which are based on correcting the neurobehavioral impairments caused by injury. The syndromes are organized into three broad categories: 1) The transient neurobehavioral syndromes; 2) the static encephalopathies; and 3) the delayed neurobehavioral sequelae of TBI (Gualtieri, 1992).

TREATMENT OF THE NEUROBEHAVIORAL SYNDROMES
Transient Neurobehavioral Syndromes

The transient neurobehavioral syndromes are disorders that arise with regularity, after mild or severe TBI. They are appropriately considered an inexorable part of the recovery process. As such, they are natural processes that deserve to be protected, and no excess of zeal should be applied to suppressing symptoms. One is better advised to allow the process to play itself out. Only in the most severe or persistent cases is it necessary to resort to pharmacologic interventions.

Postconcussion Syndrome (PCS)

Mild TBI is often the occasion of persistent impairment, notably headache, fatigue, insomnia, irritability, emotional lability, lack of concentration, and memory deficits. The symptoms usually abate over time, but the interval may be months or even years (Rimel, Giordani, Barth, Boll, and Jane, 1981). Clearly, during the first few months, the patient should be treated conservatively, perhaps with a mild analgesic for headaches and with counselling about the expected course of head injury recovery. For most patients, that is sufficient. For others, however, the problems do not abate, but may even seem to increase over the first few months. When PCS symptoms persist for 4–8 months following TBI, the physician may be inclined to prescribe a psychotropic drug.

There are two reasons to delay a psychopharmacologic intervention until at least a few months have passed after a mild TBI. One, is that most patients will recover spontaneously and drug treatment may not be necessary. The other is that drug treatment exposes the patient, and the recovering brain, to one more potential complication. Recovery from mild head trauma seems to occur best in uncomplicated circumstances.

The insomnia of PCS is typical, characterized by difficulty falling asleep because of "racing thoughts," frequent awakenings, decreased sleep time, and daytime fatigue (but not drowsiness). It is reasonable to give primacy to the treatment of insomnia because sleep has a restorative function, and the other symptoms of PCS, like fatigue and irritability, may also be relieved if the patient has slept well the night before. It is also reasonable to give primacy to the treatment of PCS insomnia because there is a very good drug for it, namely trazodone (Gualtieri, 1990). This heterocyclic antidepressant has a complex pharmacology, but it is known to be a serotonin reuptake blocker. It has never won popularity as an antidepressant, but it is a very good hypnotic. Although "hangovers" are uncommon, they may sometimes occur, and the problem is corrected by lowering the dose (the dose range is 50–300 mg qhs). Otherwise, trazodone is free of the more common side effects seen in hypnotic drugs, such as the benzodiazepines. Fatal overdose is difficult to achieve compared to the tricyclic antidepressants. It is neither anticholinergic nor cardiotoxic, and is well tolerated by elderly patients.

The only dangerous side effect is priapism, said to occur in 1 of every 6000 males treated with trazodone (Scher and Krieger, 1983). (Elderly males are said to be more prone to this side effect.) If the patient on trazodone begins to experience "unusual erections" the drug should be stopped immediately. The female equivalent of priapism, clitoral engorgement and spontaneous orgasm, is not a medical emergency of equal magnitude (Gartrell, 1986).

The alternative treatments for insomnia are amitriptyline, which is a tricyclic and thus prone to problems like weight gain, accidental overdose, anticholinergic side effects, and cardiotoxicity. The doses that usually induce sleep, however, are very low, almost homeopathic (e.g., 10–25 mg qhs). Chloral hydrate is another alternative. The hypnotic benzodiazepines may aggravate depression in the PCS patient, but they are occasionally useful.

The psychostimulants, methylphenidate, amphetamine, and methamphetamine, are extremely useful for persistent symptoms of fatigue, anergia, inability to concentrate, and memory deficits (Gualtieri and Evans, 1988). They are very good antidepressants for the anergic depression that often typifies patients with persistent PCS. They may have other, serendipitous effects: improved sleep, pain relief, restoration of sexuality. Low dose antidepressant therapy may have many of the same effects, but in our clinic the psychostimulants are preferred. The side effect profile is much better for the stimulants, compared to the antidepressants, and the clinical effects of a single dose of methylphenidate, for example, can actually be measured with neuropsychologic testing after 90 minutes.

Major depression is the most important complication of the PCS, and sertraline is probably the antidepressant of choice. It seems to be free of negative neuropsychologic effects. It lacks cardiotoxicity, it is sometimes anorexigenic (a desirable side effect for many patients), and it is, above all, an extremely effective antidepressant. It is energizing for patients with anergic depression, and it has a calming effect on patients with anguished depression or posttraumatic emotionalism. The therapeutic dose range is relatively narrow (50–200 mg/d) and its beneficial effects tend to come on quickly. Panoxetine is the primary alternative.

Akathisia is a subjective state of restlessness and dysphoria. It occurs in Parkinsonian patients and in patients treated with neuroleptic drugs. It may also be a symptom of PCS. Buspirone (5–15 mg tid) is the treatment of choice (Gualtieri, 1991).

PCS patients may also be prone to headache, neck, or back pain, or the painful symptoms of fibromyalgia. The treatment of pain frequently involves recourse to psychotropic drugs like amitriptyline, fluoxetine, and other antidepressants; benzodiazepines prescribed as muscle relaxants or mild sedatives; and anticonvulsants like carbamazepine and valproate. Treatments of this kind may also alleviate psychologic symptoms like irritability, insomnia, and depression. But any psychotrope may be expected to have an adverse behavioral or cognitive effect in a TBI patient. The first step in treatment is to carefully evaluate the positive and negative effects of the medications the patient may already be taking. The same is true for drugs like methocarbamol (Robaxan), carisoprodol (Soma), cyclobenzeprine (Flexeril), and the host of other drugs that may be brought to bear for headache or for musculoskeletal pain. Even lecithin, an acetyl choline precursor that people can buy over the counter for memory problems, may cause mental depression in some individuals.

Agitation During Coma Recovery

The patient recovering from coma usually passes through an extremely unstable state, with fluctuating levels of arousal, perceptual distortions, and difficulty understanding or complying with the demands of a therapeutic environment. Impairments in arousal, perception, cognition, and self-control may be manifest as disabling conditions like agitation, assaultiveness, screaming, wandering about, and emotional lability. Problems like this will compromise one's therapeutic program, and they may wreak havoc on a rehabilitation unit that is not well prepared. Treatment staff want compliant patients, not patients who are agitated and disorganized. If the patient slugs his therapist, resists therapy efforts, and, if he is found one evening wandering around the parking lot—well, is there not a drug you can give him, doctor?

Yes, there are several drugs, but it may not be a good idea to use any of them—at least right away. If one's goal is simply to suppress untoward behavior, you can use a neuroleptic or a benzodiazepine. They work well enough in the short run, and sometimes that is an acceptable goal. But over the long run, they are sedating drugs, and sedation is not the appropriate goal for the patient who is trying to emerge from semicoma. There is even a belief that neuroleptics may retard the course of cortical recovery (Feeney, Gonzales, and Law, 1982).

Since the state of agitation during coma recovery is usually a transient condition, it is prudent to bide one's time before prescribing a psychoactive drug. Try to maintain the patient in a *secure environment*, with only limited stimulation. Withdraw medications that may be sedating, like haloperidol or phenytoin, or drugs that may have behavioral toxicity, like baclofen or dantrolene.

If the patient has posttraumatic epilepsy, or is at extremely high risk to develop the same, the anticonvulsants to choose are carbamazepine or valproate (Gualtieri, 1990). They are both effective for states of organic agitation and for mania, so if the patient needs an anticonvulsant anyway, it is reasonable to use one that might be a psychotrope as well. (The excellence of carbamazepine and valproate as dual-purpose drugs should not obscure these facts: That they also may be sedating, that they may have behavioral toxicity, and that they are not especially good to prescribe if the patient does not need them.)

The drug of choice for agitation during coma recovery is the dopamine agonist, amantadine (Gualtieri, Chandler, Coons, and Brown, 1990). The theory behind its use is that it corrects the primary impairment that underlies the condition, an unstable, fluctuating state of arousal. Presumably, it corrects the underlying deficiency in monoaminergic neurotransmission that characterizes this stage of brain injury recovery (Bareggi, Porta, and Selenati, 1975). The psychostimulants are hardly ever of value *at this stage of recovery, because they are indirect agonists, and require an intact presynaptic neuron* (i.e., a brainstem neuron) to exercise their effect (Ross and Rush, 1981).

The other alternatives are lithium, the psychotropic anticonvulsants (carbamazepine and valproate), the β-blockers, and the benzodiazepines, especially lorazepam and clonazepam. Although medications with anticholinergic effects are to be avoided, amitriptyline has been reported to be effective during this stage of recovery. (Mysiw, et al., 1988). Clonidine is another alternative. There really is no clinical indicator, aside from a seizure diathesis, that will guide one's choice among this list; it is simply trial-and-error. Unfortunately, none of the drugs on this list has achieved the 50% success rate described for amantadine (Gualtieri, et al., 1990).

Failure to Progress

This is a common clinical dilemma: The patient is on a plateau, his recovery is going nowhere. One believes, on the basis of clinical data, that a higher level of recovery is possible, but the patient is moving slowly, or not at all. There is pressure to move him to a nursing home, where the prospects of recovery will be diminished even further.

The approach is similar to the outline given in the preceding section. First, eliminate drugs that may be sedating or that may have behavioral toxicity. Then achieve optimal anticonvulsant therapy. Then consider a trial of dopamine agonists. Even combined treatment with more than one of the dopamine agonist drugs may be considered, if the situation is desperate and something clearly must be done, to encourage the system to respond (e.g., Horiguchi, Inami, and Shoda, 1990).

The principles of pharmacologic treatment that emerge from this consideration of the transient neurobehavioral syndromes are germane to treatment in the other TBI patient groups, described below:

1) Avoid treatment if the problem is minor, or short-lived, or something that can be managed behaviorally or environmentally.
2) Before you add a new drug treatment, make sure that current treatments are necessary, and make sure they are not given to behavioral or cognitive toxicity.
3) Try to avoid polypharmacy, that is, the simultaneous use of several psychotropics. Keep the therapeutic regimen as simple as possible, and evaluate drug response as systematically as possible.
4) Whenever possible use drugs that are not anticholinergic, like the tricyclic antidepressants, or that are not sedating, like phenytoin, haloperidol, phenobarbital, dantrolene.
5) In the TBI patient every drug trial is an empirical exercise. That does not mean, however, that anything goes.

In contrast to a shotgun approach ("Let's see if this one works"), one should develop an hypothesis on the basis of the patient's physiology, and what, precisely, one expects it to do. An appropriate outcome measure with individualized behavioral experimental design (Guyatt, 1990) may be helpful in assessing a "drug's effectiveness."

6) Optimal anticonvulsant treatment for the patient with a seizure diathesis takes precedence over all but the most urgent behavioral disorders.

7) There is no such thing as a "prophylaxis" for posttraumatic epilepsy (Temkin, Dikmen, Wilensky, Keihm, Chabal, and Winn, 1990). There is, rather, antiepileptic treatment for TBI patients who may not have had a seizure yet, but who are so highly likely to have one, that treatment, as if a seizure had already occurred, is the judicious course.

Static Encephalopathies

When the neuropsychiatric sequelae of TBI are considered, especially in the classical literature, the main emphasis is given to the personality changes associated with focal areas of cortical injury; for example, the frontal lobe syndromes (Luria, 1973; Lezak, 1983) and the temporal lobe syndromes (Waxman and Geschwind, 1975). The neurobehavioral syndromes associated with static lesions of the frontal and temporal lobes are captured in the psychiatric nosology. Rather, they are described in the classical neuropsychology literature, and they refer to distinct and specific patterns of behavior, motivation, self-control and emotional response.

Although the psychiatric categories are not germane to static encephalopathic lesions, there is a developing consensus that the psychiatric drugs may be specific. It would appear that the dopamine agonist drugs are particularly useful for frontal lobe syndromes, and that the temporal lobe syndromes are well treated by mood altering psychotropics. This neuroanatomic approach to psychopharmacology is a thoroughly new idea that has not been evaluated carefully, either for its theoretic underpinnings or its success in controlled trials.

The behavioral syndrome that is associated with injury to the frontal convexity is characterized by "deficit" symptoms or disabilities—lack of initiative or motivation, low energy, lack of perseverance, attention and memory deficits, mutism. It is reasonably well treated with the dopamine agonists (Gualtieri, et al., 1990), psychostimulants for high-level cases (Gualtieri and Evans, 1988), and the direct agonist amantadine for more severely impaired cases.

The frontal lobe syndrome associated with injury to the orbital-medial service—disinhibition, socially inappropriate behavior, excitability, predatory aggression—may also be treated with the dopamine agonists. Since it is difficult, however, to damage this area without also injuring adjacent areas of the temporal lobes, temporal lobe symptoms like explosive range and affective aggression usually coexist. Therefore, treatment with the dopamine agonists may not be entirely sufficient.

There are three general categories within which to consider the behavioral syndromes associated with temporal lobe injury. First, there are the affective disorders, including panic, depression, bipolar affective disorder, anxiety and explosive rage (Altshuler, Devinsky, Post, and Theodore, 1990). Then there is the "temporal lobe personality," also known as the "interictal personality of temporal lobe epileptics" (Bear and Fedio, 1977), a peculiar constellation of traits, including hypergraphia, hyposexuality, interpersonal "stickiness," a turgid interpersonal style, hyperreligiosity and/or cosmic ruminations, and a tendency to dissociative experiences like déjà vu, out-of-body and depersonalization. The third category is the temporal lobe psychosis, a "thought disorder" in the classical psychiatric tradition, with hallucinations, delusions, paranoia, and withdrawal (Barnhill and Gualtieri, 1989).

The various temporal lobe syndromes are appropriately treated with lithium, carbamazepine, and valproate. How they come to be linked, these three disparate agents, for the treatment of such a range of disparate disorders is a mystery, since there is no common action the drugs are known to share, and there is no clinical element to share in the disorders listed above. Lithium, carbamazepine, and valproate are more or less equal in the treatment (and prevention) of manic-depression, of "organic effective disorders," and of "intermittent explosive disorder" (or "episodic discontrol") (Gualtieri, 1990). They are also equally effective when these problems are caused by a temporal lobe injury. Carbamazepine and valproate are appropriate treatments for complex partial seizures with a temporal lobe focus, and lithium, as it happens, is an effective adjunct (Jus, Villeneuve, Gautier, Pires, Cote, Jus, Villeneuve, and Perron, 1973). In fact, combinations of 2 of these 3 drugs may be effective when only 1 is insufficient. Carbamazepine and valproate are potentially therapeutic for temporal lobe psychosis, although low dose neuroleptics are often necessary, in addition (Gualtieri and Barnhill, 1989).

The wide-ranging and rather nonspecific effects of carbamazepine and valproate in temporal lobe patients may be augmented with buspirone, a serotonin 5HT1a receptor agonist (Gualtieri, 1991).

Lesions of the temporal lobe may be characterized by an extreme degree of emotional instability, variously labelled "emotionalism," emotional incontinence of pseudobulbar affect. Here, the serotonergic antidepressants are usually better than carbamazepine (Leijon and Boivie, 1989). Amitriptyline is the venerable treatment. Sertraline may be a better first choice drug, because it is not anticholinergic like amitriptyline and clomipramine. Fluoxetine is prone to a number of troublesome side effects, and its prescription requires very careful monitoring.

The serotonergic antidepressants may also be useful for treating the "thalamic syndrome," a disorder characterized by the central perception of pain, or "dysesthesia." The thalamic syndrome (of Dejerine) is seen more commonly after stroke, although it may occur after TBI (Dejerine and Roussy, 1906).

Lesions of the basal ganglia generally present as if they were frontal lobe syndromes, and are treated accordingly with dopamine agonists. Posttraumatic obsessive-compulsive disorder is rare, but it may be seen after basal ganglia lesions (Modell, Mountz, Curtis, and Greden, 1989). The treatment is similar to the treatment of the primary psychiatric disorder.

It has been our custom to treat the behavioral manifestations of lesions in the septum or the hypothalamus with dopamine agonists, because there is preclinical literature to support that practice (Marotta, Potegal, and Glusman, 1977), and because we have had modest success in a few patients. Emphasis on "modest." There have been reports of naltrexone for "organic bulimia" following hypothalamic trauma (Childs, 1986), but our success with naltrexone has been less than modest.

Delayed Neurobehavioral Sequelae

The reader is referred to a recent review of the subject (Gualtieri and Cox, 1991). There are at least 6 delayed sequelae that may arise months, or years, after TBI. Within the first 2 years, there is a posttraumatic depression and delayed amnesia. Posttraumatic epilepsy and late onset psychosis (Gualtieri and Barnhill, 1990) may occur at any time, years after the event. The incidence of Alzheimer's Disease is also increased in TBI victims, and may thus be considered a "sequela" (Shalat, Seltzer, Pidcock, and Baker, 1987). (As you know, the onset of symptoms of postconcussion syndrome may also be delayed; a higher proportion of PCS patients are symptomatic at 3 months than they are immediately after the injury (Rimel, et al., 1981).)

The diagnosis of posttraumatic depression is probably overdone in the first months after TBI, because so many of the symptoms (anergia, anhedonia, irritability, insomnia) overlap. However, by the end of the first year after TBI, patients with persistent symptoms of PCS may develop a "real" depression (in psych-speak, "Major Affective Disorder"). Their mood is more consistently sad, anguished, or hopeless, and they have less confidence that they will overcome their disability. It is hardly surprising, since they must endure a prolonged period of relative inactivity, financial hardship, the adversarial nature of "insurance" and "compensation," interpersonal failures, and medical encounters that are only occasionally helpful.

It is possible, too, that the presumed changes in neurotransmitter metabolism that occur in PCS may, over the span of months, alter the dynamics of receptor sensitivity, and this may lead to secondary changes that are "downstream" from the primary deficits.

The treatment of posttraumatic depression is similar to the treatment of the primary psychiatric disorder, but not identical. Anergic depressions probably should be treated with stimulants or dopamine agonists, while anguished depressions are better treated with serotonergic antidepressants like sertraline. The tricyclics are perfectly respectable antidepressants, but they are anticholinergic, and thus may compromise memory or motor performance (Evans and Gualtieri, 1986). They may have adverse cardiovascular side effects, which limits their utility for elderly patients, and they are fatal in overdose, which is an important consideration, because suicidal thinking is so common in the TBI population. On the other hand, posttraumatic depression may respond perfectly well to low doses of tricyclics, and their negative effects on neuropsychologic performance are by no means inevitable, so they hardly deserve an absolute prohibition.

"Delayed posttraumatic amnesia" is a clinical problem characterized by the occasional loss of memory performance during the second year after TBI, in the absence of any intervening pathology, like depression, epilepsy, drugs, etc. (Gualtieri and Cox, 1991). The phenomenon seems to be real, though it is neither well described nor is it well understood.

The only current drugs that are known to improve memory performance for cases of posttraumatic amnesia are the dopamine agonists, especially the stimulants (Evans, Gualtieri, and Amara, 1986). The cholinergics have always held center stage, though, in the literature on memory disorders for TBI and for demented patients. Tetra-amino acridine (THA) is the only cholinergic drug that will be available soon in North America, and clinical trials of THA in TBI patients are yet to be done. Lecithin is an acetylcholine precursor that is available, in health food stores, and many patients with memory deficits are tempted to give it a try, spurred on by reports in the pseudoscientific literature. It is not a completely benign agent, as patients on lecithin may experience irritability or depression.

Posttraumatic epilepsy is ideally treated with carbamazepine or valproate. The sedating anticonvulsants, like phytoin and phenobarbital, should be avoided if possible. Patients with posttraumatic epilepsy may be prone to secondary psychiatric disorders, like depression, anxiety, or psychosis. If adjunctive treatment with buspirone, amantadine, or acetazolamide does not improve the clinical situation, then appropriate psychopharmacologic treatments may be required.

Posttraumatic (or late onset) psychosis is probably the most devastating consequence of TBI. There are many types of psychosis that can arise following TBI, but in this discussion posttraumatic psychosis will refer to a schizophreniform reaction that arises 3–5 years postinjury, and is associated with significant disability. Carbamazepine is the treatment of choice based on the assumption that the source of the problem is an irritative focus in the temporal lobe. Carbamazepine alone is rarely effective, and low dose neuroleptics are usually required.

There is no intervention known to date that will diminish the likelihood of delayed posttraumatic dementia. THA will be approved soon as treatment for dementia, and it will probably work well, especially in early cases. Its toxicity profile, however, may well diminish its usefulness as a prophylactic agent. One would prefer a drug that had some neuroprotective or "prophylactic" properties, and there are some who say that deprenyl will fit that bill (Gualtieri, 1990).

Other Drugs

The β-blockers have been cited for quite some time as effective treatment for agitated and aggressive states following TBI (Yodofsky, Williams, and Gorman, 1981). They clearly have their place, though most practitioners will aver that it is in the back of the classroom. The success of clinical practice with β-blockers never seems to equal the glowing reports that appear in the psychiatric literature. The same is true for drugs like clonidine, a central α-agonist that reduces adrenergic neurotransmission in an indirect way. There is much to say on behalf of antiadrenergic treatments on the theoretical side, but there is little guidance one can offer the clinician. It is a treatment that deserves a successful indication, but it has not found one yet.

The benzodiazepines have a bad reputation in TBI: There are problems of addiction, rebound panic following withdrawal, behavioral disinhibition, and excessive sedation. There is the disorganization that might attend treatment with ultra-short-acting benzodiazepines, or even transient global amnesia. Lorazepam and clonazepam have a host of useful indications, for insomnia, agitation, anxiety, panic, akathisia, and perhaps some other problems as well. The physician should never be surprised when a patient responds well to a well selected benzodiazepine, and the problem of addiction is not nearly so formidable as you may think.

The calcium channel blockers (e.g., verapamil, nifedipine) have been cited for migraine, Tourettes syndrome, manic-depression, tardive dyskinesia, and probably for a few other conditions by the time this chapter is in print. They are extremely interesting to neuropsychiatrists because they represent a wholly new approach to treatment, and, like the β-blockers, they have an agreeable toxicity profile. The reader is advised to keep up with research that is generated over the next few years.

SUMMARY

There is more to the pharmacology of TBI than meets the eye. Neurologists and psychiatrists who treat this class of patients are at a disadvantage, because their familiarity with the psychotropics usually stems from clinical experience with "mainstream" psychopharmacology. That is not necessarily a good foundation for the treatment of TBI patients. High doses of drugs are usually not necessary for TBI patients. Reflex polypharmacy should be eschewed, and psychiatric diagnosis is only occasionally pertinent to the problems of a patient with a brain lesion.

The new epidemic of closed head injury, which accounts for the vast majority of TBI cases today, has introduced a new physiology to the study of brain injury. (See Chapter 2.) The neuropathologic injury pattern induced by closed head injury interferes with ascending neurotransmission especially of the monoamines; dopamine, norepinephrine, and serotonin. Thus, brainstem "tone" to the cerebral cortex is disrupted, and deficits in arousal compound the affliction that comes of cortical injury. This is why treatment with dopamine agonists, which plays such an important role in the foregoing disquisition, may well be a "rational" treatment for TBI patients with a wide range of behavioral disorders, from depression to amnesia.

The neuropharmacology of special populations, like TBI patients, stroke victims, demented people, and the developmentally handicapped, is not like "mainstream" psychopharmacology. It is a growing field in its own right, and the development of new treatments, like THA, deprenyl, and the calcium channel blockers, may have benefits unforeseen at this time.

References

Altschuler, L.L., Devinsky, O., Post, R.M., and Theodore, W. (1990). Depression, anxiety and temporal lobe epilepsy. Arch. Neurol. 47:284–88.

Bareggi, S.R., Porta, M., Selenati, A., et al. (1975). Homovanillic acid and 5-Hydroxyindole-acetic acid in the CSF of patients after a severe head injury. I. Lumbar CSF concentration in chronic brain post-traumatic syndromes. European Neurology, 13:528–44.

Barnhill, L.J., and Gualtieri, C.T. (1989). Late-onset psychosis after closed head injury. Neuropsychiatry, Neuropsychology and Behavioral Neurology, 2:211–18.

Bear, D.M., and Fedio, P. (1977). Quantitative analysis of interictal behavior in temporal lobe epilepsy. Arch. Neurol., 34:454–67.

Cassidy, J.W. (1989). Fluoxetine: A new serotonergically active antidepressant. J. Head Trauma Rehabil., 4:67–70.

Chandler, M., Barnhill, L.J., and Gualtieri, C.T. (1991). Amantadine: Profile of use in the developmentally disabled. In: Ratey, J.J. (ed). Mental retardation: Developing pharmacotherapies. Washington, DC: American Psychiatric Press, 139–62.

Chandler, M.C., and Gualtieri, C.T. (1990). Amantadine: A medical, neuropsychological and psychiatric profile. In: Ratey, J.J., (ed). Mental retardation: Developing pharmacotherapies. Washington, DC: American Psychiatric Press.

Childs, A. (1986; unpublished). Naltrexone in organic bulimia.

Dejerine, J., and Roussy, G. (1906). La syndrome thalamique. Rev. Neurol., 14:521–32.

Evans, R.W., and Gualtieri, C.T. (1988). Motor performance in hyperactive children treated with imipramine. Perceptual and Motor Skills, 66:763-69.

Evans, R.W., Gualtieri, C.T., and Amara, I. (1986). Methylphenidate and memory: Dissociated effects in hyperactive children. Psychopharm., 90:211-16.

Feeney, D., Gonzalez, A., and Law, W.A. (1982). Amphetamine, haloperidol and experience interact to affect rate of recovery after motor cortex surgery. Science, 217:855-57.

Gartrell, N. (1986). Increased libido in women receiving trazadone. Am. J. Psych., 143(6):781-82.

Gualtieri, C.T. (1977). Imipramine and children: A review and some speculations on the mechanism of drug action. Dis. Nerv. Sys., 38:368-75.

Gualtieri, C.T. (1990). Neuropsychiatry and behavioral pharmacology. Berlin: Springer-Verlag.

Gualtieri, C.T. (1991; unpublished). Buspirone for the neurobehavioral sequelae of temporal lobe injuries.

Gualtieri, C.T. (1991). Buspirone for the behavior problems of patients with organic brain disorders. J. Clin. Psychopharmacol., 11:280-81.

Gualtieri, C.T. (1992). Neuropsychiatric issues in head trauma rehabilitation. In: Stoudemire, A., and Fogel, B. (eds). Principles of medical psychiatry, 2nd ed. New York: Oxford University Press.

Gualtieri, C.T., Chandler, M., Coons, T., and Brown, L. (1989). Amantadine: A new clinical profile for traumatic brain injury. Clin. Neuropharm., 12:258-70.

Gualtieri, C.T., and Cox, D.R. (1991). The delayed neurobehavioral sequelae of traumatic brain injury. Brain Injury, 5:219-32.

Gualtieri, C.T., and Evans, R.W. (1988). Stimulant treatment for the neurobehavioral sequelae of traumatic brain injury. Brain Injury, 2:273-90.

Horiguchi, J., Inami, Y., and Shoda, T. (1990). Effects of long-term amantadine treatment on clinical symptoms and EEG of a patient in a vegetative state. Clin. Neuropharmacol., 13:84-88.

Jus, A., Villeneuve, A., Gautier, J., Pires, A., Cote, J.M., Jus, K., Villeneuve, R., and Perron, D. (1973). Some remarks on the influence of lithium carbonate on patients with temporal epilepsy. Internatl. J. Clin. Pharmacol., 7(1):67-74.

Leijon, G., and Boivie, J. (1989). Central post-stroke pain—a controlled trial of amitriptyline and carbamazepine. Pain, 36:27-36.

Lezak, M.D. (1983). Neuropsychological assessment. New York: Oxford University Press.

Luria, A., Naydin, V., Tsvetkova, L., et al. (1968). Restoration of higher cortical function following local brain damage. In: Vinkin, R.J., and Bruyn, G.W., (eds). Handbook of clinical neurology. North Holland: Amsterdam, 368-433.

Luria, A.R. (1973). The frontal lobes and the regulation of behavior. In: Pribran, K.H., and Luria, A.R. (eds). Psychophysiology of the frontal lobes. New York: Academic Press, 3-28.

Marotta, R.F., Potegal, M., Glusman, M., et al. (1977). Dopamine agonists induce recovery from surgically-induced septal rage. Nature, 269(6):513-15.

Modell, J.G., Mountz, J.M., Curtis, G.C., and Greden, J.F. (1989). Neurophysiologic dysfunction in basal ganglia/limbic striatal and thalamocortical circuits as a pathogenetic mechanism of obsessive-compulsive disorder. J. Neuropsychiatry, 1(1):27-36.

Rickels, K., and Schweitzer, E.E. (1987). Current pharmacotherapy of anxiety disorder. In: Meltzer, H.Y. (ed). Psychopharmacology: The third generation of progress. New York: Raven Press, 1193-1203.

Rimel, R.A., Giordani, B., Barth, J.T., Boll, T.J., and Jane, J.A. (1981). Disability caused by minor head injury. Neurosurgery, 9:221-28.

Ross, E.D., and Rush, A.J. (1981). Diagnosis and neuroanatomical correlates of depression in brain-damaged patients. Arch. Gen. Psychiatry, 38:1344–354.

Ross, E.D., and Steart, R.M. (1981). Akinetic mutism from hypothalamic damage: Successful treatment with dopamine agonists. Neurol., 31:1435–39.

Scher, M., Krieger, J., and Juergens, S. (1983). Trazadone and priapism. Am. J. Psych. 140:1362–63.

Shalat, S.L., Seltzer, B., Pidcock, C., and Baker, E.L. (1987). Risk factors for Alzheimer's disease: A case-control study. Neurol., 37:1630–33.

Temkin, N.R., Dikman, S.S., Wilensky, A.J., Keihm, J., Chabal, S., and Winn, R. (1990). A randomized double-blind study of phenytoin for the prevention of post-traumatic seizures. N. Eng. J. Med., 323:497–502.

Waxman, S.G., and Geschwind, N. (1975). The interictal behavioral syndrome of temporal lobe epilepsy. Arch. Gen. Psychiatry, 32:1580–86.

Yufodfsky, S., Williams, D., and Gorman, J. (1981). Propranolol in the treatment of patients with chronic brain syndrome. Am. J. Psych., 138:218–330.

13

Behavior Therapy in Brain Injury Rehabilitation

JOHN R. DAVIS
GERALD GOLDSTEIN

Behavioral disorders are the most enduring and socially disabling of the problems typically seen after brain injury (Rosenthal and Bond, 1990). While the specific acquisition of these disturbances is a very individual matter, they are a function of an interaction of several major factors, including the person's repertoire of premorbid cognitive and social skills, the nature of the brain injury and its consequences, and the social environment following injury (Rosenthal and Bond, 1990). It is also important to take into account the patient's stage of recovery, because time since onset may be associated to some extent with differing disorders, etiologies, treatment goals, and intervention strategies (Eames, Haffey, and Cope, 1990).

Types of disorders seen following injury can be categorized into several groups (Eames, 1988), including excesses, such as aggression and self-stimulation, deficits, such as lack of specific social skills, inappropriate stimulus control where a behavior occurs at the wrong time or place, and syndromal disorders, such as depressive or paranoid conditions. Little is known about the incidence and prevalence of behavioral disorders following brain injury, although estimates range as high as 72% following severe head trauma (Crosson, 1987). Levin and Grossman (1978) found presence of behavioral disorder to be related to severity of injury, with agitation during the acute phase of injury being related to residual behavioral problems. This relationship of behavioral disturbance to severity of injury has also been documented with a pediatric population (Fletcher, Ewing-Cobbs, Miner, Levin, and Eisenberg, 1990). Furthermore, if behavioral sequelae do occur, they are persistent unless specifically addressed with appropriate treatment (Burke, Wesolowski, and Zencius, 1988; Thomsen, 1984).

BEHAVIOR THERAPY

Behavior therapy is an applied discipline that has made increasing contributions to the field of rehabilitation generally (Fordyce, 1982), and, more recently, to the treatment of brain injury (Goldstein, 1990; Horton and Sautter, 1988; McGlynn, 1990). This field is characterized by its primary focus on measurable behavior, use of learning principles to account for behavior acquisition and change, specification of explicit treatment goals, support for the importance of defining behavior in terms of the interaction between person and environment, use of individually tailored methods, emphasis on the present, and reliance on empiricism and quantification (Masters, Burish, Hollon, and Rimm, 1987). The field displays a wealth of diversity in the problems addressed and methods employed (Bellack, Hersen, and Kazdin, 1990; Martin and Pear, 1988).

Assessment Methods

A significant goal in application of behavior methods is to generate an assessment of the target behavior as it presents itself in the individual case. This assessment describes the problem in objective terms, assists in the planning of a treatment that matches the specifics of the case, and serves as a basis for evaluating the effects of treatment (Ciminero, 1986). The exact methods used in behavioral assessment are highly varied and are modified to suit the individual case. They can be classified as either self-report, physiologic, or direct recording of behavior (Bellack and Hersen, 1988; Ciminero, Calhoun, and Adams, 1986). It is perhaps these latter approaches that are most distinctively behavioral. Included are methods such as recording the occurrence of events, duration or latency of behavior, permanent products of behavior, results of probe trials, time sampling, and occurrence or nonoccurrence of behavior during a particular interval (Van Houten and Rolider, 1991). Each of these has advantages and disadvantages and may be more or less useful in conjunction with audiotape, videotape, or automated recording methods. The important point is that behavioral assessment allows for the quantification and measurement of the target behaviors to be changed whether they are motor, verbal, cognitive, affective, or physiologic responses. These methods also lead to the behavioral formulation or functional analysis of the target behavior and its relationship to situational, cognitive, and physical factors that control its occurrence (Haynes and O'Brien, 1990; Russo, 1990). It is this formulation, in turn, that sets the stage for the development of appropriate and effective plans for intervention.

Intervention Methods

Treatment methods developed from the results of assessment are, like the assessments themselves, highly individualized. These methods are also quite diverse, depending on the response modality of the target and the principles being applied. For example, stimulus control, reinforcement, and punishment methods are associated with principles of operant conditioning while counterconditioning methods are generally associated with classical conditioning paradigms (Cooper, Heron, and Heward, 1987; Iwata, Vollmer, and Zarcone, 1990; Kazdin, 1989). More recent developments have seen the application of social learning and verbal/cognitive approaches in the use of modelling and vicarious learning techniques, and in the introduction of cognitive change methods in problem solving and self-management interventions (Bellack, et al., 1990; Masters, et al., 1987).

Evaluation Methods

Central to the method of behavior therapy is the necessary inclusion of a program evaluation component in treatment. This serves to demonstrate that clear changes occur in the target behavior and that they are caused by the introduction of treatment. While some documentation of therapeutic efficacy has been carried out using research designs that randomly assign subjects to one treatment group or another (Campbell and Stanley, 1966; Cook and Campbell, 1979), the majority of support for behavioral intervention is derived from single case experimental designs (Barlow and Hersen, 1984). The three primary single case designs are the reversal design, multiple baseline design, and alternating treatments design, each of which depends on the availability of reliable data and involves replicating treatment effects over repeated measures with the same individual (Van Houten and Rolider, 1991). The reversal design, after an initial pretreatment or baseline period, presents, then removes, and then represents treatment. In contrast, the multiple baseline design requires the collection of several different sets of baseline data, with either 2 or more individuals, settings, or behaviors. Following simultaneous collection of these several baselines, treatment is introduced sequentially to each individual, setting, or behavior. The last major design involves alternating a treatment with either no treatment or a comparison treatment while monitoring the corresponding effects on behavior. Use of these designs facilitates the identification of factors that can control or ameliorate target behaviors, and assists in the demonstration that change in behavior can be attributed convincingly to the presentation of treatment.

APPLICATIONS IN REHABILITATION

Use of behavioral approaches in brain injury rehabilitation has grown steadily in recent years with the burgeoning population of survivors. In a large number of cases, reports document the successful use of methods, but, because of experimental design flaws, it is difficult to make conclusive statements about the efficacy of treatment. An increasing number of studies using rigorous methodology with reliable measures show results of behavioral intervention that are clinically significant, generalizable, and well maintained. The present review provides a survey of problems on which behavioral interventions have focused, the treatment methods employed, and their results. The review limits itself by concentrating on the treatment of behavioral sequelae that result from acute onset brain injury, such as trauma, anoxia, and infection. Excluded are applications with patients suffering from brain injury due to complications during the perinatal period, such as asphyxia during birth, degenerative processes, or the aging process, such as stroke.

Aggression

Aggressive behavior is frequently associated with recovery from brain injury and can pose a serious obstacle to comprehensive therapeutic programming. Some case reports have noted success with programs that focus on changing antecedents of aggression by decreasing stimulation, increasing predictability by scheduling, signalling an impending event, or approaching patients from a side not affected by visual neglect (Deaton, 1990; Divack, Herrle, and Scott, 1985; Wood, 1987). One report (Turkat and Behner, 1989) explicitly takes a behavioral formulation of the patient's premorbid paranoid personality into account in developing an intervention that eliminated all sources of threat after a range of positive and aversive contingency management programs had failed. Graduated exposure with distracters and "counterconditioning" elements have also been used, for example, by Cohen (1986) who describes successfully treating screaming that occurred when a patient was accompanied to the toilet. This program also included reinforcement and modelling components. Anecdotal reports of maintenance at 12-month follow-up were encouraging. A second case (Jacobs, Lynch, Cornick, and Slifer, 1986) applied in vivo desensitization in a multiple baseline design with good success even at a 5-year anecdotal follow-up.

Most often, the emphasis of treatment has been on changing the consequences of behavior. Several reports, for example, have successfully applied programs of differential reinforcement in which aggressive behavior is selectively ignored and incompatible alternatives (Hollon, 1973) or behavior other than aggression is reinforced, either socially (Divack, et al., 1985) or with tokens (M.M. Wood, 1981; Wood, 1988). Some studies also report success with introduction of treatment into a sequence of situations (Horton and Howe, 1981; Horton and Barrett, 1988). Only one such study, however, reported long-term maintenance with a 1-year follow-up, although no supporting data are presented (Hurwitz, 1973, cited in Ince, 1976). Turner, Green, and Braunling-McMorrow (1990) used a multiple baseline across situations design to evaluate differential reinforcement of low rates of verbal and physical aggression, using token reinforcement and an increasingly stringent criterion in each situation. Although lack of interobserver agreement data somewhat compromises the results, good success was noted and, by and large, was maintained at 1-month follow-up. In contrast, however, some reports have presented cases in which reinforcement alone was ineffective and aggression responded only to a combination of reinforcement and aversive consequences (Sand, Treischmann, Fordyce, and Fowler, 1970, cited in Ince, 1976).

A number of single case studies have suggested the effectiveness of aversive methods in controlling aggressive behavior after brain injury. Many have applied either exclusionary (Goodman-Smith and Turnbull, 1983; Wood, 1984, 1986, 1987) or nonexclusionary (Wood, 1984, 1987) time out in the context of an ongoing program of positive reinforcement for nonaggressive behavior of various sorts. In addition to time out, reinforcement programs have been augmented by other aversive consequences, such as loss of tokens as a response cost (Alderman and Burgess, 1990; Wood, 1981, 1987), restitution and overcorrection (Foxx and Azrin, 1972), and negative verbal feedback and physical restraint (Deaton, 1990; Jacobs, et al., 1986; McMillan, Papadopoulos, Cornall, and Greenwood, 1990). While data from these studies appear promising, follow-up is almost wholly lacking. One report of a combined token reinforcement and exclusionary time out program showed some maintenance at 2-month follow-up (Tate, 1987), and another using restraint showed maintenance at 3-week follow-up (Jacobs, et al., 1986).

A few reports have documented some success with self-control and cognitive interventions. Burgess and Alderman (1990) taught one patient self-monitoring of anxiety levels, cognitive restructuring, and instrumental "mastery" skills to give him greater control over his personal care. At 3-month follow-up the patient's shouting showed some relapse but was still quite low relative to baseline. Another report (Burke and Wesolowski, 1988) noted that aggression in a patient occurred when he forgot something. Therefore, this memory factor was taken into account in treatment planning by developing methods to compensate for memory loss, as well as redirecting his attention early in the chain of escalating aggressive behaviors, teaching relaxation skill, and scheduling time to receive special attention from staff.

Self-control training was also a component in a broad spectrum intervention described by Burke, Wesolowski, and Lane (1988). Specifics of the self-control component were training in problem identification, generation of alternative solutions, selection of the most appropriate solution, and self-relaxation. In addition, patients received reinforcer sampling, identification of competencies and behavioral strengths, high frequency reinforcement for appropriate behaviors, reduction in environmental stimulation and demands, training in self-monitoring of appropriate and inappropriate behavior, and review of how aggression is personally inconvenient as a consequence to aggression. Following treatment implementation, results showed a dramatic decrease in aggression which was maintained at 6-month follow-up. Finally, Lira, Carne, and Masri (1983), applied a stress inoculation treatment (Novaco, 1977) that included education about the antecedents, functions, and ways to express anger, acquisition of cognitive and behavioral skills for dealing with anger eliciting situations, and training in the application of these skills with a hierarchy of actual anger related situations. In addition to positive response during the patient's hospitalization, the authors note, anecdotally, that gains were maintained 5 months after discharge.

A number of problems make qualification of these studies necessary. Use of these methods with aggressive behavior is most often presented in simple pre-post designs that do not demonstrate convincing control of the behavior by the treatment. Further, many reports are only anecdotal or fail to include documentation of interobserver agreement. Precise functional analysis is also lacking in that no reports objectively document the relationship of antecedent and consequent events to the target behavior in question. Generalization of behavior change across situations, therapists, over time, and to collateral behaviors is addressed only to a very limited extent. Some reports also present multicomponent interventions where it is difficult to determine what the necessary and sufficient elements were. Finally, few reports address the issues of relative efficacy of treatments or of matching treatments to individual cases based on a comprehensive functional analysis that includes current environmental factors as well as premorbid functioning and neuropsychologic status.

Self-Stimulation and Self-Injurious Behavior

A sequela of brain injury rarely discussed is self-stimulation or self-injury. Two reports, however, present single case investigations of hand biting (Tynan and Pearce, 1990) and leg pounding (Lewis, Blackerby, Ross, Guth, Cronkey, White, and Cook, 1986). Tynan and Pearce carried out a descriptive analysis of circumstances surrounding hand biting, providing anecdotal information that it was preceded by desire to be moved or being upset, and followed by removal to the patient's bedroom or social attention. In a pre-post design the authors used contingent restraint along with communication training, differential reinforcement of appropriate communication, and discontinuation of previously occurring changes in the patient's schedule. This intervention resulted in marked reductions in the inappropriate behavior, although no data were reported for changes in appropriate behavior. Treatment had to be reinstituted at 9-month follow-up because of relapse but at 1-year follow-up the behavior was still under control.

In a relatively well-designed study, Lewis, et al. (1986), used an alternating treatments design to evaluate the comparative efficacy of long and short durations of contingent negative practice for leg pounding. Antecedent conditions were anecdotally reported as treatment sessions and unstructured time. Treatment was applied in a counterbalanced manner concurrently with social skills training. Both intervals of negative practice showed equal success in reducing leg pounding. In spite of treatment application in several different settings by a number of therapists, generalization to a nontreatment setting did not occur until negative practice was introduced there as well.

Inappropriate Behavior

A range of inappropriate behaviors has been successfully addressed with behavioral methods following brain injury, including such nonverbal activities as throat clearing, nose picking, spitting, and hoarding, as well as verbal behaviors such as screaming, complaining, and demanding attention (Wood, 1987). Some of these reports suggest success with relatively straightforward reinforcement contingencies. For instance, Sushinsky (1970) describes the use of differential reinforcement of appropriate behavior with a patient who provoked other patients, made incessant demands of staff, and both urinated and defecated on the floor. Token reinforcers, in the form of reminder cards, were provided on a 15-minute schedule and could be exchanged for cigarettes. Although success was reported, no data are presented. Similarly, Wilson (1981) reports success with a differential reinforcement of other behavior (DRO) program involving social reinforcement to suppress yelling, but no data are presented.

Differential reinforcement was also successfully applied for low rates of manipulative behavior (Wood and Eames, 1981) and for behaviors incompatible with complaining (M.M. Wood, 1981). The long-term efficacy of these approaches has also been suggested. Hurwitz (1973, cited in Ince, 1976) used a token system to differentially reinforce behaviors incompatible with leaving the hospital, alcohol use, and wearing noninstitutional clothes. Hopewell (1983) describes applying social reinforcement for lack of symptomatic movements in a patient who developed hemichorea-hemiballismus following traumatic brain injury. Anecdotal follow-ups at 1 year and 10 months, respectively, indicated complete maintenance of change.

Positive contingencies alone may prove ineffective in some cases of inappropriate behavior. Although not specifically contrasted with reinforcement alone, several studies describe the use of decelerative approaches, in conjunction with reinforcement techniques. Time out from positive reinforcement has been successfully applied with disruptive behavior (Wood and Eames, 1981), and screaming with anecdotal reports of maintenance at 3-month follow-up (Andrewes, 1989). Wood (1984, 1987) reports cases in which aromatic ammonia was used as an aversive consequence in the context of a token economy for several inappropriate behaviors, including nose picking, throat clearing, and spitting. One of these cases presents a relatively convincing demonstration of the effectiveness of treatment by using a reversal design in the treatment of throat clearing (Wood, 1987). Whaley, Stanford, Pollack, and Lehrer (1986) evaluated the additional effectiveness of lithium medication applied in conjunction with a token reinforcement plus response cost intervention for a variety of inappropriate behaviors they related to frontal lobe damage. No additional benefit of medication was noted although the moderate suppression of behaviors that occurred with treatment was maintained at 4-month follow-up. While some success on follow-up is suggested in these studies, Wood (1987) also notes the importance of overlearning or the continued application of treatment for some time after the objectives have been reached in order for gains to be preserved.

Two innovative applications of behavioral methods are reported by Wesolowski and colleagues. Zencius and Wesolowski (1989) decreased elopement by teaching stress management skills with modelling, role playing, feedback, and homework assignments. Using these approaches, a young female patient was taught to identify stresses that had been associated with elopement, leave the immediate place where she was, go to a designated relaxation area, and once there use deep breathing and progressive muscle relaxation. At 36-week follow-up elopements were maintained at zero. A second report (Lane, Wesolowski, and Burke, 1989) treated hoarding behavior by facilitating the performance of appropriate behaviors in the same response class, in this case collecting baseball cards and picking up litter. A multicomponent treatment provided the patient with baseball cards contingent on positive behavior and taught him to organize his cards on a special board. Collecting a specified number of cards was rewarded with delivery of hats. In addition, he was taught to pick up and throw away litter with cards as a reinforcer. Staff gave him attention and social reinforcement for collecting cards and responded with a reprimand and brief time out for picking up trash at inappropriate times. Treatment effects are persuasive in this study given documentation of acceptable reliability of measures, the use of a fortuitous reversal design, and success at 1-year follow-up.

Sexual Behavior

Relatively few published reports have dealt with sexuality following brain injury (Boller and Frank, 1982; Crewe, 1984; Weinstein, 1974), although some data have suggested hyposexuality to be more frequent than hypersexuality (Zasler, 1988). Behavioral methods have thus far addressed only behavioral excesses such as touching, self-stimulation, self-exposure, and sexual comments (McMillan, et al., 1990; Turner, et al., 1990; Zencius, Wesolowski, Burke, and Hough, 1990). Functional analysis of inappropriate sexual behavior has not been described in published reports with the exception of Horton and Barrett (1988) who note the importance of integrating neuropsychologic and behavioral data in constructing a case formulation and effective plan. In this case study, the patient's touching was found to occur in situations that required him to perform in an area of relative weakness from a neuropsychologic perspective, so that touching functioned to provide an escape from what was, for him, an aversive situation.

Usually, treatment methods have been limited to pre-post designs. One exception is Turner, et al. (1990), who describe a multiple baseline design that successfully used differential reinforcement of low rates of inappropriate behavior, along with differential reinforcement of other behavior. This and other reports of differential reinforcement have used token reinforcement (Wood, 1988). Edible reinforcement (McMillan, et al., 1990) and informational feedback (Zencius, et al., 1990) have been used as well. Behavioral contracting has been described in one case (Crosson, 1987). Some cases, in addition to reinforcement methods, include aversive procedures such as time out (Wood, 1987), response cost (Crosson, 1987), and verbal reprimands (McMillan, et al., 1990). Due to the experimental designs used, it is not possible to determine the relative contribution of each component, however, Zencius, et al. (1990), report positive results using relatively novel methods such as self-monitoring, private self-stimulation, dating skills training, and scheduled acceptable touching in appropriate settings, to shift stimulus control of the behavior. In current studies, generalization data are usually absent or limited to anecdotal reports or brief follow-up assessment. However, two reports have documented maintenance of improvements following discharge from the treatment setting (McMillan, et al., 1990; Turner, et al., 1990).

Emotional Complaints

Although emotional sequelae of brain injury, such as anxiety, depression, obsessional, and paranoid disorders, are a significant concern (Rosenthal and Bond, 1990), almost no studies have been conducted to evaluate behavioral methods of intervention. One anecdotal report (Damon, Lesser, and Woods, 1979) describes a generalized decrease in social anxiety in an aphasic patient with the use of relaxation, graduated exposure, and social reinforcement. In a second report, Lysaght and Bodenhamer (1990) treated stress in four patients using relaxation training that included EMG biofeedback, autogenic exercises, imagery, deep breathing, and home practice. A self-report measure of physical and psychologic functioning documented improvements that were maintained at 4-week follow-up.

Compliance and On-Task Behavior

Persons with brain injury frequently refuse to participate in rehabilitation activities or to follow through with tasks that are necessary in order to achieve independence, even though the requisite capabilities are present. Although this domain of behavior may be seen as relating to cognitive functions, such as attention, memory, and executive functions, including initiation, it is also possible to conceptualize targets in behavioral terms. For example, anecdotal reports suggest participation in treatment increases following behavioral contracting (Crosson, 1987), and social and token reinforcement by other patients (Wilson and McCulley, 1970). Improvement has been noted in attendance at a work site following token reinforcement (Burke and Lewis, 1986), and decreases in uncooperative behavior occurred with introduction of a paradoxical intervention based on symptom prescription (Kushner and Knox, 1973). Wood (1986, 1987) presented data describing cases in which on-task behavior was operationally defined (looking at the therapist), and treated by providing token reinforcement and shaping increasingly longer durations of attention. This approach has also been successful in increasing cooperative behavior (Wood, 1988). Meyerson, Kerr, and Michael (1967), targeted attention to a typing task after informally observing that the therapist had been differentially responding to off-task behavior by paying attention to the patient primarily when he stopped working to call for help, ask a question, or complain. The patient responded to a treatment that involved moving the work to a less distracting area, making social attention contingent on a gradually increasing criterion of work completed, and ignoring off-task demands.

In contrast to earlier anecdotal reports, more conclusive demonstrations of behavioral methods in this area have appeared in recent years.

Using a reversal design, Tate (1987) reported positive changes occurred in attending treatment, trying tasks, and follow-through after sessions, with the use of token reinforcement. Generalization over time and to new situations was reported, albeit without data. It was noted that overlearning or extended application of intervention was necessary before changes were maintained in the absence of treatment.

Hegel (1988) described a noncompliant patient where treatment with goal setting, shaping of progressively more demanding goals, token reinforcement, and selective ignoring of disruptive verbalizations, was successfully implemented. The documentation of interobserver agreement and evaluation of effects in a design that combined a multiple baseline across settings with a treatment reversal allowed a convincing demonstration of treatment effectiveness.

More recently, Zencius and colleagues have used reversal designs to contrast different types of intervention for compliance problems. Zencius, Wesolowski, and Burke (1989) targeted class attendance in two TBI adolescents. They compared behavioral contracting with either a token or point system of reinforcement that provided for frequent opportunities to earn points; the point system with response cost (loss of points); and a once-daily point or "check" system. Each approach was associated with improvements, although some differential effectiveness for the point system was suggested for one client. At 2-month follow-up 100% attendance had been maintained for one client.

Antecedent control was also investigated by Zencius, Wesolowski, Burke, and McQuaide (1989) in three single-case designs. Unauthorized breaks responded best to written prompts compared to a verbal contract in one case. Use of a cane responded best to presenting the cane during the second patient's morning routine relative to either social praise, escorting a patient to get the cane if she forgot, or monetary reinforcement. Finally, attendance at sessions was shown to respond better to reviews of the patient's daily schedule prior to her first class as compared to either verbal prompts, written invitations, or monetary reinforcement. In discussing the comparative usefulness of these antecedent methods, Zencius, et al., point out the importance of taking patients' memory impairments into account.

Biofeedback

Although frequently applied with patients suffering from a variety of CNS disorders, biofeedback has been infrequently used with traumatic brain injury or other etiologies of acute onset, with the exception of cerebrovascular accidents (Brucker, 1984). This may relate to successful treatment requiring relatively intact cognitive functioning and motivation, characteristics often compromised in patients with generalized brain damage.

Reports of EMG feedback to treat spasticity, paresis, dyskinesia, and apraxia following brain injury, have noted encouraging successes (Amato, Hermsmeyer, and Kleinman, 1983; Brudny, Korein, Grynbaum, and Sachs-Frankel, 1977; Brudny, Korein, Grynbaum, Belandres, and Gianutsos, 1979), using methods involving positive and negative reinforcement, shaping, and gradual fading of treatment. In addition to changes in the activity of the specific muscle group trained, these authors note functional improvements that are maintained. However, even in this very select group of patients, some do not show gains, although this does not appear related to etiology (Brudny, et al., 1979). One novel use of EMG feedback (Frazier, 1980) focused on several targets in a 16-year-old patient following traumatic brain injury, beginning with hand movement, which led to positive response even during coma and may have contributed to eventual recovery to a level of functioning close to her premorbid status.

Coma

In addition to the report by Frazier (1980) described above, one other investigation of operant methods with coma patients has been carried out. Boyle and Greer (1983) presented music phrases contingently following response to verbal requests for three motor responses in a multiple baseline design replicated with three patients in vegetative coma. Each patient also had a withdrawal and reinstatement phase of treatment for one of the target behaviors. Positive, but limited, results were observed, with the best response occurring for the patient who had been in coma for the briefest period.

Physiotherapy

Applications of behavioral methods in the context of physiotherapy have successfully targeted increases in a variety of behaviors including duration of exercise (Lincoln, 1981), walking (Lincoln, 1978; Wood, 1984), gait pattern (Gouvier, Richards, Blanton, Janert, Rosen, and Drabman, 1985; Jarrett, Gauthier, and Olivier, 1978), transfers (Hooper-Roe, 1988; Wood, 1984, 1987), and head posture (Hooper-Roe, 1988). All of these reports, however, present only simple pre-post designs, with the exception of Gouvier, et al. (1985). Functional analysis is not explicitly presented in any of these studies, although the importance of considering memory impairment in one case is noted (Lincoln, 1981). Treatments relied primarily on reinforcement methods, including edible, social, token, activity, and publicly posted graphic feedback of performance. One case described the use of self-monitoring (Jarrett, et al., 1978) as a component of treatment.

Several cases illustrate the use of graduated task requirements ar setting, involving task analysis, chaining, and shaping togethe. ..iun prompting and reinforcement approaches (Goodman-Smith and Turnbull, 1983). The management of disruptive behavior, such as yelling and complaining during treatment, is described in one case where complaining was systematically ignored while exercise was reinforced (Lincoln, 1981). In another case, behavior incompatible with pain complaints was reinforced (Hollon, 1973). In this latter report, staff selectively ignored complaints, and used prompting and reinforcement to engage the patient in a conversation that served to distract her from potentially painful therapy activities. Punishment has also been used in conjunction with reinforcement methods during gait training by Gouvier, et al. (1985), who delivered contingent aversive sound for yelling, and by Jarrett, et al. (1978), who used brief exclusionary time out and loss of tokens as a response cost for inappropriate gait. Many of these reports indicate that improvements generalized across situations or time, although presentation of quantitative data bearing on this issue was infrequent (Hooper-Roe, 1988).

Occupational Therapy, Nursing, and Functional Skills

Not surprisingly, brain injury frequently results in serious disability in self-care skills. These functional abilities include activities of daily living such as bathing, grooming, dressing, eating, toilet use, and mobility. Typically, these have been addressed by occupational therapy and nursing staff, although more recent efforts have seen interdisciplinary collaboration involving the use of learning methods. Bathing and dressing, perhaps because they have such a large impact on burden of care and independence, have received a relatively great deal of attention. Several case x studies described successful use of task analysis of the desired activities, establishing a fixed sequence of activities, prompting, and reinforcement (e.g., social, token, edible) (Giles and Clark-Wilson, 1988; McMillan, et al., 1990; M.M. Wood, 1981; Wood, 1984). Altering the reinforcement schedule to require an increasing number of responses per reinforcer as the patient progresses has been reported (Wood, 1986, 1987). Similarly, making token earnings contingent on the number of prompts provided and fading prompts have been documented (Wood, 1986, 1987). Murphy (1976) also presented a report describing a ward-wide token economy incorporating fines that was successful with a group of "organically" impaired patients.

The few reports of this type of program for bathing and dressing that have assessed maintenance are somewhat encouraging. Giles and colleagues, for example, reported anecdotal success generalized to new situations at 6-month follow-up (Giles and Clark-Wilson, 1988; Giles and Shore, 1989). Successful maintenance at 3-month follow-up was also seen in a case that utilized spouse-delivered token reinforcement (M.M. Wood,

1981). Giles and Morgan (1989) included verbal linking phrases that were modeled by the therapist and then repeated by the patient as a cue to the next step in the sequence. This component, along with verbal and edible reinforcers, task analysis, and momentary time out for inappropriate verbalizations, was associated with washing and dressing improvements that were maintained 3 months after treatment.

Incontinence is another disability of great consequence. Treatment methods involving social, edible, and token reinforcement have been associated with improvements, and have involved scheduled checks of whether the patient currently needs to use the toilet (Papworth, 1989; Wilson, 1981) or bladder training (Papworth, 1989). These programs usually include a response cost component for accidents involving loss of tokens alone (Alderman and Burgess, 1990; Giles and Clark-Wilson, 1988) or combined with cleaning up and positive practice of appropriate toilet use (Papworth, 1989). Successful follow-up has been reported for as long as 6 months (Papworth, 1989).

Wheelchair and automobile navigation have been addressed, albeit infrequently. Wood (1988) briefly mentions using salient cues, token reinforcement, and fading to improve wheelchair placement, with apparently good generalization, to new settings. In an interesting pre-post design with a group of patients, Sivak, Hall, Henson, Butler, Silber, and Olson (1984) found that remediation of underlying visual-perceptual impairments was associated with improvements in driving. Rather than treating the hypothesized underlying problems, Kewman, Seigerman, Kintner, Chu, Henson, and Reeder (1985) compared two groups who either did or did not receive training in simulated driving exercises. Training was carried out on adapted scooters and involved visuomotor tracking, divided attention, increasingly more difficult courses, performance feedback, and social reinforcement. Compared to the group who received only unstructured opportunities to use the scooter, the treatment group markedly improved their performance driving cars, although as a group they still did not equal noninjured drivers.

Several other functional skills have responded to behavioral methods. Systematic prompting and fading after a clearly identified task analysis has been associated with improvements in shopping skills and food preparation (Giles and Clark-Wilson, 1988), and drinking from a cup (Wilson, 1987). Godfrey and Knight (1988) reported using these methods along with social reinforcement and alteration in reinforcement schedules to change a variety of self-care behaviors. Improvements in medication management and using public transportation remained at 1-year follow-up.

A small number of studies show more definitive success of behavior intervention with this category of behaviors. Reidy (1979), for example, documented reliable observations of the eating behavior of a 7-year-old patient, and then used a reversal design to evaluate the effects of a multi-component treatment involving task analysis, prompting, social reinforcement, fading, and interruption of incorrect responses. Following staff and parent training, 90% maintenance of gains was observed at 15-week follow-up at school. O'Reilly and colleagues used written checklists as self-administered prompts, along with end of session feedback, to teach self-treatment of cold symptoms (O'Reilly and Cuvo, 1989) and home accident prevention skills (O'Reilly, Green, and Braunling-McMorrow, 1990). These multiple baseline designs demonstrated the reliability and efficacy of specific and individualized checklists in contrast to generic lists. Self-treatment skills for cold symptoms were not maintained at 1-month follow-up necessitating a reapplication of treatment, however, and generalization of this skill to the home environment was not assessed. On the other hand, maintenance of accident prevention skills was seen at 1-month follow-up with some generalization to a novel assessment room. Again, however, skill use in the community was not assessed.

Vocational Skills

Specific trials of behavioral interventions to address work related behaviors have rarely been reported. However, investigation in this area is beginning, notably with the work of Wehman and colleagues (Wehman, West, Fry, Sherron, Groah, Kreutzer, and Sale, 1989). As Lewinsohn and Graf (1973) indicated, social, emotional, and behavior problems are frequent during the vocational rehabilitation of brain-injured persons, and are significantly associated with poor outcome. Wehman, et al. (1989), reported the investigation of an individual placement model of supported employment in a multiple baseline study with five subjects. The components of this model are varied, but included behavioral skill training aimed at improving work performance, social skills training, and behavioral feedback. Results showed limited but encouraging improvements, with the major problems including insubordinate, disruptive, and inappropriate social behaviors on the job site. Glisky and Schacter (1987) trained a densely amnestic patient complex knowledge and skills relating to data entry work on a microcomputer. A task analysis was done of the job components followed by training using the method of vanishing cues and extensive repetition. The patient was ultimately able to perform as quickly and accurately as experienced employees.

Speech and Communication

Given the emphasis that contemporary society places on verbal skills it is understandable that the area of speech and communication has received a great deal of attention from behavior therapists working with patients following brain trauma. An important recent development in the field of speech and language pathology has been growing interest in pragmatic aspects of communication in addition to the more formal, structural aspects of language (Prutting and Kirchner, 1987). Many brain-injured patients show intact linguistic utterances while failing to use these preserved skills to achieve effective communication (Ehrlich and Barry, 1989). While some of these pragmatic behaviors have been addressed in more general social skills training programs, such as those described below, a number of other behavioral applications have focused on more circumscribed linguistic or pragmatic targets.

Several studies of linguistic targets have evaluated antecedent events such as the specific properties of stimuli themselves (Halpern, 1965a, b) or specific cues (Yorkston, Stanton, and Beukelman, 1981). Halpern's work, for example, showed that level of abstraction, word length, word probability, and modality of presentation affect verbal perseveration and errors. Written cues with feedback have been used successfully on a verbal sequencing task with maintenance at 2-month follow-up (Yorkston, et al., 1981). Salvatore (1976) also adjusted length of pauses in the presentation of material in a study of a patient's comprehension of spoken commands where improvements were maintained 12 weeks after treatment.

Other studies have emphasized consequent events, with Wood (1987) using shaping and differential social reinforcement to improve swallowing, and token and edible reinforcement to increase polysyllabic speech. Aversive consequences have also been evaluated. Wood (1984) found exclusionary time out and token reinforcement for appropriate speech resulted in decreases in scanning dysarthria in a patient who refused to use techniques to improve the clarity of his speech in situations outside the treatment room. The effectiveness of this combination of positive and negative consequences was demonstrated in a multiple baseline across patients design which promoted use of speech techniques on the ward in patients who spoke unclearly (Wood, 1987). Examining another target, Kushner, Hubbard, and Knox (1973), contrasted the effects of time out, response cost, and aversive noise as consequences for errors on a visual paired associate matching task. While learning occurred under all conditions, the addition of a reinforcement contingency resulted in the best performance.

Several investigators have intervened with specific pragmatic components of communication. Walls (1969) used differential reinforcement to increase verbal and decrease nonverbal communication. Wood (1987) used a similar approach to decrease profanity, noting good generalization to a ward setting after using multiple therapists. Decelerative methods have also been incorporated in treatment. Jarrett, et al. (1978), used an approach that combined cuing methods and planned ignoring with a young woman who repeated herself and spoke inaudibly. Burgess and Alderman

(1990) report one case using feedback and response cost to decrease speech volume, and another using token reinforcement, response cost, and positive practice to decrease verbal perseveration (Alderman and Burgess, 1990). The second study demonstrated treatment effects in a reversal design, and showed good generalization at 3-month follow-up on a ward that continued to provide a less intensive token-based treatment.

Social Skills Training

A frequently observed sequela of brain injury is impairment of social skills (Crosson, 1987; Rosenthal and Bond, 1990; Stambrook, Moore, and Peters, 1990). These impairments can take the form of either excesses or deficits in areas such as conversational skills (Schloss, Thompson, Gajar, and Schloss, 1985), assertion (Braunling-McMorrow, Lloyd, and Fralish, 1986), nonverbal behavior (Brotherton, Thomas, Wisotzek, and Milan, 1988), amount of interaction (Deaton, 1990), personal appearance (Passler, 1987), or pragmatic features of communication (Ehrlich and Barry, 1989).

Some attempts to intervene with this category of behavior have found positive response to fairly direct treatments. For example, McMordie (1976) focused on perseverative speech using a reversal design to demonstrate the effects of relaxation and instruction on reducing the rate of perseverative remarks. Deaton (1990) used edible and activity reinforcers along with training to signal feelings of being overwhelmed to reduce classroom withdrawal in a young boy. Token reinforcers with gradually faded feedback have been used to improve fairly general categories of social behavior (Passler, 1987). They have also been used with response cost components to address several behavior excesses such as attention-seeking, laughing, and grinning (Alderman and Burgess, 1990). The latter study contrasted token reinforcement with and without response cost and found that significant changes occurred only when intervention was made more salient with the introduction of the aversive contingency. Presumably the patient's deficits were such that reinforcement alone did not address his impaired cognitive abilities. Mutism has been successfully addressed with modelling, shaping, and edible reinforcement. Anecdotal reports indicated generalization to a ward setting and maintenance at 1-year after treatment (Sabatasso and Jacobson, 1970).

Contingency management approaches with social skills have been reported by Lewis and colleagues. Burke and Lewis (1986) treated verbal outbursts, interruptions, and nonsensical talk in a multiple baseline across behaviors design. Some behaviors were found to be more responsive to treatment than others. An embedded reversal design showed that points for low rates of behavior plus feedback to be more effective than feedback alone. Some generalization to a community restaurant was found. In a second report, Lewis, Nelson, Nelson, and Reusink (1988), used an alternating treatments design to evaluate the effects of attention, systematic ignoring, and corrective feedback on socially inappropriate talk. Corrective feedback brought about the most decrease in negative behavior. Generalization and maintenance were not assessed.

Complex approaches to social skills training have been described as well. For example, Damon, et al. (1979), outline a program involving instruction, modelling, role play, feedback, and homework practice to address such targets as tone of voice, intelligibility, content of speech, pauses, interruptions, and showing interest. However, no data were presented. The methods may be beneficial, however, given their good results with other populations (Kelly, 1982). In a methodologically stronger report, Helffenstein and Wechsler (1981) used similar methods along with problem solving in a pre-post randomized controlled design with a 1-month follow-up. Results were generally positive at follow-up, with generalization seen on social validation measures, a behavioral checklist of interaction in a recreation hall, and in self-concept. However, self-reported skill and observations from videotaped simulations did not change. In addition to applying similar methods to those described above, Brotherton, et al. (1988), enlisted family participation to reinforce social skills. Nonverbal behavior, speech dysfluencies, showing interest, giving reinforcement, and making positive statements were treated in a multiple baseline across behaviors design that was replicated with four patients. In spite of positive acquisition of skills, 1-year follow-up was mixed, and no home assessment was carried out.

Hopewell, Burke, Wesolowski, and Zawlocki (1990) augmented the typical social skills training program of instruction, modelling, rehearsal, and feedback/reinforcement with self-management, relaxation, cognitive self-control, and in vivo skills training. An attempt was made to identify individualized triggers for inappropriate behavior with self-monitoring prior to treatment. A variety of behaviors was targeted including accepting criticism, accepting denial of requests, ignoring negative peer behavior, disagreeing, physical aggression, threats, absences, teasing, and touching. The relative distribution of positive and negative behaviors began to shift toward the end of a lengthy treatment, and, at 12-week follow-up, the frequency of positive behaviors exceeded that of negative behaviors.

Evaluation of the effects of one aspect of self-control skills, self-monitoring, has been carried out in two sophisticated studies by Gajar and colleagues. In the first of these, Gajar, Schloss, Schloss, and Thompson (1984) compared the effects of self-monitoring versus feedback on positive (questions, relevant comments, comments that added to the conversation, agreements and disagreements) and negative (silences, brief remarks, off topic comments, mumbles, jokes, interruptions) social skills. Both interventions were effective, with behavioral indices resulting in equivalence to a social comparison group, and generalization occurring to less structured settings. A second study (Schloss, et al., 1985) used self-monitoring in a multiple baseline across behaviors design with an embedded alternating treatments component. The targets in this case were compliments, questions, and self-disclosures. Instructions to self-monitor appeared to contribute to the success of this intervention. Positive results were seen in naturalistic situations, evaluations relative to a social comparison group, and volunteer evaluations. Results of 1-month follow-up were mixed.

In contrast to the technically complicated methods described above, Braunling-McMorrow, et al. (1986), reported the use of a game format to target compliments, social interactions, politeness, handling criticism, social confrontation, and question and answer situations. The methods included feedback, self-monitoring, reinforcement, and individualized performance criteria. In spite of training that focused primarily on verbal rehearsal during a game situation, positive generalization was found to mealtime behavior, although staff ratings did not change.

Self-Management and Problem Solving

Behavioral methods have been employed to improve functional problem solving by addressing subjects' skills in solving socially valid, real-life difficulties. In an initial study of self-control strategies to compensate for left-sided neglect, Stanton, Flowers, Kuhl, Miller, and Smith (1979) developed a self-instructional method that built on patients' intact language skills. In a control group design, this study found improvements on treatment tasks but no generalization to other tasks.

Malec (1984) reported uncontrolled case studies without supporting data, which utilized a variety of self-management approaches with apparently good success. In one case, conversational skills were targeted for change using discrimination training, rehearsal, and practice in performing complex sequences of conversation. In a second case, an attempt was made to increase a patient's attention to positive events and decrease her negative assessment of events. Although benefits were indicated, generalization was not certain.

More recently, Foxx and colleagues (Foxx, Marchand-Martella, Martella, Braunling-McMorrow, and McMorrow, 1988; Foxx, Martella, and Marchand-Martella, 1989) presented a series of studies utilizing a nonrandomized pretest-posttest control group design with a small group of patients. Four problem solving areas were targeted for training (community awareness and transportation; medication, alcohol, and drugs; stating one's rights; and emergencies, injuries, and safety). The intervention was presented in a game format that involved cue cards, response-specific feedback, modelling, self-monitoring, positive reinforcement, response practice, self-correction, and individualized performance criteria. In the first study, Foxx, et al. (1988), found that patients receiving intervention improved their problem solving skills. In contrast to untreated patients, those in the treatment group showed some improvement on measures of generalization when problem solving was assessed in phone calls, interviews, and staged interactions. The second study (Foxx, et al., 1989) replicated the results of the first, showed further evidence of generalization, and demonstrated maintenance of gains over a 6-month follow-up. Furthermore, it was found that treated patients' 6-month scores were comparable to a sample of nonhandicapped individuals.

REHABILITATIVE CONTINUA

The brain-injured population receiving rehabilitation services is heterogeneous from several standpoints. Most clearly, the severity of disability may be quite variable ranging from mild aftereffects barely clinically detectable to severe and pervasive disability. Another continuum is the variability in types of disabling disorders. As we see elsewhere in this chapter, the brain-injured patient may present a variety of different types of disorder, some of which we would describe as "behavioral," some as "cognitive," and some as "functional." Sometimes, the total disability spans several disorders, while in other cases, the disability is quite specific to one area. Therefore, it is not possible to establish a general program for brain-injury rehabilitation unless one uses the term in the sense of an umbrella framework that encompasses a variety of individualized procedures.

Program planning can be conceptualized by considering the interactions among various continua. That is, each patient may be seen as demonstrating a given degree of severity in one or more types of disorder. For example, one patient may have a severe disorder of language, while some other patient may have mild disorders of memory and behavioral self-control. Neuropsychologic and behavioral assessments are often necessary to make these determinations. Generalized severity of cognitive impairment, or level of performance, typically provides a limiting constant for the planned program. More importantly, however, it provides information as to goal formation and choice of characteristics of the rehabilitation approach taken. Type of impairment identified provides information concerning choice of appropriate content for the program. For example, the REHABIT system, developed by Reitan and collaborators, involves a choice of content based upon whether the neuropsychologic assessment reveals primarily language, visual-spatial, or conceptual difficulties (Reitan and Sena, 1983).

An extended example of these considerations is offered utilizing the case in which a single, specific deficit varies over a range of severity. The area chosen is memory. Memory impairment is a ubiquitous consequence of brain disease or injury, although its specific presentation varies widely. Its severity may range from mild forgetfulness to pervasive, global amnesia. In content, it may be modality-specific, involving, for example, only verbal or nonverbal memory, or it may pertain to only some form of memory, such as immediate recall or remote memory. Thus, patients with memory disorders may be characterized on the basis of severity and content. If rehabilitation is contemplated, the severity-content interface may be seen as the basis for program planning.

Before pursuing rehabilitation planning further, it is necessary to consider briefly the neuropsychology and clinical phenomenology of memory disorder associated with brain damage. Some patients experience only mild to moderate memory deficits that show a pattern of spontaneous recovery. Typically, the basis of this form of disorder is head trauma, immediately following which there is a period of posttraumatic amnesia (PTA). Following resolution of the PTA, many patients show no apparent sign of continued memory disorder. However, perhaps 20% of closed-head injury patients acquire a persistent memory disorder that far outlasts the PTA period (Levin, Benton, and Grossman, 1982). Sometimes this disorder is associated with attentional dysfunction, but that is not always the case. These patients often complain of forgetfulness and they may demonstrate impaired memory on tests. Another group of individuals, particularly people who sustain strokes involving the posterior cerebral arteries, acquire modality specific memory deficits. Deficits in nonverbal or verbal memory are associated with the hemisphere in which the stroke occurred. At the far end of the continuum are patients with organic amnesic disorder (Korsakoff's syndrome) who are globally and severely amnesic, generally to the point of disorientation. There are, in addition, very amnesic patients who are also generally intellectually impaired. Typically, patients with the senile dementias share this combination of disorders.

It is apparent from these considerations that some single form of memory rehabilitation would not be equally appropriate for all of these conditions. We would propose that the intervention utilized may be seen as lying on a continuum ranging from restoration to prosthetic substitution. This continuum proceeds in accordance with the extent to which the environment takes on the function in question. In restoration, there are no environmental supports and the natural healing capacity of the organism, in combination with the treatments given, lead to complete return of function. The individual is as good as he or she was before the illness or injury. An intermediate point may be characterized as environmental support in which some device is used to help in execution of an impaired function. The individual still performs the function, but is assisted in some way by an external object or device. In prosthetic approaches, the function itself is performed by some external object or device. Recently, a report prepared by the Division of Clinical Neuropsychology of the American Psychological Association made essentially the same distinctions, using the terms "restoration," "reduction of negative impact," and "compensatory aids" to describe the three points on the continuum (Matthews, Harley, and Malec, 1990).

Rehabilitation of memory can be conceptualized in this manner, but it is first necessary to concede that restoration of memory does not appear to be possible at present. We know of no cases in the literature indicating that memory impairment associated with structural brain damage can be restored to premorbid level as a result of rehabilitation efforts. However, there seems to be more hope for environmental supports and prosthetics. In memory training, environmental supports are generally strategies or techniques taught to patients to help in organizing and retaining information. Some of these techniques have been borrowed from mnemonists who used them to perform extraordinary feats of memory (Lorayne and Lucas, 1974). The peg method, method of loci, and various techniques involving use of organizing information or of visual imagery, are examples of these procedures. The current literature indicates that patients with substantial memory deficits can learn to use these procedures in the sense that they can often demonstrate remarkable improvement on memory tasks they are taught during the training process (Kovner, Mattis, and Goldmeier, 1983). Evidence that these procedures are applied in everyday life situations is less convincing. We have demonstrated that patients with dense amnesic syndromes cannot use these procedures productively (Goldstein, Ryan, Turner, Kanagy, Barry, and Kelly, 1985), although the literature concerning this matter is not without controversy. However, a prosthetic approach utilizing environmental reminders and "smart technology" would appear to be more productive for such patients. Thus, in memory training, as in other areas of rehabilitation, one can conceptualize a range of approaches extending from those that depend entirely on the natural resources of the individual, through intermediary stages, to complete dependence upon the prosthetic environment.

Another parameter discussed in the rehabilitation literature concerns the generalizability or specificity of various approaches (Goldstein, 1987). Elsewhere in this chapter there are numerous examples of rather specific behavior therapy programs; programs for reducing elopement risk, screaming, self-stimulation, work site attendance, etc. Indeed, behavior therapy as a method of treatment has focused on targeted, specific behaviors. On the other hand, traditional neuropsychologic rehabilitation has focused on training of generic skills such as memory or perceptual abilities. These skills tended to resemble the sorts of behaviors measured with neuropsychologic tests. The term generic was used to describe this form of rehabilitation in the hope that the abilities trained would generalize to a number of relevant, specific behaviors. Diller and Gordon (1981) described the more generic methods as representing psychometrist (or chemist) and biologist models, both of which involve assessment of task demands and subsequent development of optimal rehabilitation tasks. Specific approaches were described in terms of an engineer model and deal directly with the original difficulty. While some success has been reported with both methods, they share the common difficulty of relative failure to generalize to activities of daily living that extend beyond the limits of the training programs themselves. However, the generic approach has been most commonly criticized for this deficiency, particularly in those cases in which the training undertaken has no clear external behavioral referent.

While initially neuropsychologically based rehabilitation typically utilized generic training in the hope of generalization, more recently developed programs have tended to move away from that strategy. The direction taken has generally been toward the more specific-prosthetic end of the continua and has involved both supportive and prosthetic programs. Using such programs, it has been shown that severely amnesic patients can learn by rehearsal and retain items of information that may be relevant for activities of daily living (Goldstein and Malec, 1989), and can learn a series of computer-related words (Glisky, Schacter, and Tulving, 1986). The material taught has been characterized as domain specific knowledge and skills (Schacter and Glisky, 1986). Developers of these methods have speculated that they may utilize the preserved implicit or procedural memory system often found in very amnesic patients. Other than what is achieved by the training itself, these patients typically remain as amnesic as they ever were, but they have learned something that may be of some practical value in their everyday lives. Thus, there is little, if any generalization emerging from these programs but none is anticipated.

Other program developers have advocated and reported on the use of computers, reminding devices, and related "smart technologies" to provide support through the prosthetic environment. The use of lists, diaries, and other external reminders is now common in rehabilitation facilities. One of our own groups (Goldstein) is in the process of developing a memory prosthesis for severely amnesic patients. It will be a programmable device that contains a limited number of items of information. We have observed that a difficulty with prostheses that must be used voluntarily is that severely amnesic patients literally forget to use them. Therefore, part of the training program will involve a rehearsal period during which the patient will be trained to remember to use the device; for example, to put it in his pocket when he dresses in the morning.

It therefore appears that some of the behaviors dependent upon a relatively intact memory can be restored to brain-damaged patients with memory disorders of varying severity and types. While complete restoration of memory is probably never achieved, some patients may benefit from supports in the form of mnemonic strategies, while more impaired patients seem able to acquire specific knowledge through systematic training of various types. We would note that patients having the potential for supportive or "strategy teaching" programs should receive such programs rather than prosthetic interventions because of the greater likelihood of generalization with the former type of program. Appropriate neuropsychologic assessment is crucial for applying these procedures because inappropriate application may either lead to failure, or to a result that is less productive than may be possible.

EVALUATION AND FUTURE DIRECTIONS

The results of behavioral applications in brain injury rehabilitation as reviewed above are encouraging but not overwhelming. Many methodologic limitations are seen in the studies produced by this young field. A partial list includes such basic flaws as lack of reliability checks and frequent reliance on pre-post designs with single subjects that do not allow for inferences about causality. More complicated issues that need to be addressed concern generalization, long-term follow-up, social validity of behavior change, relative treatment effectiveness, and the absence of community-based studies. The integration of functional analysis and neuropsychologic data in treatment development and clinical decision making is rarely reported. Because these issues are often addressed by a range of staff involved in the implementation of treatment, it is necessary to more explicitly investigate service delivery models and staff training methods that will facilitate the effective application of behavioral methods across situations (Fuoco and Christian, 1986; Milne, 1986; Reid and Shoemaker, 1984; Rolider and Van Houten, in press). With multifaceted interventions there is a clear need to carry out component analyses to document the necessary and sufficient conditions for behavior change.

Although behavioral methods have been applied to a number of problem areas, there are other problems for which behavioral approaches have been developed that have not yet received documented clinical application in brain injury rehabilitation. Some of these areas include marital (Bornstein and Bornstein, 1986) and family therapy (Falloon, 1988), and learning based methods with educational targets (Richards, 1985). In addition, few reports are available detailing the use of learning methods to address the addictive behaviors that so often play a role in brain injury (Blackerby and Baumgarten, 1990; Sparadeo, Strauss, and Barth, 1990).

Throughout the enterprise of evaluating the application of behavioral methods with brain-injured patients, the tantalizing prospect of integrating neuropsychology's knowledge base of brain-behavior relationships with behavior therapy presents itself (Goldstein, 1984). This ambiguous specialty of behavioral neuropsychology was defined a number of years ago by Horton (1979):

> Essentially, Behavioral Neuropsychology may be defined as the application of Behavior Therapy techniques to problems of organically impaired individuals while using a neuropsychological assessment and intervention perspective (p. 20).

Some guidelines for the field have been suggested (Horton and Sautter, 1988), but its focus is principally on the rehabilitation of brain injury rather than the assessment or basic science aspects (Goldstein, 1990).

While rehabilitation within neuropsychology initially emphasized the restoration of covert generic functions, recent efforts have focused on more specific abilities. Behavioral approaches have also targeted practical and specific overt behaviors (Goldstein, 1987; Goldstein and Ruthven, 1983). The successes and failures of these approaches raise the question of whether a range of training opportunities is necessary, with behavioral neuropsychology addressing the spectrum of cognitive, behavioral, and affective processes that, in interaction, result in functional independence. Conducting program planning in a manner that considers the several continua described earlier may function to integrate behavioral and neuropsychologic approaches. Examination of patient-related continua having to do with severity, type of disorder, and time since onset will result in a profile of strengths and weaknesses in different but possibly related content areas such as those described in the World Health Organization's classification of impairment, disability, and handicap (WHO, 1980). Decisions can then be made as to where to focus rehabilitation on goal-related continua, ranging from restorative to compensatory and specific to general objectives. Depending on the content in the patient-related continua and the objective in the goal-related continua, treatment may appear more "neuropsychologic" or more "behavioral." As progress occurs, the nature of the goal may correspondingly change from a more "neuropsychologic" to a more "behavioral" one, or vice versa. In this way of approaching the integration of behavior therapy and neuropsychology, intervention methods can be viewed as based on empirically derived learning approaches, with only the type of goal differentiating whether the behavioral or neuropsychologic end of a behavioral neuropsychology continuum of rehabilitation is emphasized.

More specific points of contact between the two disciplines have also been suggested by Goldstein (1990). The first has to do with the rather direct application of behavioral learning methods to patients with brain dysfunction. Neuropsychology can provide useful input to clinical decision making here by suggesting modifications to intervention that may be necessitated by perceptual or cognitive constraints, and by recommending stimulus and response features on which to focus. The second point of contact concerns use of behavioral methods to change performance related to particular cognitive impairments. Regardless of which point of contact is considered, the issue of generalization is significant. Both response generalization from retrained underlying cognitions to functional skills, and situational generalization of specific behaviors to enduring real-life contexts, must be considered. That this generalization does not occur automatically should come as no surprise. It may be facilitated, however, by the use of prosthetic approaches in which some feature of the environment assumes responsibility or compensates for lost function, or the systematic programming of generalization in the educational efforts aiming to restore compromised abilities (Kazdin, 1989). Neuropsychology can be of assistance in deciding where rehabilitation will be most productive in this continuum of treatment (Goldstein, 1990). What is needed now is empirical verification that the integration of these two disciplines leads to effective rehabilitation.

SUMMARY

This chapter reviews the variety of behavioral problems seen following brain injury and the behavioral methods used to address them. The developing interest in this field is supported by the encouraging preliminary results. A cookbook approach to intervention with these difficult problems is inappropriate. It is important to emphasize the necessity for rigorous assessment and analysis of individual cases, using clearly documented and reproducible methods. Better designed studies of behavioral methods with brain-injured individuals are needed so that more confident conclusions can be made about their effectiveness. It will also be important to draw on the database concerning brain-behavior relationships from neuropsychology, both to articulate how it can be integrated with behavioral methods and to document its contribution. Behavioral and neuropsychologic methods may contribute jointly to the evaluation of patients along several rehabilitation continua. Finally, it is necessary to show more convincingly that behavioral change methods are capable of producing significant improvements that are relevant to the functional goals of the individual, and that these changes are preserved throughout the individual's long-term adjustment.

References

Alderman, N., and Burgess, P.W. (1990). Integrating cognition and behavior: A pragmatic approach to brain injury rehabilitation. In: Wood, R.L., and Fussey, I. (eds). Cognitive rehabilitation in perspective. New York: Taylor and Francis, 204–28.

Amato, A., Hermsmeyer, C.A., and Kleinman, K.M. (1973). Use of electromyographic feedback to increase inhibitory control of spastic muscles. Physical Therapy, 53: 1063–66.

Andrewes, D. (1989). Management of disruptive behaviour in the brain-damaged patient using selective reinforcement. Journal of Behavior Therapy and Experimental Psychiatry, 20:261–64.

Barlow, D.H., and Hersen, M. (1984). Single case experimental designs: Strategies for studying behavior change (2nd ed). New York: Pergamon Press.

Bellack, A.S., and Hersen, M. (eds). (1988). Behavioral assessment: A practical handbook (2nd ed). New York: Pergamon Press.

Bellack, A.S., Hersen, M., and Kazdin, A.E. (eds). (1990). International handbook of behavior modification and therapy (2nd ed). New York: Plenum Press.

Blackerby, W.F., and Baumgarten, A. (1990). A model treatment program for the head-injured substance abuser: Preliminary findings. Journal of Head Trauma Rehabilitation, 5:47–59.

Boller, F., and Frank, E. (1982). Sexual dysfunction in neurological disorders: Diagnosis, management and rehabilitation. New York: Raven Press.

Bornstein, P.H., and Bornstein, M.T. (1986). Marital therapy: A behavioral-communications approach. New York: Pergamon Press.

Boyle, M.E., and Greer, R.D. (1983). Operant procedures and the comatose patient. Journal of Applied Behavior Analysis, 16:3–12.

Braunling-McMorrow, D., Lloyd, K., and Fralish, K. (1986). Teaching social skills to head injured adults. Journal of Rehabilitation, 52:39–44.

Brotherton, F.A., Thomas, L.L., Wisotzek, I.E., and Milan, M.A. (1988). Social skills training in the rehabilitation of patients with traumatic closed head injury. Archives of Physical Medicine and Rehabilitation, 69:827–32.

Brucker, B.S. (1984). Biofeedback in rehabilitation. In: Golden, C.J. (ed). Current topics in rehabilitation psychology. New York: Grune and Stratton, 173–99.

Brudny, J., Korein, J., Grynbaum, B.B., Belandres, P.V., and Gianutsos, J.G. (1979). Helping hemiparetics to help themselves: Sensory feedback therapy. Journal of the American Medical Association, 241:814–18.

Brudny, J., Korein, J., Grynbaum, B.B., and Sachs-Frankel, G. (1977). Sensory feedback therapy in patients with brain insult. Scandinavian Journal of Rehabilitation Medicine, 9:155–63.

Burgess, P.W., and Alderman, N. (1990). Rehabilitation of dyscontrol syndromes following frontal lobe damage: A cognitive neuropsychological approach. In: Wood, R.L., and Fussey, I. (eds). Cognitive rehabilitation in perspective. New York: Taylor and Francis, 183–203.

Burke, W.H., and Lewis, F.D. (1986). Management of maladaptive social behavior of a brain-injured adult. Rehabilitation Research, 9:335–43.

Burke, W.H., and Wesolowski, M.D. (1988). Applied behavior analysis in head injury rehabilitation. Rehabilitation Nursing, 13:186–88.

Burke, W.H., Wesolowski, M.D., and Lane, I.M. (1988). A positive approach to the treatment of aggressive brain-injured clients. International Journal of Rehabilitation Research, 11:235–41.

Burke, W.H., Wesolowski, M.D., and Zencius, A. (1988). Long-term programs in head injury rehabilitation. Cognitive Rehabilitation, 6:38–44.

Campbell, D.T., and Stanley, J.C. (1966). Experimental and quasi-experimental designs for research. Chicago: Rand McNally.

Ciminero, A.R. (1986). Behavior assessment: An overview. In: Ciminero, A.R., Calhoun, K.S., and Adams, H.E. (eds). Handbook of behavioral assessment (2nd ed). New York: John Wiley and Sons, 3–11.

Ciminero, A.R., Calhoun, K.S., and Adams, H.E. (eds). (1986). Handbook of behavioral assessment (2nd ed). New York: John Wiley and Sons.

Cohen, R.E. (1986). Behavioral treatment of incontinence in a profoundly neurologically impaired adult. Archives of Physical Medicine and Rehabilitation, 67:883-84.

Cook, T.D., and Campbell, D.T. (eds). (1979). Quasi-experimentation: Design and analysis issues for field settings. Chicago: Rand McNally.

Cooper, J.D., Heron, T.E., and Heward, W.L. (1987). Applied behavior analysis. New York: Merrill.

Crewe, N.M. (1984). Sexually inappropriate behavior. In: Bishop, D.S. (ed). Behavior problems and the disabled: Assessment and management. Baltimore: Williams and Wilkins, 120-141.

Crosson, B. (1987). Treatment of interpersonal deficits for head-trauma patients in inpatient rehabilitation settings. The Clinical Neuropsychologist, 1:335-52.

Damon, S.G., Lesser, R., and Woods, R.T. (1979). Behavioural treatment of social difficulties with an aphasic woman and dysarthric man. British Journal of Disorders of Communication, 14:31-38.

Deaton, A.V. (1990). Behavioral change strategies for children and adolescents with traumatic brain injury. In: Bigler, E.D. (ed). Traumatic brain injury: Mechanisms of damage, assessment, intervention, and outcome. Austin, TX: PRO-ED, 231-49.

Diller, L., and Gordon, W.A. (1981). Rehabilitation and clinical neuropsychology. In: Filskov, S.B., and Boll, T.J. (eds). Handbook of clinical neuropsychology. New York: John Wiley and Sons, 641-82.

Divack, J.A., Herrle, J., and Scott, M.B. (1985). Behavior management. In: Ylvisaker, M. (ed). Head injury rehabilitation—children and adolescents. San Diego: College Hill Press, 347-60.

Eames, P. (1988). Behavior disorders after severe head injury: Their nature and causes and strategies for management. Journal of Head Trauma Rehabilitation, 3:1-6.

Eames, P., Haffey, W.J., and Cope, D.N. (1990). Treatment of behavioral disorders. In: Rosenthal, M., Griffith, E.R., Bond, M.R., and Miller, J.D. (eds). Rehabilitation of the adult and child with traumatic brain injury (2nd ed). Philadelphia: F.A. Davis, 410-32.

Ehrlich, J., and Barry, P. (1989). Rating communication behaviours in the head-injured adult. Brain Injury, 3:193-98.

Falloon, I.R.H. (ed). (1988). Handbook of behavioral family therapy. New York: Guilford Press.

Fletcher, J.M., Ewing-Cobbs, L., Miner, M.E., Levin, H.S., and Eisenberg, H.M. (1990). Behavioral changes after closed head injury in children. Journal of Consulting and Clinical Psychology, 58:93-95.

Fordyce, W.E. (1982). Psychological assessment and management. In: Kottke, F.J., Stillwell, G.K., and Lehemann, J.F. (eds). Kruser's handbook of physical medicine and rehabilitation. Philadelphia: W.B. Saunders, 124-50.

Foxx, R.M., and Azrin, N.H. (1972). Restitution: A method of eliminating aggressive-disruptive behaviour of retarded and brain damaged patients. Behaviour Research and Therapy, 10:15-27.

Foxx, R.M., Marchand-Martella, N.E., Martella, R.C., Braunling-McMorrow, D., and McMorrow, M.J. (1988). Teaching a problem solving strategy to closed head injured adults. Behavioral Residential Treatment, 3:193-210.

Foxx, R.M., Martella, R.C., and Marchand-Martella, N.E. (1989). The acquisition, maintenance, and generalization of problem solving skills by closed head-injured adults. Behavior Therapy, 20:61-76.

Frazier, L.M. (1980). Biofeedback in coma rehabilitation: Case study. American Journal of Clinical Biofeedback, 3:148-54.

Fuoco, F.J., and Christian, W.P. (eds). (1986). Behavior analysis and therapy in residential programs. New York: Van Nostrand Reinhold.

Gajar, A., Schloss, P.J., Schloss, C.N., and Thompson, C.K. (1984). Effects of feedback and self-monitoring on head trauma youths' conversation skills. Journal of Applied Behavior Analysis, 17:353-58.

Giles, G.M., and Clark-Wilson, J. (1988). The use of behavioral techniques in functional skills training after severe brain injury. American Journal of Occupational Therapy, 42:658-65.

Giles, G.M., and Morgan, J.H. (1989). Training functional skills following herpes simplex encephalitis: A single case study. Journal of Clinical and Experimental Neuropsychology, 11:311-18.

Giles, G.M., and Shore, M. (1989). A rapid method for teaching severely brain-injured adults how to wash and dress. Archives of Physical Medicine and Rehabilitation, 70:156-58.

Glisky, E.L., and Schacter, D.L. (1987). Acquisition of domain-specific knowledge in organic amnesia: Training for computer-related work. Neuropsychologia, 25:893-906.

Glisky, E.L., Schacter, D.L. and Tulving, E. (1986). Learning and retention of computer related vocabulary in memory-impaired patients: Method of vanishing cues. Journal of Clinical and Experimental Neuropsychology, 8:292-312.

Godfrey, H.P.D., and Knight, R.G. (1988). Memory training and behavioral rehabilitation of a severely head-injured adult. Archives of Physical Medicine and Rehabilitation, 69:458-60.

Goldstein, G. (1984). Methodological and theoretical issues in neuropsychological assessment. In: Edelstein, B.A., and Couture, E.T. (eds). Behavioral assessment and rehabilitation of the traumatically brain-damaged. New York: Plenum Press, 1-21.

Goldstein, G. (1987). Neuropsychological assessment for rehabilitation: Fixed batteries, automated systems, and non-psychometric methods. In: Meier, M.J., Benton, A.L., and Diller, L. (eds). Neuropsychological rehabilitation. Edinburgh: Churchill Livingstone, 18-40.

Goldstein, G. (1990). Behavioral neuropsychology. In: Bellack, A.S., Hersen, M., and Kazdin, A.E. (eds). International handbook of behavior modification and therapy (2nd ed.) (pp. 139-149). New York: Plenum Press.

Goldstein, G., and Malec, J.F. (1989). Memory training for severely amnesic patients. Neuropsychology, 3:9-16.

Goldstein, G., and Ruthven, L. (1983). Rehabilitation of the brain-damaged adult. New York: Plenum Press.

Goldstein, G., Ryan, C., Turner, S.M., Kanagy, M., Barry, K., and Kelly, L. (1985). Three methods of memory training for severely amnestic patients. Behavior Modification, 9:357-74.

Goodman-Smith, A., and Turnbull, J. (1983). A behavioral approach to the rehabilitation of severely brain-injured adults. Physiotherapy, 69:393-96.

Gouvier, W.D., Richards, S., Blanton, P.D., Janert, K., Rosen, L.A., and Drabman, R.S. (1985). Behavior modification in physical therapy. Archives of Physical Medicine and Rehabilitation, 66:113-16.

Halpern, H. (1965a). Effect of stimulus variables on verbal perseveration of dysphasic subjects. Perceptual and Motor Skills, 20:421-29.

Halpern, H. (1965b). Effect of stimulus variables on dysphasic verbal errors. Perceptual and Motor Skills, 21:291-98.

Haynes, S.N., and O'Brien, W.H. (1990). Functional analysis in behavior therapy. Clinical Psychology Review, 10:649-68.

Hegel, T. (1988). Application of a token economy with a non-compliant closed head injured male. Brain Injury, 2:333-78.

Helffenstein, D.A., and Wechsler, F.S. (1981). The use of interpersonal process recall (IRP) in the remediation of interpersonal and communication skill deficits in the newly brain-damaged. Clinical Neuropsychology, 3:139-43.

Hollon, T.H. (1973). Behavior modification in a community hospital rehabilitation unit. Archives of Physical Medicine and Rehabilitation, 54:65–72.

Hooper-Roe, J. (1988). Rehabilitation of physical deficits in the post-acute brain-injured: Four case studies. In: Fussey, I., and Giles, G.M. (eds). Rehabilitation of the severely brain-injured adult: A practical approach. London: Croom Helm, 102–15.

Hopewell, C.A. (1983). Hemichorea-hemiballismus as conversion reaction following head trauma. Clinical Neuropsychology, 5:32–35.

Hopewell, C.A., Burke, W.H., Wesolowski, M.D., and Zawlocki, R.J. (1990). Behavioral learning therapies for the traumatically brain-injured patient. In: Wood, R.L., and Fussey, I. (eds). Cognitive rehabilitation in perspective. New York: Taylor and Francis, 229–45.

Horton, A.M., Jr. (1979). Behavioral neuropsychology: Rationale and research. Clinical Neuropsychology, 1:20–23.

Horton, A. M., Jr., and Barrett, D. (1988). Neuropsychological assessment and behavior therapy: New directions in head trauma rehabilitation. Journal of Head Trauma Rehabilitation, 3, 57–64.

Horton, A.M., Jr., and Howe, N.R. (1981). Behavioral treatment of the traumatically brain-injured: A case study. Perceptual and Motor Skills, 53:349–50.

Horton, A.M., Jr., and Sautter, S.W. (1988). Behavioral neuropsychology: Behavioral treatment for the brain-injured. In: Wedding, D., Horton, A.M. Jr., and Webster, J.S. (eds). The neuropsychology handbook: Clinical and behavioral aspects. New York: Springer, 259–77.

Ince, L.P. (1976). Behavior modification in rehabilitation medicine. Springfield, IL: Charles C. Thomas.

Iwata, B.A., Vollmer, T.R., and Zarcone, J.R. (1990). The experimental (functional) analysis of behavior disorders: Methodology, applications, and limitations. In: Repp, A.C., and Singh, N.N. (eds). Perspectives on the use of nonaversive and aversive interventions for persons with developmental disabilities. Sycamore, IL: Sycamore Publishing, 301–30.

Jacobs, H.E., Lynch, M., Cornick, J., and Slifer, K. (1986). Behavior management of aggressive sequelae after Reye's syndrome. Archives of Physical Medicine and Rehabilitation, 67:558–63.

Jarrett, F.J., Gauthier, J., and Oliver, R.D. (1978). Operant management of the behavioural sequelae of Wilson's disease: A case report. Canadian Psychiatric Association Journal, 23:399–403.

Kazdin, A.E. (1989). Behavior modification in applied settings (4th ed). Pacific Grove, CA: Brooks/Cole Publishing.

Kelly, J.A. (1982). Social-skills training: A practical guide for interventions. New York: Springer.

Kewman, D.G., Seigerman, C., Kintner, H., Chu, S., Henson, D., and Reeder, C. (1985). Simulation training of psychomotor skills: Teaching the brain-injured to drive. Rehabilitation Psychology, 30:11–27.

Kovner, R., Mattis, S., and Goldmeier, E. (1983). A technique for promoting robust free recall in chronic organic amnesia. Journal of Clinical Neuropsychology, 5:65–71.

Kushner, H., Hubbard, D.J., and Knox, A.W. (1973). Effects of punishment on learning by aphasic subjects. Perceptual and Motor Skills, 36:283.

Kushner, H., and Knox, A.W. (1973). Application of the utilization technique to the behavior of a brain-injured patient. Journal of Communication Disorders, 6:151–54.

Lane, I.M., Wesolowski, M.D., and Burke, W.H. (1989). Teaching social appropriate behavior to eliminate hoarding in a brain-injured adult. Journal of Behavior Therapy and Experimental Psychiatry, 20:79–82.

Levin, H., Benton, A., and Grossman, R. (1982). Neurobehavioral consequences of closed head injury. New York: Oxford University Press.

Levin, H.S., and Grossman, R.G. (1978). Behavioral sequelae of closed head injury. Archives of Neurology, 35:720–27.

Lewinsohn, P.M., and Graf, M. (1973). A follow-up study of persons referred for vocational rehabilitation who have suffered brain injury. Journal of Community Psychology, 1:57–62.

Lewis, F.D., Blackerby, W.F., Ross, J.R., Guth, M.L., Cronkey, R.F., White, M.J., and Cook, T. (1986). Duration of negative practice and the reduction of leg pounding of a TBI adult. Behavioral Residential Treatment, 1:265–74.

Lewis, F.D., Nelson, J., Nelson, C., and Reusink, P. (1988). Effects of three feedback contingencies on the socially inappropriate talk of a brain-injured adult. Behavior Therapy, 19:203–11.

Lincoln, N.B. (1978). Behavior modification in physiotherapy. Physiotherapy, 64:265–67.

Lincoln, N. (1981). Clinical psychology. In: Evans, C.D. (ed). Rehabilitation after severe head injury. Edinburgh: Churchill Livingstone, 146–65.

Lira, F.T., Carne, W., and Masri, A.M. (1983). Treatment of anger and impulsivity in a brain damaged patient: A case study applying stress inoculation. Clinical Neuropsychology, 5:159–60.

Lorayne, H., and Lucas, J. (1974). The memory book. New York: Ballantine Books.

Lysaght, R., and Bodenhamer, E. (1990). The use of relaxation training to enhance functional outcomes in adults with traumatic head injuries. American Journal of Occupational Therapy, 44:797–802.

Malec, J. (1984). Training the brain-injured client in behavioral self-management skills. In: Edelstein, B.A., and Couture, E.T. (eds). Behavioral assessment and rehabilitation of the traumatically brain-damaged. New York: Plenum, 121–50.

Martin, G., and Pear, J. (1988). Behavior modification: What it is and how to do it (3rd ed). Englewood Cliffs, NJ: Prentice Hall.

Masters, J.C., Burish, T.G., Hollon, S.D., and Rimm, D.C. (1987). Behavior therapy: Techniques and empirical findings (3rd ed). New York: Harcourt Brace Jovanovich.

Matthews, C.G., Harley, J.P., and Malec, J.F. (1990). Guidelines for computer assisted neuropsychological rehabilitation and cognitive remediation. Washington, DC: Division 40 (Clinical Neuropsychology), American Psychological Association.

McGlynn, S.M. (1990). Behavioral approaches to neuropsychological rehabilitation. Psychological Bulletin, 108:420–41.

McMillan, T.M., Papadopoulos, H., Cornall, C., and Greenwood, R.J. (1990). Modification of severe behavior problems following herpes simplex encephalitis. Brain Injury, 4:399–406.

McMordie, W.R. (1976). Reduction of perseverative inappropriate speech in a young male with persistent anterograde amnesia. Journal of Behavior Therapy and Experimental Psychiatry, 7:67–69.

Meyerson, L., Kerr, N., and Michael, J.L. (1967). Behavior modification in rehabilitation. In: Bijou, S.W., and Baer, D.M. (eds). Child development: Readings in experimental analysis. New York: Appleton Century Crofts, 214–39.

Milne, D.L. (1986). Training behavior therapists: Methods, evaluation, and implementation with parents, nurses, and teachers. London: Croom Helm.

Murphy, S.T. (1976). Effects of a token economy program on self-care behaviors of neurologically impaired inpatients. Journal of Behavior Therapy and Experimental Psychiatry, 7:145–47.

Novaco, R.W. (1977). Stress inoculation: A cognitive therapy for anger and its application to a case of depression. Journal of Consulting and Clinical Psychology, 45:600–08.

O'Reilly, M.F., and Cuvo, A.J. (1989). Teaching self-treatment of cold symptoms to an anoxic brain-injured adult. Behavioral Residential Treatment, 4:359–76.

O'Reilly, M.F., Green, G., and Braunling-McMorrow, D. (1990). Self-administered prompts to teach home accident prevention skills to adults with brain injuries. Journal of Applied Behavior Analysis, 23:431–46.

Papworth, M.A. (1989). The behavioural treatment of nocturnal enuresis in a severely brain-damaged client. Journal of Behavior Therapy and Experimental Psychiatry, 20: 265–68.

Passler, M.A. (1987). A two-phase treatment approach for traumatically brain-injured patients: A case study. Rehabilitation Psychology, 32:215–26.

Prutting, C.A., and Kirchner, D.M. (1987). A clinical appraisal of the pragmatic aspects of language. Journal of Speech and Hearing Disorders, 52:105–19.

Reid, D.H., and Shoemaker, J. (1984). Behavioral supervision: Methods of improving institutional staff performance. In: Christian, W.P., Hannah, G.T., and Glahn, T.J. (eds). Programming effective human services: Strategies for institutional change and client transition. New York: Plenum Press, 39–61.

Reidy, T.J. (1979). Training appropriate eating behavior in a pediatric rehabilitation setting: Case study. Archives of Physical Medicine and Rehabilitation, 60:226–30.

Reitan, R.M., and Sena, D.A. (August, 1983). The efficacy of the REHABIT technique in remediation of brain-injured people. Paper presented at the annual meeting of the American Psychological Association, Anaheim, California.

Richards, C.S. (1985). Work and study problems. In: Hersen, M., and Bellack, A.S. (eds). Handbook of clinical behavior therapy with adults. New York: Plenum Press, 557–71.

Rolider, A., and Van Houten, R. (in press). The interpersonal treatment model: Teaching appropriate social inhibitions through the development of personal stimulus control by the systematic introduction of antecedent stimuli. In: Van Houten, R., and Axelrod, S. (eds). Effective behavioral treatment: Issues and implementation. New York: Plenum Press.

Rosenthal, M., and Bond, M.R. (1990). Behavioral and psychiatric sequelae. In: Rosenthal, M., Griffith, E.R., Bond, M.R., and Miller, J.D. (eds). Rehabilitation of the adult and child with traumatic brain injury (2nd ed) Philadelphia: F.A. Davis, 179–92.

Russo, D.C. (1990). A requiem for the passing of the three-term contingency. Behavior Therapy, 21:153–65.

Sabatasso, A.P., and Jacobson, L.I. (1970). Use of behavioral therapy in the reinstatement of verbal behavior in a mute psychotic with chronic brain syndrome: A case study. Journal of Abnormal Psychology, 76:322–24.

Salvatore, A.P. (1976). Training an aphasic adult to respond appropriately to spoken commands by fading pulse duration within commands. Clinical Aphasiology Conference Proceedings, 172–91.

Schacter, D.L., and Glisky, E.L. (1986). Memory remediation: Restoration, alleviation, and the acquisition of domain-specific knowledge. In: Uzzell, B.P., and Gross, Y. (eds). Clinical neuropsychology of intervention. Boston: Martinus Nijhoff, 257–82.

Schloss, P.J., Thompson, C.K., Gajar, A.H., and Schloss, C.N. (1985). Influence of self-monitoring on heterosexual conversational behaviors of head trauma youth. Applied Research in Mental Retardation, 6:269–82.

Sivak, M., Hill, C.S., Henson, D.L., Butler, B.P., Silber, S.M., and Olson, P.L. (1984). Improving driving performance following perceptual training in persons with brain damage. Archives of Physical Medicine and Rehabilitation, 65:163–67.

Sparadeo, F.R., Strauss, D., and Barth, J.T. (1990). The incidence, impact, and treatment of substance abuse in head trauma rehabilitation. Journal of Head Trauma Rehabilitation, 5:1–8.

Stambrook, M., Moore, A.D., and Peters, L.C. (1990). Social behaviour and adjustment to moderate and severe traumatic brain injury: Comparison to normative and psychiatric samples. Cognitive Rehabilitation, 8:26–30.

Stanton, K.M., Flowers, C.R., Kuhl, P.K., Miller, R.M., and Smith, C.H. (1979). Language-oriented training program to teach compensation of left side neglect. Archives of Physical Medicine and Rehabilitation, 60:540.

Sushinsky, L.W. (1970). An illustration of a behavioral therapy intervention with nursing staff in a therapeutic role. Journal of Psychiatric Nursing and Mental Health Services, 8:24-26.

Tate, R.L. (1987). Behaviour management techniques for organic psychosocial deficit incurred by severe head injury. Scandinavian Journal of Rehabilitation Medicine, 19:19-24.

Thomsen, I. (1984). Late outcome of very severe blunt head trauma: A 10-15 year second follow-up. Journal of Neurology, Neurosurgery, and Psychiatry, 47:260-68.

Turkat, I.D., and Behner, G.W. (1989). Behaviour therapy in the rehabilitation of brain-injured individuals. Brain Injury, 3:101-02.

Turner, J.M., Green, G., and Braunling-McMorrow, D. (1990). Differential reinforcement of low rates of responding (DRL) to reduce dysfunctional social behaviors of a head injured man. Behavioral Residential Treatment, 5:15-27.

Tynan W.D., and Pearce, B.A. (1990). Head injury and self-injury: Treatment of self-injurious behavior in a head injured adolescent male. The Behavior Therapist, 13:158-59.

Van Houten, R., and Rolider, A. (1991). Applied behavior analysis. In: Matson, J.L., and Mullick, J.A. (eds). Handbook of mental retardation (2nd ed). New York: Pergamon Press, 569-85.

Walls, R.T. (1969). Behavior modification and rehabilitation. Rehabilitation Counselling Bulletin, 13:173-83.

Wehman, P., West, M., Fry, R., Sherron, P., Groah, C., Kreutzer, J., and Sale, P. (1989). Effect of supported employment on the vocational outcomes of persons with traumatic brain injury. Journal of Applied Behavior Analysis, 22:395-405.

Weinstein, E.A. (1974). Sexual disturbances after brain injury. Medical Aspects of Human Sexuality, 8:10-31.

Whaley, A.L., Stanford, C.B., Pollack, I.W., and Lehrer, P.M. (1986). The effects of behavior modification and lithium therapy on frontal lobe syndrome. Journal of Behavior Therapy and Experimental Psychiatry, 17:111-15.

Wilson, B. (1981). A survey of behavioural treatments carried out at a rehabilitation centre for stroke and head injuries. In: Powell, G.E. (ed). Brain function therapy. London: Gower, Great Britain, 256-75.

Wilson, B. (1987). Single-case experimental designs in neuropsychological rehabilitation. Journal of Clinical and Experimental Neuropsychology, 9:527-44.

Wilson, E.D., and McCulley, C. (1970). The use of patient-teachers in a maximum security psychiatric unit. Hospital and Community Psychiatry, 21:37-38.

Wood, M.M. (1981). Behavioural methods in rehabilitation. In: Dinning, T.A.R., and Connelley, T.J. (eds). Head injuries: An integrated approach. Brisbane: Wiley, 224-30.

Wood, R.L. (1984). Behaviour disorders following severe brain injury: Their presentation and psychological management. In: Brooks, D.N. (ed). Closed head injury: Psychological, social, and family consequences. Oxford: Oxford University Press, 195-219.

Wood, R.L. (1986). A neuro-behavioural approach in the rehabilitation of severe brain injury. In: Mazzucchini, A. (ed). Neuropsychological rehabilitation. Italy: I.L. Mulino.

Wood, R.L. (1987). Brain injury rehabilitation: A neurobehavioural approach. Rockville, MD: Aspen.

Wood, R.L. (1988). Management of behavior disorders in a day treatment setting. Journal of Head Trauma Rehabilitation, 3:53-61.

Wood, R.L., and Eames, P. (1981). Application of behaviour modification in the rehabilitation of traumatically brain-injured patients. In: Davey, G. (ed). Applications of conditioning theory. London: Methuen, 81-101.

World Health Organization. (1980). International classification of impairment, disability, and handicaps: A manual of classification relating to the consequences of disease. Geneva: Author.

Yorkston, K.M., Stanton, K.M., and Beukelman, D.R. (1981). Language based compensatory training for closed head injured patients. In: Brookshire, R.H. (ed). Clinical aphasiology. Minneapolis, MN: BRK Publishers, 293–300.

Zasler, N.D. (1988). Sexuality issues after traumatic brain injury. Sexuality Update, 1:1–3.

Zencius, A., and Wesolowski, M.D. (1989). Using stress management to decrease inappropriate behavior in a brain-injured adult. Behavioral Residential Treatment, 5:61–64.

Zencius, A., Wesolowski, M.D., and Burke, W.H. (1989). Comparing motivational systems with two non-compliant head-injured adolescents. Brain Injury, 3:67–71.

Zencius, A., Wesolowski, M.D., Burke, W.H., and Hough, S. (1990). Managing hypersexual disorders in brain-injured clients. Brain Injury, 4:175–81.

Zencius, A., Wesolowski, M.D., Burke, W.H., and McQuaide, P. (1989). Antecedent control in the treatment of brain-injured clients. Brain Injury, 3:199–205.

14

Prevention of Brain Injuries by Improving Safety-Related Behaviors

RON VAN HOUTEN, AHMOS ROLIDER,
LOUIS MALENFANT, and JOY VAN HOUTEN

Each year between 420,000 and 470,000 Americans sustain preventable traumatic head injuries (Kalsbeek, McLaurin, Harris, and Miller, 1980). The most frequent victims being young males, with motor vehicle collisions being the primary cause. Even with the best available care, survivors are faced with years of rehabilitation and life-long disabilities.

Brain injuries typically result from a collision between a person's head and an object. Many of these collisions could be avoided or rendered less dangerous if the individuals involved had engaged in one or more safety related behaviors. Some safety related behaviors, such as not driving after consuming alcohol or drugs that could impair functioning and driving at speeds that are safe for road conditions, can reduce the probability that a person will become involved in a collision. Other safety related behaviors, such as wearing a seat belt or a bicycle helmet, can reduce the probability that an injury will occur following a collision.

Modifying safety related behaviors has led to increases in the length and quality of life. For example, the connection between safety related behavior and disease has long been known. Changes in community sanitation related behaviors and the supply of clean drinking water has reduced the incidence of cholera and dysentery. Behavioral practices that reduce the number of vermin has all but eliminated bubonic plague. Draining swamps and implementing mosquito control programs has reduced the incidence of malaria. Improved personal hygiene, washing clothes in very hot water, or having fresh changes of clothing has all but eliminated typhus. Changes in the way food is preserved and prepared has reduced instances of salmonella, botulism, and other food related diseases.

In the area of brain injury, the connection between safety related behaviors and the incidence of the problem is even more easily observed than is the case between safety related behavior and disease. Yet, many people are willing to take risks in regard to injury that they are not willing to take in regard to disease. There are at least two reasons why it is often more difficult to alter physical risk taking behavior. First, many people consider injuries resulting from collisions as being accidental, and hence more dependent on chance and luck. Such a view discourages taking action to reduce the risk of an injury. Second, many safety related behaviors are perceived to reduce enjoyment, or to be more uncomfortable or inconvenient than more risky behavior. For example, people might find wearing helmets, or seat belts, inconvenient or uncomfortable. Similarly they might find alternatives to drinking and driving less attractive than engaging in drinking and driving. A similar problem exists in persuading people to engage in several other health related behaviors, such as using condoms, and refraining from smoking. In both cases adoption of safety related behavior is perceived as associated with reductions in enjoyment.

CAUSES OF BRAIN INJURY
Transportation Related Causes

Epidemiologic data indicate that most brain injuries result from transportation related collisions. For example, it is estimated that about 50% of brain injuries are the result of motor vehicle related collisions, and an additional 4% are related to bicycle related crashes, for a total of 54%. Accurate data collected in San Diego County, California, in 1981 (Kraus, Black, Hessol, Ley, Rokaw, Sullivan, Bowers, Knowlton, and Marshall, 1984), indicated that 48% of all brain injuries resulted from transportation related causes. This same study reported that 20.6% of brain injuries were caused by falls, 12% were caused by assaults, and 9.7% were caused by sports and recreation related collisions. Kraus, et al. (1984), also found that males had a higher incidence of brain injury, particularly males between the ages of 15–24. It is reasonable to conclude that a high percentage of this discrepancy is the result of higher male involvement in motor vehicle crashes.

Although automobile collisions are the major cause of brain injury for older teens and young adults, bicycle related falls were the leading cause of brain injury in children up to age 15 (Ivan, Choo, and Ventureyra, 1983). Head trauma is the most frequent reason for hospitalization following bicycle mishaps (Guichon and Myles, 1975; Selbst, Alexander, and Ruddy, 1987), and the incidence of brain injury is 3 times higher for males than females (Kraus, Fife, and Conroy, 1987). Kraus, et al. (1987), reported that only 1/3 of bicycle-related brain injuries involved collision with a motor vehicle, but brain injuries resulting from this cause tended to be more severe than those resulting from falls from a bicycle. These authors also reported that over half of bicyclists aged 15 and older tested for alcohol use were found to be legally intoxicated.

Crashes involving pedestrians is another cause of brain injury. Kraus found that 11.7% of all persons receiving brain injury from motor vehicle collisions were pedestrians. Children are highly represented in these figures. Up to 40% of all pedestrian-motor vehicle crashes involve children under 9 years of age (Ross and Seefeldt, 1978), and children were pedestrians in 73% of the motor vehicle crashes in which they were involved (Ivan, et al., 1983).

It is clear that efforts to prevent brain injury resulting from transportation related causes need to concentrate on reducing the frequency of, and damage resulting from, motor vehicle collisions, collisions between motor vehicles and bicycles, collisions between motor vehicles and pedestrians, and bicycle falls.

Falls

Falls represent another major cause of brain injury. Kraus, et al. (1984), present data showing that falls, including falls from bicycles, accounted for 20.6% of brain injuries in San Diego, California. Half of these falls occurred from the person's height, while half occurred from a greater height. The distribution of falls causing brain injury across age showed a U-shaped function, with the greatest numbers of such falls in children and senior citizens. Although more males received brain injuries from falls than females, the difference was not nearly as great as that shown for transportation collisions.

Approximately 2/3 of brain injuries in children result from falls (Ivan, et al., 1983). Ivan (1983) reported that 19% of falls were from a bicycle; 14% each from furniture, play, and down stairs; 11% during sports; 9% from a height; and 3% or less, on ice, from playground equipment, from a horse, or accidentally dropped.

Sports and Recreation

Brain damage in sport and recreation account for nearly 10% of all brain injury (Kraus, et al., 1984). Kraus (1984) also reported that the incidence of brain injury from this cause was 6 times higher among males than among females. Contact sports show a high risk for brain injury, with boxing, football, and rugby associated with relatively high risk.

PREVENTION OF BRAIN INJURY

There are three basic approaches to preventing the occurrence of brain injury. First, one can design or redesign the environment to reduce the probability or severity of collisions between peoples head and objects. Examples of this approach would be to twin highways to reduce the likelihood of a head on crash, or to install air bags on all new vehicles to reduce the risk of brain injury should a crash occur. Second, one can change the behavior of a person to reduce the probability or severity of a collision. Examples of this approach would be programs designed to reduce the probability of a person drinking while impaired to reduce the likelihood of a crash, or programs designed to get people to wear their seat belts to reduce the probability of brain injury in the event of a crash. Third, one can change behavior so that people will incorporate into their environment safety devices that reduce the probability or severity of a collision. Examples of this approach would be programs designed to persuade people to purchase anti-lock brakes when they purchase a new car, thereby reducing the likelihood of a crash, or influencing children to wear approved helmets whenever they ride their bicycle, thereby reducing the severity of injuries resulting for crashes.

Designing a Safe Environment

A good deal of research in the area of traffic safety has focused upon designing safer roads and vehicles. Two lane roads have higher fatality and injury rates than divided highways (Evans, 1991). This difference holds up even after controlling for urban-rural differences, and is related to the reductions in head-on crashes, striking trees close to the roadway, intersection crashes, and pedestrian impacts on divided highways.

Vehicle design is also an important factor in determining the probability of a vehicle having a crash, as well as the likelihood that a crash will cause injury. For example, after an experiment with fleet vehicles (Kohl and Baker, 1978) demonstrated that center high mounted brake lights reduced the frequency of rear impact crashes by 54%, the installation of this type of brake light was made mandatory on all North American cars. A follow-up study conducted by Kahane (1989), after the lights had become mandatory, indicated that they resulted in reductions in property damage that were nine times as great as the cost of the devices. It is also likely that the adoption of this device reduced the incidence of neck injuries.

Vehicle mass is also an important factor. Both mass and the amount of crushable material have an effect on the risk of injury in a crash. Campbell and Reinfurt (1973) found that when cars of dissimilar mass crash into each other the risk of injury is substantially greater in the lighter car. Other data show that if cars of equal mass collide, the greater the mass the less the risk of injury (Evans and Wasielewski, 1987). Data for single vehicle crashes with (Partyka, 1989) and without rollover (Partyka and Boehly, 1989) yield similar results. Taken together these data suggest that people can greatly reduce the risk of injury by driving cars with a greater mass. Data also indicate a higher ejection rate associated with two-door vehicles than four-door vehicles. Other design factors that have contributed to improved safety are energy absorbing steering columns (Kahane, 1982a), improvements in the instrument panels (Kahane, 1988), and side door beams (Kahane, 1982b).

Further safety gains could be achieved by installing air bags in all front seat positions. However, air bags alone will not solve the problem of safe driver restraint. Evans (1990a) provides data indicating that the combination of a lap belt, shoulder belt, and air bag yields a 47% effectiveness level, which is 8.5% more effective than the lap belt plus shoulder belt without the air bag. However, the data further indicate that the use of the air bag alone provides 17% effectiveness.

Accident reduction has also been obtained by replacing two-way with four-way stop signs (Hauer, 1985), lighting crosswalks (Polus and Katz, 1978), and introducing speed limits. Since selected speed has a large effect on the probability of crash, injury, and death (Nilsson, 1990), and is a major contributor, along with alcohol to serious injuries and fatalities, reducing driver speed can lead to the prevention of brain injury. It is interesting to note that the injury rate is proportional to the square of the speed. The introduction of the 55 mph speed limit in the United States led to a 34% reduction in the crash rate and increasing the speed limit led to an increase in the crash rate (Garber and Graham, 1990).

Although much has been done to make roadways and cars safer, data indicate that the largest single factor contributing to crashes are not engineering factors, but the driver (Rumar, 1985). Therefore, one effective way to reduce crashes, and the incidence of brain injury, would be to produce a change in driver behavior. Before discussing how one can produce such a change, it is first necessary to address which aspects of driver behavior require modification. The next section will identify several target behaviors for change.

Selection of Target Behaviors

Research into the causes of serious crashes have identified several important human factors. The two most significant factors resulting in serious collisions are alcohol and excessive speed. Reducing impaired driving and speeding will reduce the probability of a severe crash, and will also reduce the severity of any injuries sustained should a crash occur. Another set of target behaviors is increasing the use of protective equipment, such as seat belts and helmets. This approach will not reduce the probability of a severe collision but will reduce the severity of any injuries that would result should such a crash occur.

Studies have shown that nearly half of all traffic fatalities were caused, at least in part, by alcohol use (Donaldson, Beirness, Hass, and Walsh, 1989; Evans, 1990b). Data indicates that a driver with a blood alcohol level (BAC) of .05%–.099% is nearly 3 times as likely of causing a crash as a driver with a zero BAC, while a driver with a BAC over .10% is 6 times as likely to cause a crash. Reducing the occurrence of drinking and driving would thereby reduce the number of serious crashes as well as the number of brain injuries.

Another important target behavior is to reduce speeding. Driving at 65 mph when the speed limit is 55 mph increases the risk of involvement in a fatal crash by a factor of 2.0, which is nearly as much as the increase produced by driving with a BAC between .05%–.09% (Evans, 1991). Speeding is particularly dangerous because the amount of damage resulting from a crash is proportional to the square of the vehicle's velocity. For this reason it is important to focus on means to reduce speeding.

The use of safety equipment can also reduce the severity of crashes of automobile, motorcycle, and bicycle crashes. Safety equipment can also reduce the incidence of serious injury in sports and recreation.

Campbell (1987) provided good evidence that lap/shoulder belts reduced serious injuries by 52% for the driver, and by 44% for the front right passenger. The use of motorcycle helmets have been found to be 28% effective in preventing fatalities (Evans and Frick, 1988) and 76% effective in preventing head injuries (NHTSA, 1980) in motorcycle riders. Several studies have examined the efficacy of helmets for bicyclists (Friede, Azzara, and Gallagher, 1985; Rivara, 1985). One recent study provided evidence that safety helmets could reduce the risk of head injury among bicyclists by as much as 80% (Thompson, Rivara, and Thompson, 1988). The effectiveness of helmets should be even higher for skate boarders, ice skaters, and people involved in contact supports, because of the lower velocities involved. It might also be valuable to teach children protective tightening of the head and neck muscles if a crash is eminent (May, Fuster, Newman, and Hirschman, 1976).

BEHAVIOR CHANGE STRATEGIES

A wide variety of behavior change strategies have been employed in isolation as well as in a variety of combinations in order to change safety related behaviors. Each of these techniques will be outlined in this section of this chapter.

Education

A variety of educational methods have been employed in order to influence safety related behaviors. One educative approach is to provide people with appropriate models for prosafety behaviors. Particularly, such models could promote safety related behavior on television and in movies. Studies have shown that most prime time broadcasting in the United States models irregular driving acts (Atkin, 1989; Greenburg and Atkin, 1983).

Little data exists on the efficacy of television modelling in changing safety related behaviors.

Modelling can also be carried out in an in vivo setting with a person modelling and demonstrating relevant safety related behavior. However, little data exists to support the effectiveness of this approach.

Another educational method is to provide new drivers with driver training courses. However, the data from the largest evaluation of driver education indicate that it has no effect on the crash rate typical of the person taking the course (Lund, Wiiliams, and Zador, 1986). Hence the main effect of such programs is to allow younger, high risk drivers to obtain a license earlier than if they did not take the course. This results in more fatality and injuries than if driver education were not available. A better way to address the problems associated with young drivers might be to provide them with conditional licenses that restrict use to daytime hours.

Health education counselling is another approach to changing safety related behaviors. Several studies have demonstrated that face-to-face encounters between the pediatrician and parents can influence the use of child restraints (Bass and Wilson, 1964; Kantor, 1976). Although some support exists for the value of face-to-face counselling, the support for large group educational programs is less positive. For example, a program supported by the Oregon Neurosurgical Society (Neuwelt, Coe, Wilkinson, and Avolio, 1989), did not produce a change in attitude or behavior (observed shoulder belt use), even though it did produce a change in knowledge about the problem. This program failed to change the behavior of high school students even though the program involved the showing of an award winning film about the causes of head injury, young speakers who had experienced head injury, and a paramedic presentation about appropriate bystander action.

Another educational technique, termed bibliotherapy, involves the use of written materials designed to motivate increased use of safety related behaviors. This approach, when employed alone, has not typically proven effective (Gielen, Eriksen, Daltroy, and Rost, 1984). However, it should be noted that researchers have not performed a careful behavior analysis in order to determine the variables that might lead to more effective results. One factor that makes this approach attractive is the low cost associated with its use.

Rule Setting

Another approach to changing safety related behavior is to make rules, either informally in the case of sports and recreation, or more formally as in the case of legislation.

Rules, such as requiring the use of helmets in contact sports, are one way to reduce the incidence of brain injury. Persons could be excluded from organized participation unless they wear the prescribed safety equipment. Rules could also be changed in sports, such as football and hockey, to eliminate the likelihood of behaviors that could result in brain injury.

Legislative interventions have proven effective in increasing safety belt use. Mandatory seat belt laws have increased average wearing rates from 40% to 65% after legislation (Marburger, 1985), and reductions in fatalities and injuries have also been reported (Hedlund, 1985). Seat belt laws that empower officers to directly stop vehicles when they observe occupants who are not wearing their belts, are the most effective. In the U.K., the introduction of a direct seat belt law led to an increase in belt use from 40% to 90% (Mackay, 1985). Even though high compliance rates are often produced by mandatory belt use legislation, the number of lives saved is often less than would be computed according to theory. One reason for this discrepancy is that drivers that take the most risks often are the least likely to respond to the legislation. Hence, if 90% of the population complies with a mandatory seat belt law, but the 10% who do not are also the ones most likely to drink and drive, or to speed, the reductions in fatalities and injuries will be less than expected.

Legislation has proven effective in other safety areas as well. Motorcycle helmet laws have reduced fatalities and injuries resulting from motorcycle crashes (Chenier, and Evans, 1987), and municipal laws requiring bicyclists to wear helmets are also likely to be somewhat effective in promoting bicycle helmet use. Legislation of drunk driving laws has proven somewhat effective in New South Wales, Australia, when backed up by frequent random breath testing.

Prompts

The use of prompts is another way to influence behavior. To be maximally effective, prompts should occur just before the opportunity to engage in a safety related behavior, and should be relatively specific. For example, Van Houten and Van Houten (1987) found that a sign prompting motorists to "BEGIN SLOWING HERE" was more effective than a sign that indicated that the speed zone was reduced ahead. In another study, Malenfant and Rolider (1985) found that a sign posted at crosswalks that prompted pedestrians to extend an arm before crossing the street, produced a modest increase in the percentage of pedestrians extending their arm at crosswalks. Signs at exits to malls and other locations might be effective in increasing seat belt use as well.

In another series of studies Van Houten (1988), and Van Houten and Malenfant (in press), demonstrated that a simple prompt could reduce the risk to pedestrians being struck in crosswalks on multilane roads. Often pedestrians are struck in a crosswalk on a multilane highway by a vehicle after another vehicle has yielded to the pedestrian, thereby blocking the vision of the motorist approaching in the outside lane. One way to avoid this type of collision is to get motorists to yield farther back from the crosswalk so that other motorists have a better view of the pedestrian crossing the street. In the Van Houten (1988) study, a sign that read "STOP HERE FOR PEDESTRIANS" and that had an arrow pointing down toward the road at an angle of 45° below the horizontal, was placed 50 feet before the beginning of the crosswalk. The data from one of the roads presented in Figure 14.1, shows that the motorists stopped further back from the crosswalk when the sign was in place. The data presented in Figure 14.2 shows that the number of motor vehicle-pedestrian conflicts, or near collisions (a measure believed to be related to the collision rate), showed a marked decline when the sign prompt was introduced. Similar results were obtained on highways with pedestrian activated lights in the Van Houten and Malenfant (in press) study.

Checklists are another prompt procedure that can be effective in improving the occurrence of safety related behaviors. Checklists are employed with great success in aviation, and have recently been adapted for use with adults with brain injuries. For example, O'Reilly, Green, and Braunling-McMorrow (1990), used written checklists to teach home accident prevention skills to 4 adults with brain injuries. The results indicated that the checklist alone was sufficient to improve home safety related behaviors.

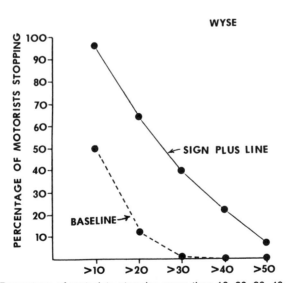

Figure 14.1. Percentage of motorists stopping more than 10, 20, 30, 40, and 50 feet behind the crosswalk. From Van Houten, R. (1988). The effects of advance stop lines and sign prompts on pedestrian safety in a crosswalk on a multilane highway. Journal of Applied Behavior Analysis, 21:249. Reprinted with permission.

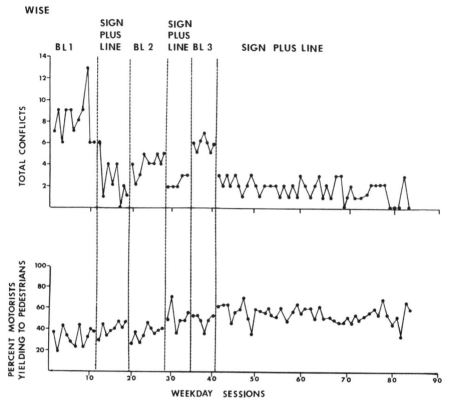

Figure 14.2. Total number of conflicts (*upper frame*) and percent of motorists yielding to pedestrians (*lower frame*) during each condition of the experiment. From Van Houten, R. (1988). The effects of advance stop lines and sign prompts on pedestrian safety in a crosswalk on a multilane highway. Journal of Applied Behavior Analysis, 21:248. Reprinted with permission.

Feedback Interventions

Another approach to changing safety related behaviors is to provide feedback on the percentage of persons engaging in safety related behavior. Van Houten, Nau, and Marini (1980), demonstrated that publicly posting the percentage of drivers not speeding could result in large reductions in speeding behavior. It was also demonstrated that the criterion selected to define speeding had an impact on the magnitude of the effect produced by the sign (Van Houten and Nau, 1983). Specifically, the selection of a lenient criterion which allowed for the posting of high percentages of drivers not speeding was more effective in reducing speeding than the use of a stringent criterion. Several studies have demonstrated the effects posting the percentage of drivers not speeding can persist for years (Van Houten, Rolider, Nau, Freidmann, Becker, Chalodovsky, and Scherer, 1985).

Posted feedback has also been employed to increase safety belt use. Grant, Jonah, Wilde, and Ackersville-Monte (1986), found that the use of a large feedback sign at the exits of a parking lot resulted in a 10% increase in seat belt use that was maintained for 12 weeks. Nau and Van Houten (1982) reported that a similar sign was effective when placed at the start of a high speed highway, but that it was not effective when placed on an urban road.

Feedback can also be provided on a more individualized basis with the assistance of electronic recording equipment. For example, Larson, Schnelle, Kirchner, Carr, Domash, and Risley (1980), employed tachographs to directly monitor the emergency driving behavior of police officers. The tachographs monitored driver speed and were placed in locked black boxes in the trunk of the vehicles. The number of police vehicle collisions was reduced when the section supervisors monitored speeding behavior from the tachograph records.

Feedback has also been employed, along with instructions, to teach parents of young children to make the home environment more safe (Mathews, Friman, Barone, Ross, and Christophersen, 1987). This type of an approach could be selectively employed with children identified as being at risk for injury.

Punishment Procedures

The use of punishment has long been part of the strategy to reduce dangerous behaviors. Police give summary offense tickets for speeding behavior, failure to yield at traffic lights and stop signs, and, more recently, for failing to wear seat belts. Police frequently set up radar checkpoints and charge motorists travelling over the speed limit. However, a number of studies have demonstrated that this approach has limited success in reducing the percentage of speeding motorists (Carr, Schnelle, and Kirchner, 1980; Cirillo, 1968; Van Houten and Nau, 1980). One reason the traditional method of enforcement may not be effective is that the large number of motorists speeding on most roads precludes the charging of all but a small percentage of the total number of violators involved.

One alternative to charging motorists is to issue special warning tickets or give verbal warnings to all first offenders. This approach saves time in two ways. First, it takes less time to collect information and write a warning ticket than to charge a motorist, and second the issuance of a warning ticket does not require the police officer to appear in court.

Van Houten and Nau (1983) employed such warning program in order to reduce speeding on several urban roads. During the warning intervention each motorist stopped received a warning ticket, along with a flyer explaining the number and types of accidents on the road during the past year, and asking the motorist's cooperation in making his or her street a safer place. The introduction of the standard enforcement program on two of the roads, Portland Street and Raymond Street, had little effect on speeding behavior, while the introduction of the warning program on all three streets was very effective in decreasing speeding behavior. It is important to note that the standard enforcement program was in effect for the same amount of time each day as the warning program.

There are a number of reasons why the warning program was more effective than the traditional enforcement program. First, the number of vehicles stopped during the warning program was considerably greater than during the standard enforcement program. For example, the police stopped 6.7 times as many drivers on Portland street during the warning campaign. Thus, officers made personal contact with many more speeding motorists during the warning program. Second, many more drivers were pulled over by the police at one time because it did not take long to write the ticket. As a result motorists were able to observe many more people being stopped for speeding. It is also possible that the information flyer given to the drivers had an effect on the efficacy of the program.

Van Houten and Malenfant (1989), and Van Houten, et al. (1985), employed a similar warning procedure to punish failing to yield to pedestrians. One advantage of giving warning tickets for failing to yield to pedestrians is that it is very difficult for the police officer to obtain sufficient evidence to charge a motorist with failing to yield in all but the most flagrant cases.

A similar approach could be employed to increase safety belt use. Malenfant and Van Houten (1988) reported the results of a study where a nighttime seat belt enforcement campaign was conducted in conjunction with signs posted in all taverns and drinking establishments indicating that seat belt laws were enforced day and night. A combination of verbal warnings, written warnings, and charges were given out for failing to wear seat belts with 90% of the contacts involving warnings. The results of this study indicated that the enforcement program increased seat belt use by tavern patrons (a high risk group) but the effects of the enforcement campaign declined over time once the campaign ended. The failure of the effects of a brief program to endure with this population is not surprising given that nearly half of drivers leaving drinking establishment have been shown to be impaired (Van Houten, Nau, and Jonah, 1985).

Warning enforcement programs could also be employed to promote helmet use by bicyclists. This would allow a high rate of contact with violators without dedicating a disproportionate amount of police resources.

Although punishment programs can be effective in decreasing unsafe behavior, as well as establishing safe behavior to avoid unpleasant consequences, this does not always imply that more severe punishment will always prove more effective. Because of the way the criminal justice system operates, more severe punishment is often associated with a lower probability that punishment will be delivered following a specific instance of a behavior (Ross, 1991). The enforcement of drunk driving laws is a good example. The probability of being caught for impaired driving in Canada has been estimated to be one in 514 drinking-driving occurrences or .002 (Jonah and Wilson, 1983).

There are several reasons why the probability of being caught for impaired driving is so low. Both reasons are related to the severity of the penalty. First, the criminal justice system requires police officers to follow very precisely specified and time-consuming procedures. Thus, the delivery of just one impaired driving charge can mean removing one or more officers from an enforcement site for 2 hours or more, making it difficult to charge a large number of violators without markedly increasing the number of police (Vingilis, Blefgen, Colbourne, Reynolds, Solomon, and Wasylyk, 1983). Second, punishing even a small proportion of the violators would overwhelm the criminal justice system. This is, perhaps, the reason why it is relatively easy to plea bargain, pleading guilty to a first offense, when caught for subsequent offenses of impaired driving.

Of course a warning in the case of impaired driving would be perceived as too mild a penalty and would likely prove ineffective in deterring this behavior. However, administrative consequences, such as immediate license suspension and revocation on the spot, have proven to be highly effective in deterring impaired driving (Nichols and Ross, 1989). Perhaps it is time to consider decriminalizing impaired driving in order to provide more certain punishment for those who drink and drive.

Positive Reinforcement

Roberts and Turner (1986) have demonstrated that reinforcement programs can increase child safety seat and seat belt use in children in preschool and elementary school settings. In another study, Campbell, Hunter, and Strutts (1984), increased seat belt use by high school students from 25% to 65% using incentives such as a lottery, coupons worth $5.00, and a group incentive ($100 toward the senior prom when the school achieved a level of seat belt use of 60% for two consecutive days). Other studies have shown that reinforcement programs can also increase seat belt use in community settings with adults (Geller, Paterson, and Talbott, 1982; Geller, Rudd, Kalsher, Streff, and Lehman, 1987; Hagenzieker, 1991).

Although a good deal of evidence indicates that safety related behaviors can be increased through the use of specific psychologic procedures, it is, however, likely that programs employing a combination of such procedures will produce the largest changes in safety behavior. The final section of this chapter will examine the efficacy of broad communitywide, multifaceted treatment programs in promoting safety related behaviors.

MULTIFACETED TREATMENT APPROACHES

One example of a multifaceted treatment approach was employed in the city of Haifa, Israel, to reduce speeding behavior (Scherer, Freidmann, Rolider, and Van Houten, 1985; Van Houten, Rolider, Nau, Freidmann, Becker, Chalodovsky, and Scherer, 1985). The treatment program was applied to traffic travelling in one direction on each of 14 streets identified as having serious speeding problems. The treatment procedures included: Feedback signs on each street providing information on the percentage of drivers not speeding each week, as well as the record for each street; the use of a warning enforcement program that involved giving warning tickets and information flyers to speeders; employing university students to assist the police in giving out warning tickets; media publicity; and an incentive program, where a pen engraved with the message "Thank you for driving within the speed limit—Haifa Police" was given to some motorists who were driving within the speed limit. The results of the study indicated that the intervention package was effective in the reducing speeding behavior of motorists driving in the direction that the program was applied on all 14 streets. More significantly these reductions in speeding resulted in large reductions in injuries.

During the first 6 months following the erection of signs and the beginning of the enforcement program, there were 13 injury accidents on the side of the streets where the signs were placed and the warning programs were employed. These 13 injury accidents resulted in 2 serious injuries and no fatalities. During the same 6 month period of the preceding year there were 37 injury accidents resulting in 6 serious injuries and 1 fatality. No decreases in injury accidents were observed on the side of the streets where the program was not introduced. These injury data are presented in Table 14.1.

Another multifaced safety program designed to increase pedestrian safety in three Canadian cities was reported by Malenfant and Van Houten (1989). This program was designed to alter the safety related behaviors of both motorists and pedestrians. The program contained the following components. First, public education through the use of flyers, large feedback signs reporting the percentage of motorists yielding to pedestrians each week on a citywide basis, schoolwide training programs in pedestrian safety, and media attention. Second, improved engineering through the use of advance stop lines at crosswalks, along with signs requesting motorists to yield further back behind the crosswalk, and signs at problematic crosswalks instructing motorists how to safely cross the street.

Table 14.1.
The number of people injured in accidents in the direction that the sign and enforcement program were introduced during the 6 months following the program and during the same 6-month period during the preceding 2 years along with equivalent data for injuries that occurred in the opposite direction.

STREET	DIRECTION OF THE SIGN			OPPOSITE DIRECTION (CONTROL)		
	BEFORE PROGRAM		AFTER PROGRAM	BEFORE PROGRAM		AFTER PROGRAM
	1981	1982	1983	1981	1982	1983
Hagiborim	10	2	2	3	2	3
Hatzionut	2	3	0	2	5	2
Guela	2	1	0	0	0	0
Hankin	3	2	0	1	1	2
Yad-Labanim	2	1	1	2	2	6
Hashmal-West	2	0	0	1	0	1
Allenby-East	2	10	5	3	9	9
Allenby-West	3	3	2	0	0	0
Abba Hushie	6	10	4	5	4	5
International	2	3	0	1	0	0
Haganah	2	5	0	5	2	3
Hameginim	9	4	2	9	1	3
Tchernichovsky	6	1	0	2	2	5
Golomb	2	0	0	0	2	2
Total	53	45	16	34	30	41

Third, an intensive police enforcement campaign consisting of giving out warning flyers and warning tickets to motorists who failed to yield and small incentives such as a pen and bumper sticker to motorists yielding to pedestrians.

The introduction of this program resulted in a marked increase in the percentage of motorists yielding to pedestrians in each city, and a modest increase in the percentage of pedestrians signalling their intention to cross the street. The introduction of the program was also associated with a 50% reduction in the number of pedestrians struck in crosswalks in the two cities where this data was available.

The results of the two above mentioned studies demonstrate that large scale changes in safety related behavior can be achieved when a number of behavioral principles are applied together in a comprehensive program. Perhaps the failure to achieve large rapid changes in safety related behavior in the past is related to the piecemeal manner that safety programs are often employed.

SUMMARY

The results of epidemiologic studies indicate that the major cause of brain injury in transportation is related to collisions. It follows then, that changes in safety related behaviors that lead to a reduction in both the number of transportation related collisions and the amount of damage produced by such collisions is the most effective way to prevent brain injury.

An examination of the safety factors related to transportation related collisions suggests that the following goals should be addressed. First, efforts should be made to reduce the incidence of drinking and driving, and speeding behavior. Second, programs should be developed to increase seat belt use by motorists, and helmet use by motorcyclists. It is important to note that those at greatest risk are often least likely to wear these devices. Third, efforts should be coordinated to promote the use of helmets by bicyclists.

An examination of the treatments available to influence safety related behavior show that education, rule setting, prompts, feedback, punishment, and reinforcement have all proven somewhat effective at influencing the occupance of safety related behaviors. Finally, it is recommended that comprehensive, multifaceted programs be developed to maximize the impact on safety related behavior.

References

Atkin, C.K. (1989). Television, socialization and risky driving by teenagers. Alcohol, Drugs and Driving, 5:1-11.

Bass, L.W., and Wilson, T.R. (1964). The pediatrician's influence in private practice measured by a controlled seat belt study. Pediatrics, 33:700.

Campbell, B.J. (1987). Safety belt injury reduction related to crash severity and front seated position. Journal of Trauma, 27:733-39.

Campbell, B.J., and Reinfurt, D.W. (1973). The relationship between driver crash injury and passenger car weight. Chapel Hill, NC: Highway Safety Research Center, University of North Carolina.

Campbell, B.J., Hunter, W.W., and Stutts, J.C. (1984). The use of economic incentives and education to modify safety belt use behavior of high school students. Health Education, 15:30-33.

Carr, A.F., Schnelle, J.F., and Kirchner, R.E. Jr. (1980). Police crackdowns and slowdowns: A naturalistic evaluation of charges in police traffic enforcement. Behavioral Assessment, 2:33-41.

Chenier, T.C., and Evans, L. (1987). Motorcyclist fatalities and the repeal of mandatory helmet wearing laws. Accident Analysis and Prevention, 19:133-39.

Cirillo, J.A. (1968). Interstate system accident research, study 2, interim report 2. Public Roads, 35:71-754.

Donaldson, A.C., Beirness, D.J., Hass, G.C., and Walsh, P.J. (1989). The role of alcohol in fatal traffic crashes: British Columbia, 1985-1986. Ottawa, Canada: Traffic Injury Research Foundation of Canada.

Evans, L. (1990a). Restraint effectiveness, occupant ejection from cars and fatality reductions. Accident Analysis and Prevention, 22:167-75.

Evans, L. (1990b). The fraction of traffic fatalities attributable to alcohol. Accident Analysis and Prevention, 22:587-602.

Evans, L. (1991). Traffic safety and the driver. New York: Van Nostrand Reinhold, 83-85.

Evans, L., and Frick, M.C. (1988). Helmet effectiveness in preventing motorcycle driver and passenger fatalities. Accident Analysis and Prevention, 20:447-58.

Evans, L., and Wasielewski, P.F. (1987). Serious or fatal driver injury rate versus car mass in head-on crashes between cars of similar mass. Accident Analysis and Prevention, 19:119-31.

Friede, A.M., Azzara, C.V., and Gallagher, S.S. (1985). The epidemiology of injuries to bicycle riders. Pediatric Clinicians of North America, 32:141-51.

Garber, S., and Graham, J.D. (1990). The effects of the new 65 mile-per-hour speed limit on rural highway fatalities: A state by state analysis. Accident Analysis and Prevention, 22:137-49.

Geller, E.S., Patterson, L., and Talbott, E. (1982). A behavioral analysis on incentive prompts for motivating seat belt use. Journal of Applied Behavior Analysis, 15: 403-15.

Geller, E.S., Rudd, J.R., Kalsher, M.J., Streff, F.M., and Lehman, G.R. (1987). Employer-based programs to motivate safety belt use: A review of short-term and long-term effects. Journal of Safety Research, 18:1-17.

Gielen, A.C., Erikson, M.P., Daltroy, L.H., and Ross, K. (1984). Factors associated with the use of child restraint devices. Health Education Quarterly, 11:195-206.

Grant, B.A., Jonah, B.A., Wilde, G.J.S., and Ackerville-Monte, M. (1986). The use of feedback to encourage seat belt wearing. Unpublished manuscript.

Greenburg, B., and Atkin, C. (1983). The portrayal of driving on television, 1975-1980. Journal of Communication, 33:44-45.

Guichon, D.M., and Myles, S.T. (1975). Bicycle injuries: One year sample in Calgary. Journal of Trauma, 15:504-46.

Hagenzieker, M.P. (1991). Enforcement or incentives? Promoting safety belt use among military personnel in the Netherlands. Journal of Applied Behavior Analysis, 24:23-30.

Headlund, J. (1985). Casualty reductions resulting from safety use laws. In: Working papers for OECD workshop on effectiveness of safety belt use laws: A multi-national examination. Washington, DC: U.S. Department of Transportation, 92-113.

Ivan, L.P., Choo, S.H., Ventureyra, E.C.G. (1983). Head injuries in childhood: A 2-year survey. Journal of the Canadian Medical Association, 128:281-84.

Jonah, B.A., and Wilson, R.J. (1983). Improving the effectiveness of drinking-driving enforcement through increased efficiency. Accident Analysis and Prevention, 15:463-81.

Kahane, C.J. (1982a). Evaluation of current energy-absorbing steering assemblies. SAE Paper 820473. Warendale, PA: Society of Automotive Engineers.

Kahane, C.J. (1982b). An evaluation of side structure improvements in response to Federal Motor Vehicle Safety Standard 212. Washington, DC: National Highway Safety Administration, Report DOT HS 806314.

Kahane, C.J. (1988). An evaluation of occupant protection in frontal interior impact for unrestrained front seat occupants of cars and light trucks. Washington, DC: National Highway Safety Administration, Report DOT HS 807203.

Kahane, C.J. (1989). An evaluation of center high mounted stop lamps based on 1987 data. Washington, DC: National Highway Traffic Safety Administration, Report DOT HS 807442.

Kalsbeek, W.P., McLaurin, R.L., Harris, B.S.H., and Miller, J.D. (1980). The national head and spinal cord injury survey: Major findings. Journal of Neurosurgery, 53:513-31.

Kantor, H.A. (1976). Car safety for infants: Effectiveness of prenatal counselling. Pediatrics, 58:320.

Kohl, J.S., and Baker, C. Field test evaluation of rear lighting systems. Washington, DC: National Highway Traffic Safety Administration, Report DOT HS 803456.

Kraus, J.F., Black, M.A., Hessol, N., Ley, P., Rokaw, W., Sullivan, C., Bowers, S.,

Knowlton, S., and Marshall L. (1984). The incidence of acute brain injury and serious impairment in a defined population. American Journal of Epidemiology, 119:189-201.

Kraus, J.F., Fife, D., and Conroy, C. (1987). Incidence, severity, and outcomes of brain injuries involving bicycles. American Journal of Public Health, 77:76-78.

Larson, L.D., Schnelle, J.F., Kirchner, R., Jr., Carr, A.F., Domash, M., and Risley, T.F. (1980). Reduction of police vehicle accidents through mechanically aided supervision. Journal of Applied Behavior Analysis, 13:571-81.

Lund, A.K., Williams, A.F., and Zador, P. (1986). High school driver education: Further evaluation of the DeKalb County study. Accident Analysis and Prevention, 18:349-57.

Mackay, M. (1985). Seatbelt use under voluntary and mandatory conditions and its effect and casualties. In: Evans, L. (ed). Human behavior and traffic safety. New York: Plenum Press, 259-78.

Malenfant, L., and Van Houten, R. (1988). The effects of nighttime seat belt enforcement on seat belt use by tavern patrons: A preliminary analysis. Journal of Applied Behavior Analysis, 21:271-76.

Malenfant, L., and Van Houten, R. (1989). Increasing the percentage of drivers yielding to pedestrians in three Canadian cities with a multifaceted safety program. Health Education Research, 5:275-79.

Marburger, E.A. (1985). Safety usage rates. In: Working papers for OECD workshop on effectiveness of safety belt use laws: A multi-national examination. Washington, DC: U.S. Department of Transportation, 17-37.

Mathews, J.R., Friman, P.C., Barone, V.J., Ross, L.V., and Christophersen, E.R. (1987). Decreasing dangerous infant behaviors through parent instruction. Journal of Applied Behavior Analysis, 20:165-69.

May, P.R.A., Fuster, J.M., Newman, P., and Hirschman, A. (1976). Woodpeckers and head injury. Lancet, 454-55.

National Highway Traffic Safety Administration. (1980). A report to Congress on the effect of motorcycle helmet use repeal—A case report for helmet use. Washington, DC: National Highway Traffic Safety Administration, Report DOT HF 805312.

Nau, P.A., and Van Houten, R. (1982). The effects of prompts, feedback and an advertising campaign on the use of safety belts by automobile drivers in Nova Scotia. Journal of Environmental Systems, 11:351-61.

Neuwelt, E.A., Coe, P.H., Wilkinson, A.M., and Avolio, A.E.C. (1989). Oregon head and spinal cord injury prevention program and evaluation. Neurosurgery, 24:453-58.

Nichols, J., and Ross, H.L. (1989). The effectiveness of legal sanctions in dealing with drinking drivers. In: Office of the Surgeon General, Surgeon General's workshop on drunk driving: Background papers. Rockville, MD: U.S. Department of Health and Human Services, 33-60.

O'Reilly, M.F., Green, G., and Braunling-McMorrow, D. (1990). Self-administered written prompts to teach home accident prevention skills to adults with brain injuries. Journal of Applied Behavior Analysis, 23:431-46.

Partyka, S.C. (1989) Registration-based fatality rates by size from 1978 through 1987. Papers on car size-safety and trends. National Highway Traffic Safety Administration, Report DOT HS 807 444, 45-72.

Partyka, S.C., and Boehly, W.A. (1989). Passenger car weight and injury severity in single vehicle nonrollover crashes. Paper ESV 89-2B-0-005, presented to the Twelfth International Technical Conference on Experimental Safety Vehicles, Gothenburg, Sweden.

Rivara, F.P. (1985). Traumatic deaths of children in the United States: Currently available prevention strategies. Pediatrics, 75:456-62.

Roberts, M.C., and Turner, D.S. (1986). Rewarding parents for their children's use of safety seats. Journal of Pediatric Psychology, 11:25-36.

Ross, H.L. (1991). Decriminalizing drunk driving: A means to effective punishment. Journal of Applied Behavior Analysis, 24:89–90.

Ross, S.P., and Seefeldt, C. (1978). Young children in traffic: How can they cope? Young Children, 33:68–73.

Rumar, K. (1985). The role of perceptual and cognitive filters in observed behavior. In: Evans, L., and Schwing, R.C. (eds). Human behavior and traffic safety. New York: Plenum Press, 151–65.

Selbst, S.M., Alexander, D., and Ruddy, R. (1987). Bicycle-related injuries. American Journal of the Disabled Child, 141:140–44.

Scherer, M., Freidmann, R., Rolider, A., and Van Houten, R. (1985). The effects of saturation enforcement campaign on speeding in Haifa, Israel. Journal of Police Science and Administration, 12:425–30.

Thompson, R.S., Rivara, F.P., and Thompson, D.C. (1988). Prevention of head injury by bicycle helmets: A field study of efficacy. American Journal of the Disabled Child, 142:386.

Van Houten, R. (1988). The effects of advance stop lines and sign prompts on pedestrian safety in a crosswalk on a multilane highway. Journal of Applied Behavior Analysis, 21:245–51.

Van Houten, R., and Malenfant, L. (in press). The influence of signs prompting motorists to yield 50 feet (15.15m) before marked crosswalks on motor vehicle-pedestrian conflicts at crosswalks with flashing amber. Accident Analysis and Prevention.

Van Houten, R., Malenfant, L., and Rolider, A. (1985). Increasing driver yielding and pedestrian signalling with prompting, feedback, and enforcement. Journal of Applied Behavior Analysis, 18:103–10.2

Van Houten, R., and Nau, P.A. (1981). A comparison of the effects of posted feedback and increased police surveillance on highway speeding. Journal of Applied Behavior Analysis, 14:261–71.

Van Houten, R., and Nau, P.A. (1983). Feedback interventions and driving speed: A parametric and comparative analysis. Journal of Applied Behavior Analysis, 16:251–81.

Van Houten, R., Nau, P.A., and Jonah, B. (1985). Effects of feedback on impaired driving. In: Kaye, S., and Meier, G.W. (eds). Alcohol drugs and traffic safety. Washington, DC: U.S. Government Printing Office, 1375–94.

Van Houten, R., Rolider, A., Nau, P.A., Freidmann, R., Becker, M., Chalodovsky, I., and Scherer, M. (1985). Large-scale reductions in speeding and accidents in Canada and Israel: A behavioral ecological perspective. Journal of Applied Behavior Analysis, 18:87–93.

Van Houten, R., and Van Houten, F. (1987). The effects of a specific prompting sign on speed reduction. Accident Analysis and Prevention, 19:115–17.

Vingilis, E., Blefgen, H., Colbourne, D., Reynolds, D., Solomon, R., and Wasylyk, N. (1983). Ontario police survey on DWI enforcement. Paper presented at the Ninth International Conference on Alcohol, Drugs and Traffic Safety, San Juan, Puerto Rico.

15

Family Adjustment Following Traumatic Brain Injury: A Systems-Based, Life Cycle Approach

MICHAEL STAMBROOK, ALLAN MOORE,
DARYL GILL, and LOIS PETERS

"... More and more disabled persons, salvaged because of a more efficient treatment, [are] bringing home the truth that a major head injury can be a disaster not only to the victim but also to his family and dependents, as well as being a heavy charge on the community and its over-strained hospital services" (Potter, 1967, p. 576).

"The consequent result has been a saving, and then a prolonging of life, but with little attention paid to the quality of such life, that which most profoundly effects patients, their families, and the social network they are immersed in" (Stambrook, Peters, and Moore, 1989, p. 87).

Unfortunately, despite the fact that Potter's (1967) statement dates back almost a quarter of a century, it is an unpleasant reality to report that the situation for patients and families of head injury victims remains largely unchanged.

In this chapter we present a heuristic conceptual model outlining a systems-based, developmental perspective of family adjustment following traumatic brain injury (TBI) that identifies major themes related to development on a number of levels. Specifically, we will focus on exploring the use of the Family Life Cycle model (Carter and McGoldrick, 1989) as a conceptual basis for understanding the wide range of changes, stresses, and challenges that families confront in dealing with both the acute and long-term sequelae of TBI.

A practical and comprehensive approach to understanding family dynamics and development following TBI requires a model that: 1) is sensitive to the unfolding of the recovery process; 2) recognizes that individual development of family members takes place within a larger dynamic family process; and 3) integrates illness related crises with normative family developmental tasks. Because such a model is developmental, multidimensional, and dynamic, a "one time" family assessment for clinical or research purposes provides only a snapshot of an otherwise changing, evolving family. Clinical assessment and research designs that do not specifically attend to factors such as systemic life cycle changes and influences, unwittingly "averages" potentially significant effects. This may underestimate the real burden on family functioning that may be modified by factors such as the patient's recovery stage, role and position in the family, and age and sex of the patient.

This chapter will not comprehensively review the growing literature on family functioning following TBI, as a number of excellent reviews have recently been made available (see Brooks, 1991; Jacobs, 1989; Florian and Katz, 1991; Florian, Katz, and Lahav, 1989; Lezak, 1986, 1988; Livingston and Brooks, 1988). While the research has generated a rich database, there is a need for an organizing theoretical framework to guide work in the area for research and clinical practice. This chapter will provide the beginnings of a conceptual framework for this analysis.

RATIONALE FOR SYSTEMS-BASED LIFE CYCLE APPROACH

The central thesis of this chapter is that the occurrence of a TBI imposes specific challenges the family system must confront, that are over and above its normative developmental tasks. The patient and family system's ability to successfully navigate the wide range of family and individual patient developmental challenges is determined by a unique blend of patient and family-specific variables. These include 1) premorbid factors, 2) injury related variables, 3) stage-of-life factors, 4) family and social support factors, 5) family financial considerations, 6) general societal factors that are related to the family's place of residence and community resources, and 7) the kinds of intervention strategies that can be mobilized to assist.

TBI primarily affects individuals who are in the early stages of their lives. Unfortunately, the risk factors related to sustaining TBI are also risk factors for family discord and dysfunction, and, even in the absence of a TBI, a variety of academic, psychologic, and social problems (Haas, Cope, and Hall, 1987). Frequently, a TBI patient is a male in late adolescence or early adulthood, who may have a history of academic difficulties, interpersonal conflict, or problems with authority (Bond, 1986; Parkinson, Stephenson, and Phillips, 1985). As well, suggestive data exists indicating that, among families of children who sustain TBI and other accidental injuries, there is a higher percentage of discord and parents with psychopathology (Rutter, Chadwick, and Shaffer, 1983). Long-term cognitive deficits, personality changes, and associated social dependency have been consistently documented in the outcome literature, and have been specifically addressed by Bond (1986) and Lezak (1978, 1988). Lezak described the "characterologically altered brain injured patient" who has impaired social perception, impaired social awareness, impaired self-control, and increased dependency, impulsivity, and egocentricity, as well as the substantial implications of these changes on a variety of roles within the family.

There is increasing attention in the family coping literature on 1) understanding the family as a system in adaptation to chronic illness, 2) appreciating the multiple developmental factors which influence the patient's psychosocial recovery and integration, and 3) examining the family's adjustment and coping with particular disabilities and chronic illnesses (Drotar, Crawford, and Bush, 1984; Tritt and Esses, 1986; Whitt, 1984). In this analysis, TBI is a unique disability, since it represents a specific challenge to the family system over and above that imparted by other substantial life altering, catastrophic injuries or illnesses (DeDompei, Zarski, and Hall, 1987). The patient and family must not only deal with the physical aftermath, but also with: 1) the primary emotional and neuropsychologic deficits caused by actual damage to the brain; 2) changes in the patient's emotional functioning secondary to difficulty with TBI related coping deficits; and 3) changes in the family system's adaptation to the fallout of TBI secondary to the changed family roles and the patient's frequent inertia.

The family unit must be placed within the larger milieu of interacting, interrelated systems, hierarchically arranged within the broader socioeconomic and sociocultural context, evolving over an individual's life cycle (Walsh, 1982). This family-centered approach (Drotar, Crawford, and Bush, 1984) attempts to understand the complex, hierarchic relationships as they are moderated and changed by transitory and situational stresses, and by longer lasting and permanent stressors that may be caused by irreversible changes in a family member's brain functioning.

UNDERSTANDING THE FAMILY FOLLOWING TBI

Family Response to Normative Development

One approach to understanding the dynamic changes that follow a traumatic brain injury is to place the injury within the Family Life Cycle (FLC) perspective. This model "views symptoms and dysfunctions in relation to normal functioning over time and views therapy as helping to reestablish the family's developmental momentum. It frames problems within the course the family has moved along in its past, the task it is trying to master, and the future towards which it is moving" (Carter and McGoldrick, 1989, p. 4). The FLC model sees several events in the family's developmental course as critical transition points with developmental challenges to be overcome. Specifically, Carter and McGoldrick (1989) identify the major normative developmental challenges facing the family system as time driven and associated with stages of life consisting of:

1) the family with young children, 2) the family with adolescents, 3) launching children and moving on, 4) between families: young and unattached adults, 5) joining of families through marriage, and 6) the family in later life.

Figure 15.1 illustrates this spiral of development, as well as the many factors that impinge upon the cycle's unfolding, specific to a brain injury. Here, FLC model focuses on an interactional/transactional perspective, where causation is not seen simply as linear or unidirectional. In addition, it is important to consider the individual's life cycle in terms of their physiologic maturation and their cognitive, social, and psychologic development.

Normally, the family deals with life stresses and developmental crises throughout the stages of the life cycle. Some of these challenges have the effect of creating greater cohesion (i.e., centripetal forces) while others have the effect of creating dissension and emotional distance between family members (i.e., centrifugal forces; Combrinck-Graham, 1985). In the

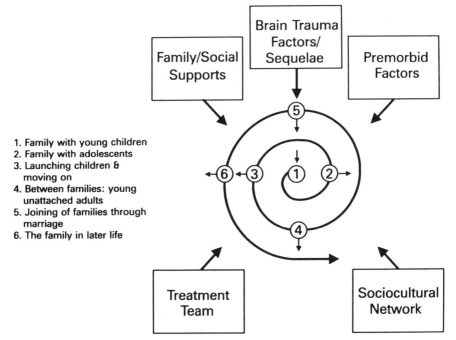

Figure 15.1. Stages of the Family Cycle (adapted from concepts presented by Carter and McGoldrick, 1989). The major stages in a life cycle are outlined as are the multiple influences on the family as the crises of the TBI is superimposed upon their life cycle. The *arrows* correspond to the hypothesized direction of stressors with *inward directed arrows* reflecting centripetal forces and *outward directed arrows* reflecting centrifugal forces.

case of TBI, the injured family member experiences cognitive deficits—particularly those related to executive functioning and the related changes in emotional modulation, insight, judgment, planning, social relatedness, and in the ability to empathize and to read the nonverbal cues of other family members. These lead to substantive alterations in the patient's ability to play a role in the give-and-take of family life, and, thus, the roles of family members within the system. The magnitude and quality of this ripple effect is moderated by the individual developmental stage the patient is in, and the roles the injured member plays in the family system. For example, a pediatric brain injury has qualitatively different implications in contrast to a brain injury that occurs in later life when cognitive schemas, linguistic skills, and procedural knowledge have been laid-down and are well integrated prior to brain damage.

Family Response to TBI

Understanding family adjustment following TBI benefits from knowledge of the FLC in relation to the brain injury and an appreciation of how disability-specific developmental issues impact on the family system. These issues have been examined by Lezak (1986, 1988), Spanbock (1987), and Stambrook, Peters, and Moore (1989).

An analysis of the psychologic adjustment to any disability or illness requires an understanding of the multiple factors that influence both the TBI patient's reactions during initial recovery and the adaptation of the patient and family to the long-term effects of TBI (Stambrook, et al., 1989). These factors relate to the patient, treatment team, family, and sociocultural network systems (Table 15.1). The factors are complex and interact, in any individual case, in unique ways, developmentally and cumulatively, to determine patient and family outcome from TBI at any one point in time.

Recovery Crises

Figure 15.2 presents a timeline perspective of what can be considered three major medical/psychologic/social "crises" that the patient and family confront throughout the course of survival and recovery from TBI. Figure 15.3 outlines three perspectives on the disability-specific developmental path. While there is substantial commonality between the models, an important difference separating the Spanbock (1987) and Lezak (1988) models from the Stambrook, et al. (1989), model, is that the latter is specifically tied to some of the environmental and situational factors that confront families. Previous models have used time-based stage concepts that are descriptive of some of the emotions that families may feel, with the obvious implication that not all families go through stages in the man-

Table 15.1.
Factors that Influence Brain Injury Outcome[a]

PATIENT	FAMILY	TREATMENT TEAM	SOCIAL/ CULTURAL NETWORK
Premorbid factors			
	Support	Roles	Prejudice
Age	Conflict	Expectations	Public apathy
Roles	Status	Ego investments	"Sick role"
Competence	Empathy	Transference/ counter- transference	"Body beautiful ethic"
Status	Power and roles		Architectural barriers
Coping style	Life cycle stage	Conflicts	Transportation barriers
Life cycle stage	Expectations	Resources	Financial disincentives
Education Psychological stability	Flexibility		Lack of resources
Brain trauma factors			
Severity and extent of injury Location Neurological sequelae Restrictions in activities of daily living Cognitive deficits			

[a]Reprinted by permission of the publisher from Stambrook, M., Peters, L.C., and Moore, A.D. (1989). Issues in the rehabilitation of severe traumatic brain injury: A focus on the neuropsychologists' role. *Canadian Journal of Rehabilitation,* p. 89. Copyright 1989 by the Canadian Association for Research in Rehabilitation.

ner outlined. The three crises in the Stambrook, et al. (1989), model relate to: 1) events surrounding the head injury itself; 2) discharge from post-acute hospitalization; and 3) the eventual discharge from hospital or community-based ongoing outpatient resources. Because of the complexity of the developmental course involved in family adjustment to TBI, a complete inventory of the potential paths of adjustment is beyond the scope of this brief review. We will focus on some major developmental crises, and highlight common issues for families, as the patient with severe TBI moves through the cycle of emergency resuscitation, intensive care, stepdown unit care, early rehabilitation, postacute rehabilitation, hospital discharge, discharge from outpatient therapies, and community living.

The issues for mild and moderate TBI are no less complex and problematic for families, as patients frequently report postconcussional symptoms that may well have neuropsychologic and neurologic bases long after they have normal neurologic exams and normal imaging studies (Binder, 1986; Levin, Eisenberg, and Berton, 1989; Levin, Mattis, Ruff, et al.,

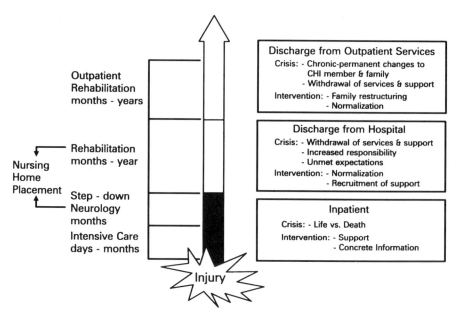

Figure 15.2. Disability Specific Time-Line of the Crises facing the family.

1987). Patients and families confront a range of problems related to reduced information processing speed, decreases in attention and concentration, mental flexibility, recent memory, frustration tolerance, noise tolerance, and dizziness, for example, as well as fatigue, irritability, anxiety, and depression, all of which they are unprepared for. These are frequently silent disabilities, as the patient looks "normal" and hence has expectations imposed on him or her that may exceed his or her skill levels. A sizable minority of mild and, in larger proportions, moderate TBI patients, and their families, deal with posthospital issues, outlined in this chapter, similar to the severe TBI patients (Canboy, Barth, and Boll, 1986). The mild and moderate TBI patients, who are at higher risk for problems, may be older, have histories of substance abuse, and/or have a previous record of TBI's (Binder, 1986; Canboy, et al., 1986).

Inpatient

Life vs. Death

At the time of the initial injury, the family faces a crisis related to the life or death of the patient. Common reactions include shock, disbelief, denial, and anger. If the family members' acts of either omission or com-

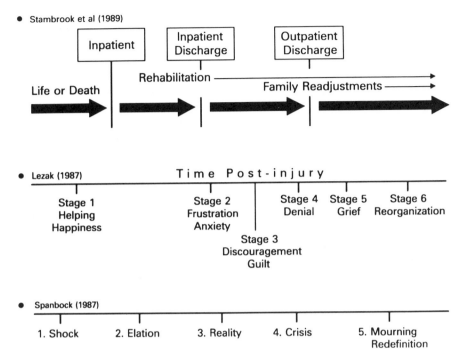

Figure 15.3. Models of Family Adjustment Following TBI.

mission are related to the actual injury, feelings of substantive guilt may be present. The family members need support and concrete, repeated information during this time, preferably from a single health care provider who serves as a liaison and interpreter between the family and the health care team.

Coma vs. Consciousness

Following the resolution of the life or death crisis, families are commonly elated by the survival of their loved one, and become invested in the rehabilitation of the injured family member. At this time, families frequently believe that their prayers, pacts to themselves, bargains, and other responses used during the earlier crisis, have cleared the way for a "full" recovery. At times, family members believe they can take professional advice with skepticism. However, excitement fades as it becomes apparent that the sequelae are substantial, permanent, and relatively pervasive. Reactions to this include frustration, anxiety, and anger towards staff (Stern, Sazbon, Becker, and Costeff, 1988).

Unfortunately for patients who may remain in a vegetative state, some families maintain beliefs in a positive prognosis and higher functioning than can be objectively supported by the extent of brain damage (Romano, 1974). Family members may become extremely angry with staff over perceived lack of therapy, insufficient nursing care, and "abandonment" of the patient, despite the objective presence of adequate nursing care and therapeutic intervention. Family members often interpret the reflexive and, at times, random movement of vegetative patients as purposeful movement, provoking confrontations between staff and families over the actual status of the patient.

As coma lifts, families are confronted with patients who typically go through stages of confusion, disorientation, marked cognitive dysfunction, and disinhibited behavior. Comas of greater than 24 hours are consistently associated with postcoma agitation, lasting from a few days to several weeks (Gill, Sparadeo, and Parziale, 1988). This period is frequently difficult for families since their expectations, following resolution of coma, typically involve a rapid resolution of symptoms and return to normalcy. In fact, Willer (1990) reports that over one-third of the general public believes that there will be no long lasting ill-effects when an individual emerges from a coma. During this stage, family members can be important in the management of the patient, since they are well placed to provide a structured and predictable environment, reality testing, and soothing, concrete, and repetitive conversation that can help to settle the patient.

Discharge from Hospital

The second major crisis arises with discharge home. The family must deal with the responsibility for total patient care, together with their increasing recognition that recovery will be incomplete. While hospital discharge is usually a happy event, and is a goal vigorously pursued by the patient, it is also an anxious time for caregivers, and the onset of heavy challenges for the family system. The family must face and deal with major changes in many areas of the patient's life, particularly with personality changes. In fact, the mental sequelae, including personality change, are more problematic than physical changes for families following TBI (Lishman, 1973). Recent research from our laboratory indicates that the psychosocial, family, and marital fallout from TBI far outweigh those from nonbrain-injured but wheelchair dependent spinal cord injured patients (Stambrook, Moore, Peters, Zubek, and Friesen, 1991). Thus, there are unique effects of injury to the brain and the consequent disruption of cognitive and personality functioning, over and above the sequelae attributable to substantial physical disability.

Psychosocial vs. Physical Deficits

Family members experience a variety of anxiety-based and depressive symptoms, including rapid fatigability, increased social isolation, and increased frustration with the patient's personality change and their lack of insight into their situation. Family members consider the mental and interpersonal sequelae most troubling, in contrast to physical sequelae, in their everyday life for all grades of severity of TBI (Jennett, Snoek, Bond, and Brooks, 1981). More severe injuries, however, are associated with more personality-based changes. Oddy, Humphrey, and Uttley (1978a and b), and Oddy and Humphrey (1980), indicated that the highest level of stress for relatives was within the first month following an injury, but decreased only minimally over a 1-year follow-up. The stress level for relatives leveled-off by 6 months postinjury, and was directly related to the relative's perception of the severity of personality changes in the survivor. As well, spouses and parents of TBI patients did not seem to differ in their level of stress. McKinlay, Brooks, Martinage, and Marshall (1981), noted that relatives have specific concerns over the patient's mental slowness, emotional changes, irritability, and poor memory. Panting and Merry (1972) found that 60% of the relatives in their sample were taking "supportive treatment," such as a tranquilizer or sleeping pill, and they felt that they had insufficient information on the nature of TBI aftermath. Thompson (1974) has also identified a number of problematic patient-based personality changes that included irritability, "hot temper," aspontaneity, restlessness, emotional regression, lability, and stubbornness.

Lishman (1973) has stated that "what is virtually certain is that the mental sequelae out-strip the physical as a source of difficulty with relationships, hardship of work, and social capacity generally, and in terms of the strain thrown on families to whom the head injured patient's return" (p. 304). This continues to be the case even 5 years postinjury (Brooks, Campsie, Symington, Beattie, and McKinlay, 1986).

Marital vs. Parental Issues

Married partners of brain-injured adults face specific developmental challenges. The husband/wife dyad has been hypothesized to be less stable following TBI than the parent/head-injured child dyad (Panting and Merry, 1972; Thompson, 1974). The speculation has been that the instrumental and emotional burdens and role changes following TBI are easier for parents to accommodate as they have previously experienced this type of parent-child, care giving relationship with the TBI patient (Thomsen, 1974). In contrast, this is a new and unexpected role for a spouse, who may be less able to accept, accommodate, and cope with the changed, and frequently regressed, role of the TBI patient. Panting and Merry (1982) have also speculated that the uninjured spouse's role may be more difficult because they become the only adult family member, as contrasted to the dual parent family system. A dual parent family system has the advantage of including mutual supports for each other in dealing with the long-term personality-based and behavioral changes that the TBI sets in motion.

The stress to marriages following TBI has been well documented. The initial study in this area demonstrated convincingly that wives of head injured patients face dramatic life changes, including major role shifts in parenting, in family management, and in finances, and that spouses of TBI patients reported significantly more loneliness, isolation, and depression, in contrast to spouses of male spinal cord injured patients (Rosenbaum and Najenson, 1976). There were decreases in perceived marital sharing, care of children, and in satisfaction with life.

Livingston, Brooks, and Bond (1985a), have documented higher rates of anxiety, insomnia, and social dysfunction in family members following TBI. Specifically, they note that marital functioning and family system functioning is substantially worse following severe TBI, in contrast to "minor" TBI, but no difference was noted in anxiety, depression, or health related concerns between wives and mothers of head injured patients. A 6 and 12 month follow-up of the same group (Livingston, Brooks, and Bond, 1985b) documented that the family's "social maladjustment" increased between 3–6 months postTBI and remained stable at 12 months postinjury. Wives tended to perceive their burden to be greater than that perceived by mothers. Mothers were found to view their perceived burden as decreasing over time. The patient's level of subjective complaints was found to be the strongest predictor of psychologic problems in the family.

Peters, Stambrook, Moore, and Esses (1990), have noted that wives whose partners have suffered severe TBI report significantly more depressed affect than wives of mildly and moderately injured patients. Wives of severe TBI husbands perceive less dyadic consensus, less affective expression, and lower dyadic adjustment following the injury, and their reports of depression increased with increasing severity of TBI and patient's postinjury psychopathology. Perceived marital adjustment worsened as injury severity and family financial strain increased. Comparisons between spousal ratings from wives of spinal cord injured patients who were wheelchair dependent, and demographically matched ambulatory severe TBI patients, indicated that wives of the TBI patients reported marriages characterized by less affective expression, less dyadic adjustment, less cohesion, and less overall marital satisfaction (Peters, Stambrook, Zubek, Moore, and Dubo, 1989). Wives of TBI patients must deal with not only any potential physical sequelae, but, as well, the neuropsychologic, emotional, and interpersonal deficits following their spouses' injury. Also,

Lezak (1978) has argued that the spouse is in "social limbo," because he/she cannot effectively mourn the loss of the spouse due to social prohibitions that usually are in place to preclude the active mourning of individuals who remain alive.

Family coping style may serve as a moderator of the quality of marital adjustment following TBI. Moore, Stambrook, Peters, and Lubusko (1991), demonstrated that, following TBI, families differ in both quality and quantity of coping strategies used. Families who make high use of strategies, like acquiring social support, reframing, seeking spiritual support, mobilizing family resources, and reappraisal, appear to experience greater degrees of marital satisfaction.

Intervention

The specific kinds of intervention that are useful at the time of hospital discharge include normalization of feelings and thoughts, as well as assisting the family in recruiting social supports. Helping the family to define realistic expectations, and providing individual treatment with family members, as well as brief couple and marital therapy, may be critical. Specific environmental and behavioral programming that assists the family in managing the patient's behaviors in the home and in the community may be more important. It is also important to have a clear understanding of the developmental trend related to the evolution of family reactions, and assessment of the family system for counselling and therapy, to resolve the disruption of roles and patterns of communication following TBI. "Psychological counselling will not protect family members from the pain that marks these stages. However, psychologists [and other care providers] who understand how head injury disrupts families can help them work through these stages more rapidly and with less distress than they might without such help" (Lezak, 1986, p. 224). The harsh reality is that the family is confronting real changes in the patient that will possibly, in some form, be permanent changes, and that their task is to face these, integrate them, develop a new family "order," and move beyond.

Lezak (1986) has outlined a conceptual developmental scheme of the family's adaptation to the head injury (Fig. 15.3). She focussed on the tension between the patient's behaviors, relative recovery, and the expectations the family has for recovery at each stage. As indicated in Figure 15.3, following discharge from the hospital, the family goes through stages marked by frustration and anxiety, discouragement and guilt, denial, grief, and, in her model, reorganization. The family alternately approaches and avoids confronting the real life implications of the patient's changes and behavior. Her model is predicated upon the fact that, despite professionals' efforts in educating and assisting families to cope with major changes, it is only through day-to-day experience with the patient and their impaired executive functions that the family can actually come to know and face the reality of the multifaceted and pervasive nature of the deficits. It should be emphasized, as Lezak does note, that not all families go through this cycle in the way it is presented as "the stages tend to overlap and they can shift back and forth" (Lezak, 1986, p. 244). However, the family may not survive. Some authors have commented on the increased divorce rate following TBI (Anderson-Parente, DeCesare, and Parente, 1990; Panting and Merry, 1972; Thompson, 1974) although this was not demonstrated by Oddy, et al. (1978).

Discharge from Outpatient Services

The third major crisis occurs when the TBI patient is discharged from all the therapies and supports that were initially available to him or her. At the point that the family are beginning to appreciate the real life significance of the major psychosocial, interpersonal, and neuropsychologic changes, they are also forced to confront the reality of long-term changes in family functioning on their own. Family members frequently feel overwhelmed, abandoned, and isolated, as they now assume some degree of responsibility for the head injured family member without resources that were previously available to them.

Productivity vs. Inertia

An important source of strain is the behavioral and ideational inertia that many severely injured TBI patients experience, and the consequent need for external supports that are not generally available. There is often a lack of appropriate day programming, a relative absence of family respite services, and limited means to reduce the known hardship that TBI patients, particularly severely injured patients, have in returning to employment (Brooks, McKinlay, Symington, et al., 1987; Stambrook, Moore, Peters, Deviaene, and Hawryluk, 1990). Financial distress is a crucial family stressor after TBI (McMordie and Barker, 1988; Moore, Stambrook, and Peters, 1991; Peters, Stambrook, and Moore, 1988). The family's coping resources, particularly when a spouse/parent sustains a TBI, may become overwhelmed on many levels at a time when they have less access to helping resources. The social support network may not appreciate some of the changes that the spouse confronts on a daily basis. Society views the TBI spouse as physically intact and, therefore, "normal," and fails to appreciate the largely "silent" problems that are an integral part of life after TBI.

THEORETICAL INTEGRATION

The sequence of disability-specific events and family reactions represents one strand of development that needs to be considered in a complete model of family adjustment. These factors must be nested within the larger framework of the patient and family life cycle. The impact of a TBI will depend on the stage of the family system within its developmental life cycle, the developmental stage of the individuals in the family, the relationship of each family member to the TBI victim (e.g., spouse, child, parent, sibling), and on the structural and interactional shifts the family is able to make in coping with the strain of combined normative and injury related changes. These system modifications include role changes and alterations in communication patterns, and may be moderated by the social supports and coping strategies that the family can mobilize. Adjustment also depends on interactions between the family's developmental stage and the position/role of the injured member. Lezak (1988) has discussed the experience of being a patient's parent, a patient's minor child, a patient's sibling, or a patient's spouse. There were qualitative differences between these family roles, in terms of interpersonal connectedness, emotional supports, independence, financial strain, and the altered developmental challenges at each stage.

Child as Patient

Despite the devastating and tragic nature of pediatric TBI in terms of developmental, cognitive, social, and personality implications, the injury in the FLC perspective does not, in isolation, impose significant "role" changes for the family. Parents have a caretaking role with the child, and the child's contribution to the family is as a dependent member. The family system at this stage is normatively under the influence of centripetal forces that unite it (i.e., the birth and early development of the infant and child). Family stressors precipitated by the TBI are also centripetal. TBI thus results in additive sets of pressures that amplify and reinforce inward interactional forces (Rolland, 1989). There is no major role change within the family system although the family system may become impeded in later transitions in the family's life cycle when the normative forces shift to centrifugal forces (e.g., navigating a child's adolescence; Rolland, 1989).

Although no forces are hypothesized at this level to pull the family apart, Patterson and McCubbin (1983) state that alterations in family functioning do occur when a child has illness or disability. These include increases in strained family interactions, modified activities and goals, competing time demands, increased financial burdens, social isolation, continuing medical concerns, and grief for the loss of the child who was.

The parents are typically young adults who may not have developed emotional maturity and/or a repertoire of coping resources to allow them to manage the substantive stresses in dealing with a life threatening injury to an infant or young child (Karpel and Straus, 1983). Also, the young parents may not have developed the community roots, life experience, or permanence in their sense of identity and career to prepare them to withstand the substantial stresses facing them. As well, acts of omission or commission that might have led to the TBI can be an added source of guilt and stress. These forces may be modified by factors related to the individual developmental cycle of the parents and the life cycle of the grandparents who are, at a different level of analysis, a family in a later stage in their life cycle.

TBI is a stressor that will continue to require major adjustments throughout the life cycle. If the infant survives as a multiply disabled child, long-term, multidimensional deficits will ripple throughout the family's life cycle and impose challenges at each developmental stage. Normative expectations are for developmental progression on many levels, and for time-based changes in family functioning and roles when preschoolers enter school, adolescents become independent, begin to date, develop their own relationships, and subsequently move away from home, for example. The family system of a child with a TBI will confront implications of this injury at every stage in their development (Wortman and Silver, 1987). Additionally, the TBI of a family member will substantially alter the individual life cycle of each family member. For example, parents, in later life, may confront the fact that they now have a very disabled adult and they, themselves, cannot progress to the next stage, appropriate to their age level—that of an "empty nest" family with grown children.

Sibling as Patient

Sibling reaction to the changes in the family system, and to their disabled brother or sister, will depend in large part on the parents' reactions, and on their own level of understanding, which will be limited by their cognitive level. Frequently, the siblings of disabled children are inadvertently neglected, particularly early in the course of recovery from the injury, because the most attention is paid to the patient. While the patient may have his or her developmental cycle arrested (Spanbock, 1987), there is potential for the healthy siblings to be pushed to assume roles beyond their developmental level (Florian, et al., 1989; Florian and Katz, 1991). Siblings may have expectations for support and instrumental roles that may exceed their skill level and resources. Paradoxically, while the expectations for the siblings may increase, parental support for them may decline as attention focuses specifically on the disabled child.

Parent as Patient

The developmental implications of the pediatric TBI are very different from those of injury to a parent in this early stage of the family life cycle, and, in turn, are very different from the issues that would confront a family in later life. Rolland (1989) stated that:

> "if the disease affecting a parent is more debilitating (e.g., traumatic TBI or cervical spinal cord injury), its impact on the child rearing family is two-fold. The ill parent becomes, for the family, like another child with special needs competing with the real children for potentially scarce family resources. Second, a parent is lost and the semblance of a single parent family is created. For acute onset illnesses, both events can occur simultaneously. In this circumstance family resources may be inadequate to meet the combined child rearing and caretaking demands. This situation is right for the emergence of a parentified child or the re-enlistment into active parenting of a grandparent" (p. 449).

In examining this issue in a sample of families with an adult male head injured victim, Moore, Stambrook, and Peters (1991), reported that the variable most associated with decreased quality of life appeared to be increased perceived financial strain, a centrifugal variable. In addition, having younger children, a centripetal variable, was also associated with increased difficulties. When these results were considered together, the stage of the family with young children may be particularly difficult to navigate, especially if there are financial difficulties. This point has been made in a different context by Peters, Stambrook, and Moore (1988), in documenting that financial strain was related to increased spousal level of depression and increased marital difficulty.

Advances in medical science have resulted in increased survival of individuals who are severely disabled. In contrast, the families of these patients have not received the assistance they need to increase their survival—the tools for coping with the long-term changes that TBI provokes. It is the responsibility of those who design health care systems targeting this TBI population to move beyond the initial neurosurgical and general medical management of these patients. A complete intervention program must also target preservation of the integrity of the family and provide the support needed to cope, adjust, and move beyond the initial injury. A broad system-based developmental model is necessary in structuring clinical and research efforts, and to develop appropriate systems to assist the family system to adjust to the TBI and its long-term sequelae.

SUMMARY

This review of a life cycle perspective has underscored the need to conceptualize patients with TBI and their families in a systemic, developmentally structured, and multidimensional manner. It is important to consider the developmental unfolding of adaptation and change in the patient's own developmental cycle, the disability specific developmental cycle, and the larger family life cycle. The greatest challenges for families relate specifically to the mental sequelae that include executive functioning deficits, personality changes, behavioral disorganization, and disinhibition. These changes markedly alter the pattern, quality, and quantity of social interactions, both within a family and within the patient's and family's social network. The decreased social independence of patients has educational, financial, social, and vocational implications that resonate in the immediate family, into the extended family, and over generations. The FLC approach highlights the importance of identifying patients, spouses, and families who are at high risk, or who are in distress, to prevent or immunize the family system against what the research literature has identified as substantial fallout or, if this proves not to be possible, to moderate the effects of the TBI on long-term family functioning. The family life cycle developmental approach is a powerful one, not only in terms of its conceptual breadth, but also in its potential practical applications. The model provides a tool for understanding the tasks to be accomplished in normal development, and in identifying factors that may lead either to developmental success, or developmental failures. As well, the model provides a theoretical framework to guide future clinical research efforts and to integrate what, at times, seems to be a wide array of diverse research findings.

Thus, the new challenge facing the health care team is not only to increase survival rates of individual patients but to increase the survival rate, and the quality of life of the family unit.

Acknowledgements

The preparation of this paper was partially supported by the Manitoba Mental Health Research Foundation, the Manitoba Health Research Council, the Medical Research Council of Canada, and the National Health Research and Development Program, Health and Welfare Canada. Appreciation is extended to Cheryl Deviaene, Dell Ducharme, and Gordon Sones for their careful reading, and to Elaine Breedon for her assistance in manuscript preparation.

References

Anderson-Parente, J.M., DeCesare, A., and Parente, R. (1990). Spouses who stay. Cognitive Rehabilitation, 8(1):22-25.

Bond, M.R. (1986). Neurobehavioral sequelae of closed head injury. In: Grant, I., and Adams, K.M. (eds). Neuropsychological assessment of neuropsychiatric disorders. New York: Oxford University Press, 347-73.

Brooks, D.N. (1991). The head-injured family. Journal of Clinical and Experimental Neuropsychology, 13:155-88.

Brooks, D.N., and McKinlay, W. (1983). Personality and behavioral change after severe blunt head injury—a relative's view. Journal of Neurology, Neurosurgery, and Psychiatry, 46:336–44.

Brooks, D.N., McKinlay, W., Symington, C., et al. (1987). Return to work within the first seven years of severe head injury. Brain Injury, 1:5–19.

Carter, B., and McGoldrick, M. (1989). The changing family life cycle: A framework for family therapy (2nd ed). Boston: Allyn and Bacon.

Combrinck-Graham, L. (1985). A development model for family systems. Family Process, 23:139–50.

Canboy, T.J., Barth, J., Boll, T.J. (1986). Treatment and rehabilitation of mild and moderate head trauma. Rehabilitation Psychology, 31(4):203–15.

DePompei, R., Zarski, J.J., and Hall, D.E. (1987). A systems approach to understanding CHI family functioning. Cognitive Rehabilitation, 5(2):6–10.

Drotar, D., Crawford, P., and Bush, M. (1984). The family context of childhood chronic illness: Implications for psychosocial intervention. In: Eisenberg, M.G., Sutkin, L.C., and Janzen, M.A. (eds). Chronic illness and disability through the life span: Effects on self and family. New York: Springer, 103–29.

Florian, V., and Katz, S. (1991). The other victims of traumatic brain injury: Consequences for family members. Neuropsychology, 5(4):267–79.

Florian, V., Katz, S., and Lahav, V. (1989). Impact of traumatic brain damage on family dynamics and functioning: A review. Brain Injury, 3:219–33.

Gill, D., Sparadeo, F., and Parziale, J. (1988). Agitation and acute head injury rehabilitation. (Abstract). Archives of Physical Medicine and Rehabilitation, 69:722.

Hass, J.F., Cope, D.N., and Hall, K. (1987). Premorbid prevalence of poor academic performance in severe head injury. Journal of Neurology, Neurosurgery, and Psychiatry, 50:52–56.

Jacobs, H.E. (1989). Long-term family intervention. In: Ellis, D.W., and Christensen, A.L. (eds). Neuropsychological treatment after brain injury. Boston: Kluwer, 297–316.

Jennett, B., Snoek, J., Bond, M.R., and Brooks, N. (1981). Disability after severe head injury: Observations on the use of the Glasgow Outcome Scale. Journal of Neurology, Neurosurgery, and Psychiatry, 44:285–93.

Karpel, M.A., and Straus, E.S. (1983). Family evaluation. Boston: Allyn and Bacon.

Levin, H.S., Eisenberg, H.M., and Berton, A.L. (1989). Mild head injury. New York: Oxford University Press.

Levin, H.S., Mattis, S., Ruff, R.M., et al. (1987). Neurobehavioral outcome following minor head injury: A three centre study. Journal of Neuropsychology, 66:234–43.

Lezak, M.D. (1978). Living with the characterologically altered brain injured patient. Journal of Clinical Psychiatry, 39:592–98.

Lezak, M.D. (1986). Psychological implications of traumatic brain damage for the patient's family. Rehabilitation Psychology, 3:57–69.

Lezak, M.D. (1988). Brain damage is a family affair. Journal of Clinical and Experimental Neuropsychology, 10:111–23.

Lishman, W.A. (1973). The psychiatric sequelae of head injury: A review. Psychological Medicine, 3:304–18.

Livingston, M.G., and Brooks, D.N. (1988). The burden on families of the brain injured: A review. Journal of Head Trauma Rehabilitation, 3:6–15.

Livingston, M.G., Brooks, D.N., and Bond, M.R. (1985a). Three months after severe head injury: Psychiatric and social impact on relatives. Journal of Neurology, Neurosurgery, and Psychiatry, 48:870–75.

Livingston, M.G., Brooks, D.N., and Bond, M.R. (1985b). Patient outcome in the year following severe head injury and relatives' psychiatric and social functioning. Journal of Neurology, Neurosurgery, and Psychiatry, 48:876–81.

McKinlay, W.W., Brooks, D.N., Bond, M.R., Martinage, D.P., and Marshall, M.M. (1981).

The short-term outcome of severe blunt head injury as reported by relatives of the injured persons. Journal of Neurology, Neurosurgery, and Psychiatry, 44:527–33.

McMordie, W.R., and Barker, S.L. (1988). The financial trauma of head injury. Brain Injury, 2:357–64.

Moore, A.D., Stambrook, M., and Peters, L.C. (1991). Centripetal and centrifugal family life cycle factors in long-term outcome following traumatic brain injury. Brain Injury, (in press).

Moore, A.D., Stambrook, M., Peters, L.C., and Lubusko, A. (1991). Family coping and marital adjustment after head injury. Journal of Head Trauma Rehabilitation, 6(1):83–89

Oddy, M., and Humphrey, M. (1980). Social recovery during the year following severe head injury. Journal of Neurology, Neurosurgery, and Psychiatry, 43:798–802.

Oddy, M., Humphrey, M., and Uttley, D. (1978a). Subjective impairment and social recovery after closed head injury. Journal of Neurology, Neurosurgery, and Psychiatry, 41:611–16.

Oddy, M., Humphrey, M., and Uttley, D. (1978b). Stresses upon the relatives of head-injured patients. British Journal of Psychiatry, 133:507–13.

Panting, A., and Merry, P. (1972). The long-term rehabilitation of severe head injuries with particular reference to the need for social and medical support for the patient and family. Rehabilitation, 38:33–37.

Parkinson, D., Stephesen, S., and Phillips, S. (1985). Head injuries: A prospective, computerized study. Canadian Journal of Surgery, 28:79–83.

Patterson, J.M., and McCubbin, H.I. (1983). Chronic illness: Family stress and coping. In: Figley, C.R., and McCubbin, H.I. (eds). Stress and the family I: Coping with catastrophe. New York: Brunner/Mazel, 21–36.

Peters, L.C., Stambrook, M., and Moore, A.D. (1988). Stress related adjustment problems in the wives of head injury patients. Canadian Journal of Rehabilitation, 1(4):71.

Peters, L.C., Stambrook, M., Moore, A.D., and Essess, L. (1990). Psychosocial sequelae of closed head injury: Effects on the marital relationship. Brain Injury, 4(1):39–47.

Peters, L.C., Stambrook, M., Moore, A.D., Zubeck, E., and Blumenschein, S. (1992). Differential effects of spinal cord injury and head injury on marital functioning. Brain Injury, 6. (5), 461–467.

Potter, J.M. (1967). Head injuries today. Postgraduate Medical Journal, 43:574–81.

Rolland, J.S. (1989). Chronic illness and the family life cycle. In: Carter, B., and McGolderick, M. (eds). The changing family life cycle: A framework for family therapy (2nd ed). Boston: Allyn and Bacon, 433–56.

Romano, M.D. (1974). Family response to traumatic head injury. Scandinavian Journal of Rehabilitation, 6:1–4.

Rosenbaum, M., and Najenson, T. (1976). Changes in life patterns and symptoms of low mood as reported by wives of severely brain-injured soldiers. Journal of Consulting and Clinical Psychology, 44:881–88.

Rutter, M., Chadwick, O., and Shaffer, D. (1983). Head injury. In: Rutter, M. (ed). Developmental Neuropsychiatry. London: Guilford Press, 83–111.

Spanbock, P. (1987). Understanding head injury from the families' perspective. Cognitive Rehabilitation, 5:12–14.

Stambrook, M., Moore, A.D., Peters, L.C., Deviaene, C., and Hawryluk, G.A. (1990). Effects of mild, moderate, and severe closed head injury on long-term vocational status. Brain Injury, 4(2):183–90.

Stambrook, M., Moore, A.D., Peters, L.C., Zubek, E., and Friesen, I.C. (1991). Head injury and spinal cord injury: Effects on psychosocial functioning. Journal of Clinical and Experimental Neuropsychology, 13:521–30.

Stambrook, M., Peters, L.C., and Moore, A.D. (1989). Issues in the rehabilitation of severe traumatic brain injury: A focus on the neuropsychologist's role. Canadian Journal of Rehabilitation, 3:87-98.

Stern, J.M., Sazbon, L., Becker, E., and Costeff, H. (1988). Severe behavioral disturbance in families of patients with prolonged coma. Brain Injury, 2(3):259-62.

Thomsen, I.V. (1974). The patient with severe head injury and his family. Scandinavian Journal of Rehabilitation Medicine, 6:180-83.

Tritt, S.G., and Esses, L.M. (1986). The effects of childhood chronic illness on the family: Implications for health care professionals. Canadian Journal of Community Mental Health, 5:111-27.

Walsh, F. (1982). Conceptualizations of normal family functioning. In: Walsh, F. (ed). Normal family processes. New York: Guilford Press, 3-44.

Whitt, J.K. (1984). Children's adaptation to chronic illness and handicapping conditions. In: Eisenberg, M.G., Sutkin, L.C., and Janzen, M.A. (eds). Chronic illness and disability throughout the life span: Effects on self and family. New York: Springer, 69-102.

Willer, B. (November, 1990). Brain injury research needs to confront policy issues. Paper presented to the National Institute on Disability and Rehabilitation Research.

Wortman, C.B., and Silver, R.C. (1987). Coping with irrevocable loss. In: Vanderbos, G.R., and Bryant, B.K. (eds). Cataclysms, crises, and catastrophes. Washington: American Psychological Association, 189-235.

COMMUNITY INTEGRATION

16

Community Integration and Barriers to Integration for Individuals with Brain Injury

BARRY WILLER RICHARD LINN KAREN ALLEN

What are the goals of rehabilitation? It seems unnecessary that one should have to ask. There are ever increasing numbers of rehabilitation programs and rehabilitation beds in hospitals brought on by the demands of an aging population with an increased number of individuals with disabilities. The increase in programs naturally leads to an increased need for rehabilitation professionals. With all this, the question of purpose or *goal* of rehabilitation remains largely unanswered.

There are at least four different perspectives to be considered in any discussion of the goal(s) of rehabilitation: the professional, the policy maker, the payer, and the consumer (see the edited text by Fuhrer, 1987). The family of the consumer might easily represent a fifth perspective. Earlier chapters in this volume generally reflect the focus or perspective of the professionals. Professionals in brain injury rehabilitation are trained to assess and treat medical problems (see Chapter 5), physical problems (Chapter 6), speech and communication disorders (Chapter 8), cognitive deficits (Chapters 9 and 10), and behavior problems (Chapter 13). The inference one may draw is that the *goal* of rehabilitation is the effective elimination or reduction of deficits in each of these areas of functioning. This inference is supported by the development of functional assessment approaches (described in Chapters 4 and 7) that purport to assess function and recovery of function in the individual as a result of brain injury rehabilitation.

Payers and policy makers have somewhat similar interests in the outcome of rehabilitation (DeJong and Hughes, 1982). They, too, are interested in the recovery of physical and cognitive functioning, but they add the variable of cost to the outcome equation. Payers, in particular, want rehabilitation outcomes to be achieved in the least costly manner (Mullins, 1989). Related to this interest in cost containment is the element of time. The time it takes to achieve the desired rehabilitation outcome is directly related to the cost to achieve that outcome. It is important to point out that the cost to provide rehabilitation services to individuals with severe brain injury is substantial and is, in fact, greater than most other trauma-related causes of disability, including spinal cord injury (MacKenzie, Shapiro, and Siegel, 1988; MacKenzie, Shapiro, Moody, Siegel, and Smith, 1986). In the interest of cost containment, payers may wish to limit the level of functional outcome to those that can be achieved in some (arbitrarily) defined time or dollar limit. The other cost and time related *goal* for both payers and policy makers is the reduced dependency of the individual on costly long-term health care or social services. The ideal outcome from the perspective of the payers and policy makers is for the individual with brain injury to attain or regain the ability to be either totally self-sufficient or dependent upon only natural (i.e., low cost) support systems, such as their families. Payers have the expectation that their involvement in rehabilitation will not be ongoing throughout a person's life, but rather clearly defined and finite.

The consumer and family's perception of the rehabilitation *goal* is probably the least understood. The differences in perception of the rehabilitation goal between consumers and professionals was brought to our attention when we conducted research on the long-term outcomes of married individuals with brain injury (Willer, Allen, Liss, and Zicht, 1991). While we did not specifically ask about goals, we did ask these men and women (2-years and more postinjury) and their partners about the problems they faced. Through open-ended discussions we learned that memory deficits and other disabilities presented as difficulties but were ranked considerably behind problems of living, such as altered relationships and restrictions of autonomy. The conclusion we drew from this research is that the *goal* of rehabilitation for the individual with brain injury is to become an active and contributing member of his or her family and of the community. Individuals with brain injury are not very different from the rest of us, with quality of life and self-esteem being derived largely from successful social relationships and the feeling that one is contributing to the well being of others.

On the surface there appear to be few conflicts between the goals of the rehabilitation professional, the payer, the policy maker, and the consumer. This is especially true during the phase of intensive (inpatient) rehabilitation that follows soon after the injury. Everyone is focused on the recovery of physical and cognitive function and everyone wants the recovery to occur as quickly as possible. Problems in goal discrepancy become apparent when the individual leaves the inpatient rehabilitation setting and begins to focus on recovery of life skills and relationships. The problems associated with reintegration of the individual into the family and social setting are magnified for those with brain injury. There are few professional programs that assist the individual with brain injury to cope with problems of reintegration. The functional assessment approaches and other indices of rehabilitation outcome rarely include any indicators of reintegration. Third-party payers rarely support intervention programs which aim to facilitate integration, and professionals receive little training in how to increase levels of integration.

In order to address some of the problems of definition and measurement of community integration identified above, we have developed an instrument to assess community integration for individuals with brain injury. This chapter describes the development of the Community Integration Questionnaire (CIQ) and its rationale. The CIQ represents the end product of a search for a measure of rehabilitation outcome that more closely reflects the values and goals of individuals who have disabilities. A discussion of community integration would be incomplete without some articulation of the barriers to integration experienced by individuals with disabilities. Although the CIQ and its conceptual framework was developed and tested on individuals who experienced brain injury, we believe that the concept and measurement applies equally to all individuals with disabilities.

THE WHO MODEL OF REHABILITATION

Our search for a measure of long term rehabilitation outcome measure began naturally with consideration of the World Health Organization's (WHO) description of handicap. The impairments and disabilities components of the International Classification of Impairments, Disabilities and Handicaps (ICIDH) (World Health Organization, 1980) is described in detail in Chapters 4 and 7. The WHO's description of disease and impairments is widely accepted and led directly to the development of the international coding scheme. The International Classification of Diseases is now in its 9th revision but, ironically, does not include a code for brain injury.

The WHO's description of disabilities, that is, limitation in activities of daily function as a result of impairment(s), is also widely accepted. However, the issue of how to measure disabilities is still controversial. For example, in preparing for a major disability study in Canada, investigators Bindor and Morin (1988) found that some areas of daily functioning were not adequately defined by the WHO descriptions. Areas poorly defined included cognitive functioning, memory, attention, and emotional problems. Clearly, these complex areas of function are important disability issues for individuals with brain injury.

Another Canadian group, committed to clarifying ICIDH issues, also points out that the WHO's description of disabilities neglects life habits, such as personal care, nutrition, communication, etc. The Quebec group (Fougeyrollas, St. Michel, and Blouin, 1989) suggests that these types of disabilities exist at a different level than motoric or sensory disabilities. They further suggest that these life habits be included in a broader definition of handicap. While we agree that life habits need to be included in the ICIDH definitions, we support the WHO distinction where disabilities represent problems at the personal level and handicap represents problems of the person as a member of society. The life habits outlined by the Quebec group are largely at the individual level and might be better viewed as a second level of disabilities.

Whatever weaknesses one may find in the WHO's ICIDH model and description, the fact remains that it is widely accepted and has contributed in a substantial way to international communication on disability. The model also served to focus the attention of professionals on a higher level of concern and purpose for rehabilitation, namely the elimination of handicap. Handicap is defined by the WHO as "a disadvantage for a given individual, resulting from an impairment or a disability, that limits or prevents fulfillment of a role that is normal (depending on age, sex, and social and cultural factors) for that individual" (World Health Organization, 1980, p.183). The WHO description of handicap identifies six areas of role performance that can be interfered with by impairment or disability: Orientation, Physical Independence, Mobility, Occupation, Social Integration, and Economic Self-Sufficiency.

The most notable attempt to develop measurable indices of handicap, as defined by WHO, is that of Whiteneck (1987), who did so for evaluation of rehabilitation outcomes for individuals with spinal cord injury. Whiteneck (1987) points out that most of the measures of handicap employed by the National Spinal Cord Injury Database were eliminated because of the difficulty they pose for reliability and cost of data collection. He also points out that measures of orientation are not really necessary for individuals with spinal cord injury. What is left unstated is that orientation does not describe a role, and is probably better viewed as a disability since it is more reflective of individual difficulties rather than interpersonal difficulties that characterize role performance. This only serves to illustrate the difficulties investigators have had with developing measures of handicap.

Our search for a long term rehabilitation outcome measure did not end with *handicap*. As widely accepted as the ICIDH is, the term handicap appears to have taken on a variety of meanings to different people. Through personal communication with Philip Wood (1989), the principal author of the ICIDH, we learned that the WHO's ICIDH was intended as a draft, and the concept of handicap was the factor least satisfactorily described because most of the discussants and authors were health care professionals, whose primary focus is impairment and disability. In addition to being surrounded by considerable ambiguity, the term *handicap* is potentially pejorative. It appears to have derived from the concept of begging *with cap in hand*. Regardless of various semantic concerns, our aim was to develop an outcome measure and accompanying concept that described a goal for rehabilitation that is acceptable to consumers (i.e., individuals with disabilities). The term community integration appeared most acceptable.

CONSTRAINTS ON ASSESSMENT OF COMMUNITY INTEGRATION

Our search for a definition and measure of community integration was directed partially by our role in the development and maintenance of the Model Systems database. The Model Systems database currently has five participating hospital programs, from various regions of the United States, which compile the same data on each patient from the point of entry into the program to regular follow-up after discharge from rehabilitation (Thomas 1988). One purpose for the development of the CIQ was to serve as a principal measure of rehabilitation outcome for the Model Systems database.

A community integration measure that would be suitable for use in the Model Systems database had to meet certain criteria. First, and foremost, the instrument had to be brief. The Model Systems database is comprehensive, covering many aspects of demography, impairment, disability, and treatment. Individual data elements have undergone considerable scrutiny by rehabilitation experts to determine if the measure used is the most precise and efficient means to assess that aspect of medical need or care. The database is not a medical record system and, therefore, is not intended as a comprehensive representation of an individual's medical needs and treatment. Instead, the database is intended for research and, therefore, includes *minimal* data on individuals with maximum reliability for data analysis.

The community integration assessment component of the Model Systems database was to occur during follow-up and this provided further constraints on the community integration measure. In addition to being brief, the questions had to make sense in a telephone interview with the individual with brain injury, since not all former patients would be able to return to the hospital for follow-up. To increase the reliability of the questions during a telephone interview, questions were aimed at assessing behaviors, as opposed to feeling states. This eliminated questions about satisfaction or psychologic well-being even though we perceive these as important aspects of integration.

A further constraint on the assessment of community integration is the tremendous heterogeneity represented by individuals with brain injury. It is important that a community integration measure should not show undue bias to age (although the Model Systems database is limited to adults), sex, or economic status. It must also be sensitive to the wide variety of situations that an adult with brain injury may live in. For example, the community integration assessment had to be applicable to someone living in a nursing home or living independently. Hence, the home integration questions had to assess activities that can be performed in every living situation.

REVIEW OF CURRENT DEFINITIONS AND MEASURES

Commonly used expressions which describe the goal of rehabilitation are "community integration," "community reintegration," and "community re-entry." Despite numerous articles and several books devoted to the topic of community integration, there appears to be an absence of a clear definition of the concept. The terms are used as if completely understood by all concerned, but they are rarely clarified or anchored operationally.

An edited text by Ylvisaker and Gobble (1987) on community re-entry for adults with brain injury, does an excellent job of describing various interventions that increase practical outcomes for patients. However, throughout the book community re-entry is inferred rather than defined. The most common index of successful re-entry is placement into competitive employment, as described in the chapter by Wachter, Fawber, and Scott (1987). For individuals with brain injury, however, competitive employment outcomes are not necessarily possible. Gobble, Dunson, Szekeres, and Cornwall (1987), describe programs to improve avocational outcomes which are further described as substitutes for competitive employment. Avocational activities are "meaningful, productive, interesting—and fun—activities" (Gobble, et al., 1987, p. 377) and are an important aspect of integration.

Condeluci, Cooperman, and Seif (1987), discuss outcome in terms of independent living. Independence is defined as control over one's life "based on choice of acceptable options that minimize reliance on others" (p. 302). The authors then proceed to outline the various independent living options on a continuum of dependency, from institutions to living independently. Articles about this continuum (Cervelli, 1990; Seaton, 1988), however, have identified the fact that the type or name of a residential setting does not describe adequately the level of independence experienced. Individuals may live in group settings but have the opportunity to move about, carry out daily functions, work or go to school, have privacy in their homes, and have control over their lives, while someone living alone may be dependent on others for many activities and in the absence of their support may live the life of a recluse.

Two additional texts provide a compendium of articles on various approaches to facilitating community integration for individuals with brain injury. Kreutzer and Wehman's text, "Community Integration Following Traumatic Brain Injury" (1990), is divided into chapters addressing areas of vocational, family, and community integration. One can infer that these represent three broad areas of community integration. In a separate book, Williams and Kay (1991) look specifically at family issues and, while the focus is not specifically on community integration, the various chapters outline the impact on the family and some of the impediments to re-entry. In one chapter, for example, Kneipp (1991) describes the role and function changes that must occur to allow reintegration of the individual with disabilities. Again, one is left to infer that successful integration into the family or home setting is represented by the degree to which the individual with disabilities fulfills age appropriate roles and functions.

The problem of defining and measuring community integration has been approached by several investigators as part of research on outcome of rehabilitation. Rappaport, Herrerro-Backe, Rappaport, and Winterfield (1989), designed a simple 4-item scale that rates the impact of physical impairments and changes in mood and frustration tolerance on work and living situation. However, the psychometric properties of this scale were not presented. In addition, the scale was not designed to assess the situation where someone is limited in work and living situations for reasons other than physical impairment, mood or frustration.

Another assessment instrument of note is the Reintegration to Normal Living (RNL) Index (Wood-Dauphinee, Opzoomer, Williams, Marchand, and Spitzer, 1988) which was designed as an outcome measure for rehabilitation from chronic disease. The instrument is composed of 11 items which include measures of disability (mobility, self care), role performance (productive daytime activities, recreational activities, and family roles), interpersonal relationships, comfort with self, and self confidence. The RNL Index presents promise as a measure of reintegration, but not does comply with the ICIDH distinction of the World Health Organization, which separates disability from handicap and further separates these from psychologic well-being and other indicators of feeling states.

The literature has provided us with considerable insight into integration issues and through inference, a description of integration itself. The literature on community re-entry makes broad reference to what appears to be three general categories of role function: home (and family), social networks (friends, leisure activities), and productive activities (work, school). In our search for a measure of community integration we decided to attempt a clearer description of these three areas of role performance.

DEVELOPMENT OF THE COMMUNITY INTEGRATION QUESTIONNAIRE
Initial Selection of Items

A 2-day conference was attended by a group of nine experts with experience in various aspects of research on rehabilitation of individuals with traumatic brain injury. The purpose of the conference was to develop a brief questionnaire to assess integration related to the following: 1) activities performed in the home, 2) social activities, and 3) productive activities. The experts were assigned to one of three groups, and each group focused on one aspect of community integration (i.e., home, social roles, or productive activity). In addition to the members of each subgroup, the conference was attended by four individuals who represented consumers and advocates, and provided reactions and feedback to each of the groups throughout the item selection process.

Conferees were asked to spend the first day developing a minimum set of questions to be presented to the whole group for possible inclusion into the final questionnaire. Each group reached its list of items by identifying and conceptualizing broad issues of importance within the specified domain, and then discussed ways in which such issues could be included as items in a brief questionnaire. On the second day, all conferees participated in a consensus process of selecting critical items from within the three domains of interest while eliminating redundant or irrelevant information.

The initial version of the CIQ, developed during the consensus conference of experts, consisted of 47 questions. These questions included items directed at assessing integration into the current living situation, social activities, performance of household duties, family decision making, use of transportation, employment, and school-related activities. The panel of experts recommended that these items undergo pilot study to enhance selection of items for inclusion in a briefer, final version of the CIQ.

Pilot Study

The purpose of the pilot study was to assess the internal consistency of the items identified by the panel of experts, and to assist with deletion of items that were redundant or that had little relationship to the construct of community integration. In this section, we briefly describe the pilot study results and look at the influence of some demographic variables on community integration.

Subjects

To date, information on the initial version of the CIQ has been obtained from a sample of 49 individuals who experienced severe brain injury. This information was obtained from three sources: 1) the Family

Studies project at the Rehabilitation, Research and Training Center on Community Integration of Persons with Traumatic Brain Injury at the State University of New York at Buffalo (N = 22); 2) the Model Systems project at the Rehabilitation Institute of Michigan (N = 16); and, 3) the Model Systems project at the Santa Clara Valley Medical Center (N = 11). Since the main purpose of obtaining pilot information was to assist in item selection, the information from the three samples was combined into one data set (N = 49).

Procedure

All subjects were administered the 47-item version of the CIQ developed by the expert panel. The questionnaires were then scored and the data was entered into a DEC VAX/VMS system running SPSS-X. Initially, all items were intercorrelated (Pearson product-moment correlations). Based upon these initial results, items were grouped into one of three integration domains: home, social activities, and productive activities. Subscale scores were derived by adding together all items within the same domain, and a total score was developed by adding the three subscores together. Test items were correlated with other items within the same subscale, and were also correlated with each of the three subscale scores and with the overall score. Items having little or no association with a particular subscale (r <.30) were correlated to the subscale score of a different domain; those having no association with any other subscale or with the overall score were dropped from the questionnaire.

Results

Using these procedures, a group of 15 items was derived. Three of these items, concerned with productive activities (e.g., employment, school, and volunteer activities) were combined into one variable (Job/School). Statistical analysis was then performed using the final 13 variables. Correlations between the items, the three subscales, and the overall score are displayed in Table 16.1. The CIQ itself is attached to this chapter as Appendix A.

The pilot CIQ data were subjected to a principal components analysis using varimax rotation. As depicted in Table 16.2, this analysis yielded three factors which corresponded closely (although not perfectly) with our initial constructs of integration into home, social, and productive activities. Factor I (Home Integration) consisted of items associated with domestic activities such as housework, caring for the children, shopping, and preparing meals, but also included an item associated with making social plans. Factor II (Social Integration) consisted of items related to shopping, visiting friends, or engaging in leisure activities. In addition, this

Table 16.1.

Pearson Product-Moment Correlations Between CIQ Items, Subscales, and Total Score

ITEM CONTENT	SUBSCALE			CIQ TOTAL
	HOME	SOCIAL	PRODUCTIVITY	
1. Grocery shopping	.70***	.03	−.01	.43**
2. Meal preparation	.74***	.15	.14	.56***
3. Housework	.83***	.22	.21	.67***
4. Personal finances	.64***	.54***	.10	.65***
5. Childcare	.89***	.28*	.15	.71***
6. Social plans	.64***	.23	.14	.53***
7. Shopping (Times/month)	.38**	.68***	.23	.60***
8. Leisure activities	.32*	.75***	.42**	.67***
9. Visiting others	.28	.67***	.21	.53***
10. Socialization (with whom)	.06	.57***	.11	.32*
11. Best friend	.18	.69***	−.03	.39**
12. Use of transportation	.17	.21	.59***	.40**
13. Job/school (Combination of three questions assessing work, school activities, and volunteer activities)	.13	.21	.96***	.51***

*p <.05
**p <.01
***p <.001

Table 16.2.

Principal Component Analysis of the Community Integration Questionnaire with Varimax Rotation (N=49)

VARIABLE	FACTOR I (HOME)	FACTOR II (SOCIAL)	FACTOR III (PRODUCTIVITY)
Child Care	.866	.223	.100
Housework	.824	.081	.291
Grocery Shopping	.815	−.036	−.183
Meal Preparation	.801	.049	−.004
Social Plans	.555	.131	.288
Visiting Others	.097	.757	.030
Personal Finances	.384	.695	.019
Best Friend	.040	.662	−.188
Leisure Activities	.082	.623	.599
Shopping (Times/Month)	.231	.564	.397
Socialization (With Whom)	−.145	.494	.240
Use of Transportation	.118	−.064	.787
Job/School	.037	.084	.667

factor contained an item reflecting management of personal finances. We had originally included this item in the Home subscale, so its higher loading on the Social factor was somewhat unexpected. Inspection of Table 16.1, however, does demonstrate a significant correlation between the personal finances item and the Social subscale. Factor III (Productivity) represents items involved with work, school, and volunteer activities, as well as an item reflecting use of transportation.

The principal components analysis was performed using a small sample size, so the results reported here must be interpreted with caution. Nonetheless, the presence of three relatively distinct integration factors which correspond well with the domains outlined at the start of this investigation is encouraging, and indicates that collection of further data is warranted.

The coefficient α of the overall CIQ for this sample was .76, indicating reasonably good internal consistency of the overall scale. Coefficient α was also calculated for the Home and Social subscales as derived from the principle components analysis, yielding results of .84 and .73, respectively. Coefficient α for the Productivity subscale was low (.35), but since only two items enter into this subscale the size of this measure is limited to the size of the correlation between the items. These results, coupled with outcome of the factor analysis, suggest that the 15-item CIQ can be used both as a measure of overall community integration and to evaluate integration into several discrete domains.

Factor scores were derived by applying the results of the principle components analysis and adding the scores of each item that loaded on a particular factor. The relationship between age, gender, and these specific factors, as well as overall community integration, was analyzed by assigning subjects to groups and using independent samples t-tests. These results are displayed in Tables 16.3 and 16.4, and are discussed below.

Age

Cases were assigned to one of two age groups: Younger (16–34 yrs; N = 25) or Older (35+ yrs; N = 24). Group comparison indicated that younger brain-injured subjects showed significantly higher overall CIQ scores than older subjects: $t(47) = 2.21$, $p < .033$. None of the subscale comparisons reached significance, but possible trends were present for the Social and the Productivity subscales: $t(47) = 1.84$, $p < .072$; $t(47) = 1.93$, $p < .06$, respectively. For both subscales, the trend was for younger individuals to demonstrate greater integration.

Gender

The male-to-female ratio in the pilot sample was slightly greater than 2:1 (35 males, 14 females), a ratio consistent with that reported in the

Table 16.3.

Relationship Between Age and Community Integration

	AGE GROUP[a]	
VARIABLE	YOUNGER (N = 25)	OLDER (N = 24)
Home Integration	4.1 (2.3)	3.4 (3.0)
Social Integration	8.3 (2.5)	6.8 (3.1)
Productivity	3.8 (1.7)	2.8 (2.0)
Total Community Integration	16.3 (3.8)	13.1 (6.1)*

[a]Scores are presented as mean score within a group, with standard deviation in parentheses.
*p < .05

Table 16.4.

Relationship Between Gender and Community Integration

	GENDER[a]	
VARIABLE	MALE (N = 35)	FEMALE (N = 14)
Home Integration	3.4 (2.5)	4.8 (2.9)
Social Integration	7.8 (2.9)	7.0 (2.7)
Productivity	3.5 (1.9)	2.9 (1.8)
Total Community Integration	14.7 (5.4)	14.8 (5.2)

brain injury incidence literature (Willer, Abosch, and Dahmer, 1990). Females demonstrated higher mean scores on the Home integration subscale, and males demonstrated higher mean scores on the Social and Productivity subscales (see Table 16.4). None of these differences reached significance, but a possible trend was present for the Home integration subscale: $t(47) = 1.80$, $p < .078$. Overall CIQ scores were very similar between males and females, and did not differ significantly.

DISCUSSION

Our search for a definition and measure of community integration has not come to an end. Although we have reached the conclusion that community integration is measurable, further work is needed to clarify the role functions that an individual with disabilities might fulfill. We have arbitrarily defined three role function areas: home/family, social, and productive activities. The results of our pilot investigation suggest that the fairest assessment of community integration comes when all three areas of integration are taken as part of the whole. For example, some individuals who manage to become integrated into productive activities (the most difficult area for individuals with brain injury to integrate into), may demonstrate less integration in the other domains. Others who are unsuccessful at integration into productive activities, have the option of greater role performance in home and social activities. Thus, it is our recommendation that all three domains of role function of the individual be considered when evaluating the degree of integration.

The CIQ was constructed by following guidelines set for the development of outcome indices in the field of rehabilitation. The initial principal components analysis lends some support to the decision to separate the assessment of community integration into the three domains of home, social, and productive activities. However, these results require validation through the evaluation of larger sample sizes. The internal consistency of the entire questionnaire in this sample was high enough to indicate that the total CIQ score represents a reasonably homogenous measure of community integration.

When the CIQ was being developed, it became clear that community integration might be affected by background variables such as age or gender. Our analysis of the pilot data indicates that older individuals demonstrate lower overall community integration than do younger individuals. Analysis of the subscales did not provide a precise answer as to the source of this effect, but did raise the possibility that for individuals with acquired brain injury, increased age may place a limit on involvement in social and productive activities. With respect to gender, male and female participants in our study did not differ on the overall measure of community integration. This result suggests that the overall CIQ score is relatively independent of the effects of gender, and does not reward traditional male and female roles in a discriminatory manner. Subscale analysis did indicate a possible trend of females demonstrating higher scores on the Home subscale, but this difference was balanced by slightly higher scores for the males on the other subscales. These results reinforce the notion that, in order for the construct to be useful, community integration must be considered from multiple rather than unitary vantage points.

It is our belief that the CIQ holds promise as an outcome measure in rehabilitation. There are, however, some problems with its use that may require modification and may perhaps limit its use to certain situations. First, and foremost, the instrument does not serve as a thorough evaluation of community integration for an individual. It was designed for program evaluation and for this reason is brief and not responsive to the wide variety of living, working, and leisure situations that individuals want or have available to them. Consequently, the CIQ would not help substantially in preparing individual program plans as part of a community re-entry program. Instead, the CIQ is best used as a measure of outcome for an aggregate of individuals, and as such could be used to perform evaluations of rehabilitation program effectiveness. We are currently carrying out studies which employ the CIQ in program evaluation.

The major concern we have for the CIQ in its present form is that feeling states, such as the individual's level of satisfaction with integration, are not assessed. Similarly, the instrument does not assess the degree to which the individual *chooses* to be integrated. We hope to overcome this problem somewhat by collecting normative data on individuals who have not experienced brain injury. With normative data we assume that the number of individuals who would opt out of integrative activities on the basis of choice alone, would be the same as for a brain-injured group. We recognize, however, that this only partially deals with the issue of choice.

Another problem with the CIQ, which would exist with any measure of handicap or rehabilitation outcome, rests upon the *reason* for the lack of integration. Just as we cannot assess the degree to which the individual decides not to become integrated, we cannot determine whether the individual is prevented from integrating because of his or her disabilities or because of other factors in the environment. According to the rehabilitation model, environmental barriers to integration can range from familial overprotectiveness to architectural barriers. As the next step to assessment of community integration, we are now searching for a definition and measurement of environmental barriers to community integration. This chapter concludes with the first stage of this search.

BARRIERS TO COMMUNITY INTEGRATION

The rehabilitation model allows for consideration of alternative explanations for increased handicap, or using our terminology, decreased integration into the community. Usual practice is to relate the level of community integration to the individual's disabilities. The rehabilitation model takes a broader view and suggests that barriers within the individual's social and physical environment may also contribute to low levels of integration into the community.

In addition to providing a conceptual framework from which to approach the *measurement* of community integration, the factors of the CIQ can be used to consider the barriers encountered in *realizing* community integration as well. In this section we will discuss how various barriers influence degree of integration in home, social, and productive activities.

Family as a Barrier to Community Integration

Although, at first, it may seem counterintuitive to think of the family as a barrier, closer examination reveals several ways that family members may indirectly and directly influence community integration of an individual with traumatic brain injury. For example, it is often much easier and more efficient for nondisabled family members to do most things for (rather than with) the injured family member. Families can be overprotective, they can be patronizing, and they can just be in a hurry to get things done (Turnbull, Turnbull, Bronicki, Summers, and Roeder-Gordon, 1989).

Family members may truly believe that they are keeping the person with brain injury safe by limiting options and choices that nondisabled individuals take for granted. We do not often think of the satisfaction we derive from the control we have over what we choose in the grocery store, what we buy to wear, or how we take care of our own financial matters. Although we may sometimes fantasize about how marvelous it would be to have someone else doing everything else for us, in reality the personal control we would lose would not be worth the tradeoff. Not encouraging or allowing the person with brain injury to engage in everyday home activities also reduces chances of gaining skills necessary for independent living.

In our research about family adjustment to traumatic brain injury, family members have told us about many creative ways to involve individuals with brain injury into home activities. The most important message we have heard is that the person with brain injury does not want to be left out of home activities and feels frustrated because it may take him/her a little longer to accomplish certain tasks. The families have also told us that using creative flexibility with traditional roles within a family has often helped increase the brain-injured person's self-esteem and confidence. For example, a person with a brain injury could take on the task of managing family finances or social engagements; it may take some extra time to accomplish, but such arrangements have worked out very successfully and have contributed to a happier family environment.

Just as the family may sometimes unknowingly interfere with the brain-injured person's integration into home activities, family overprotectiveness and concern may limit his/her choices for an age-appropriate social life. In their attempts to protect, families often create a very restricted environment that allows little freedom and virtually no chance for independence. Often people who experience brain injury are perceived by their families as perpetual adolescents; that is, they are thought of as wanting independence, but needing nurturing, guidance, and permission to do things. Individuals with brain injury and their families have told us that talking about creating a balance in a family between nurturing and encouraging independence is very important.

Integration into productive activities outside the home (e.g., paid employment or volunteer work) also can be impeded by the family of a brain-injured individual. Our research with married couples (Willer, et al., 1991) has produced some interesting and thought provoking results in this area.

We have found a negative relationship between the psychologic well-being of the spouses of individuals with brain injury and the fact that the injured person in the marriage goes to work. Spouses have reported that when their husbands and wives with head injury leave the house they worry about them constantly. What this indicates to us is that increased emphasis should be focused on the role of the whole family in vocational rehabilitation counseling and programs.

Architectural Barriers to Community Integration

The average family home is not barrier-free and accessible to individuals with a variety of disabilities, and such architectural barriers can make it impossible for persons with traumatic brain injury to become integrated into normal home and family activities. The physical barriers in most homes actually make it more likely than not that family members will do things for, rather than with, the person with brain injury. The height and location of stoves, refrigerators, counters, closets, and other daily necessities make them inaccessible to anyone with mobility and balance problems, especially individuals who must use wheelchairs (Lewis, 1987).

Architectural barriers to integration into social and work activities are numerous as well. The newly enacted Americans With Disabilities Act may eventually remedy some of these problems, but currently it is difficult to find office buildings, movie theaters, restaurants, sports arenas, concert halls, churches, and stores that have easy access to their services for people with physical disabilities. Participants in our research have told us that even when access technically exists (e.g., a ramp outside of a restaurant), the access is not often functional because of design limitations. In other words, some businesses and restaurants may comply with the letter of the law, but not with the spirit of the law, by making the experience of using their facilities difficult and unpleasant for people with disabilities.

Most individuals with brain injury do not have physical problems but rather have cognitive problems and difficulty managing sensory input. Individuals we interviewed indicated that ambient noise severely impaired their ability to function. We may have to expand our definition of architectural barriers when considering the needs of individuals with acquired brain injury.

Service Access Problems

Ability to participate in home, social, and work activities also can be diminished by the lack of appropriate services or the high cost of such services when they are available. For example, an individual with brain injury who wishes to live independently may encounter several obstacles in attempting to shop for daily necessities. Even if only minimal help is needed to accomplish everyday tasks, often such assistance comes with a high price tag. According to the Medical-Rehabilitation Department of the American Re-Insurance Company (1990), someone with moderate brain injury can expect costs between $6,700 and $23,340 per year. That estimate does not include transportation or therapy longer than 180 days after injury.

In our society it is much easier to qualify for funding for a life support system than for a *quality of life* support system. Many people with brain injury could manage in the community very well with just a little assistance in organization of time, shopping, and meal preparation, but such help is usually perceived as a luxury, and consequently very difficult to qualify for.

Integration into social activities may be similarly difficult because of high costs of cultural and sports events. In some rural areas cost may not be an issue, but rather the fact that such events are nonexistent. Our research about people with brain injury and their families indicates that the most important predictor of psychologic well-being and satisfaction is a life that includes getting out of the house and engaging in social activities with friends (Willer, Allen, Durnan, and Ferry, 1990; Willer, et al., 1991). This research clearly demonstrates many important human qualities and aspirations that are not changed or diminished by the experience of traumatic brain injury.

Transportation Barriers

For a large percentage of individuals with brain injury, the lack of appropriate transportation can make integration into home, social, and work activities only a dream. If no public transportation is available, and driving is not an option, even shopping for everyday necessities becomes a challenge. Even if an individual with brain injury manages to find an appropriate job, a reliable and cost effective way of getting to the job is vital. Unlike most European cities, communities in North America depend almost exclusively on private transportation. We place an extremely high value on independence, and such an ideology is most unfortunate for anyone living with a disability (Robinault, 1980).

Social Attitudes and Stigma

The barriers to community integration that are perhaps the most difficult of all to surmount are those that are more subtle than lack of transportation, and more difficult to document than lack of a wheelchair ramp. Social beliefs and the attitudes that fuel them can insure that a person with a disability will never live independently, never be accepted in social situations, and never become employed.

For decades social psychologists have been researching and accumulating vast support for something called the "just world" hypothesis (Lerner, 1965). Simply stated, this hypothesis suggests that people generally believe that fate and merit are closely aligned, and that justice and fairness inevitably prevail in human affairs. Despite overwhelming evidence to the contrary, people cling to the notion that the world is an orderly place, and that if something bad happens to someone, that person somehow must have done something to deserve it. By maintaining a belief in a "just world," and by blaming the victim, we also maintain the illusion that bad things will not happen to us.

It is possible to apply the idea of belief in a just world to increasing understanding of social attitudes about individuals with brain injury, and how such attitudes influence community integration. For example, blame and guilt are often powerful factors in family dynamics, and individuals with brain injury may have to live with the knowledge that family members blame them for the accident that caused the injury, as well as for the many changes in family life that have occurred. It is easy to see how such a situation could make it difficult for the person with brain injury to become involved in family and home activities.

Perhaps more harmful than blame by family members, however, is the blame society places on people with disabilities. The just world hypothesis suggests that as severity of illness increases, victims will receive increased derogation by others. That is, as a disease or condition becomes more serious and frightening, it is self-protective for us to distance ourselves from the possibility that it could ever happen to us. Recent research has demonstrated, however, that the way in which blame is placed is very complex and is related to the type of disability (physical vs. mental) and the degree to which the condition is perceived as avoidable (Gruman and Sloan, 1983).

Of direct application to people with brain injury and integration into the work force is the research of Bordieri and Drehmer (1987, 1988, 1986), demonstrating that *type* of disability appears to influence the reactions of potential employers to an applicant. In general, job applicants with cognitive problems are judged less favorably than those with physical problems. The reason most often given for such a judgment is that a mental or cognitive problem is perceived as something an individual is responsible for, and can improve upon with effort, whereas a physical disability is not. Bordieri and Drehmer (1987) also have demonstrated that social acceptance of disabled workers by nondisabled workers can be predicted by perceived responsibility for the disability.

While research evidence in support of belief in a just world certainly fosters a dismal view of possibilities for community integration and acceptance of individuals with brain injury, such research can also be used to educate the public. The more that people understand the reasons for some of their irrational fears and beliefs, the more likely they are to modify their views.

SUMMARY

The fact that few alternate measures of community integration exist made it difficult to compare our measure and definition of community integration to an accepted standard. It is our contention that few measures exist because the concept of community integration has not adequately been assumed within the goals and purpose of rehabilitation programs. Other constraints on development of measures of community integration may include the complexity of the concept.

Development of a measurable definition of community integration should serve as an impetus for subsequent research. For individuals with acquired brain injury, what disability factors serve as primary impediments to integration: motoric, sensory, behavioral, cognitive, or emotional? What environmental factors impede integration the most: family, architectural, transportation, or stigma? What interventions or combination of interventions are the most effective at increasing community integration outcomes? A measurable definition of community integration should ultimately increase our understanding of the impact of brain injury on the lives of individuals affected. Ideally we hope that subsequent research could assist in reducing the handicapping effects of brain injury.

Acknowledgment

We wish to express our appreciation to Mitchell Rosenthal, Ph.D., and his staff at the Rehabilitation Institute of Michigan, and Jeffrey Englander, M.D., and his staff at the Santa Clara Valley Medical Center, for providing us with pilot data on the Community Integration Questionnaire.

We also wish to thank the panel of rehabilitation experts who participated in the CIQ development conference: Drs. Mitchell Rosenthal, John Noble, Gale Whiteneck, Harvey Jacobs, Thomas Kay, Byron Hamilton, William Haffey, Rodger Wood, Catherine Bontke, Ray Rempel, Sherry Watson, and Gary Wolcott.

The research on community integration was made possible by a grant from the National Institute on Disability and Rehabilitation Research of the U.S. Department of Education to the Rehabilitation Research and Training Center at the State University of New York at Buffalo.

Finally, the authors wish to acknowledge the procedural and conceptual support of J. Paul Thomas, Ph.D., Director of Medical Sciences Programs at the National Institute of Disability and Rehabilitation Research.

References

Binder, D., and Morin, J. (1987). Use of questions on activities of daily living to screen for disabled persons in a household survey. The Canadian Journal of Statistics, 16:143–56.

Bordieri, J.E., and Drehmer, D.E. (1987). Attribution of responsibility and predicted social acceptance of disabled workers. Rehabilitation Counseling Bulletin, 30:218–26.

Bordieri, J.E., and Drehmer, D.E. (1988). Causal attribution and hiring recommendations for disabled job applicants. Rehabilitation Psychology, 33(4):239–47.

Bordieri, J.E., and Drehmer, D.E. (1986). Hiring decisions for disabled workers: Looking at the cause. Journal of Applied Social Psychology, 16:199–210.

Cervelli, L. (1990). Re-entry into the community and systems of posthospital care. In: Rosenthal, M., Griffith, E.R., Bond, M.R., and Miller, J.D. (eds). Rehabilitation of the adult and child with traumatic brain injury (2nd ed). Philadelphia, PA: F.A. Davis Co., 463–75.

Condeluci, A., Cooperman, S., and Seif, B.A. (1987). Independent living: Settings and supports. In: Ylvisaker, M., and Gobble, E.M.R. (eds). Community re-entry for head injured adults. Boston, MA: Little, Brown and Company, 301–48.

DeJong, G., and Hughes, J. (1982). Independent living: Methodology for measuring long-term outcomes. Archives of Physical Medicine and Rehabilitation, 63(2):68–73.

Fougeyrollas, P., St. Michel, G., and Blouin, M. (1989) Consultation: Proposal for a revision of the third level of the ICIDH: The handicap. International ICIDH Network Canadian Society on the ICIDH, 2:(1).

Fuhrer, M.J. (1987). Rehabilitation outcomes: Analysis and measurement. Baltimore, MD: Paul H. Brookes Publishing Co.

Gobble, E.M.R., Dunson, L., Szekeres, S.F., and Cornwall, J. (1987). Avocational programming for the severely impaired head injured individual. In: Ylvisaker, M., and Gobble, E.M.R. (eds). Community re-entry for head injured adults. Boston, MA: Little, Brown and Company, 349–80.

Gruman, J.C., and Sloan, R.P. (1983). Disease as justice: Perceptions of the victims of physical illness. Basic and Applied Social Psychology, 4(1):39–46.

Kneipp, S. (1991). Family and community re-entry. In: Williams, J.M., and Kay, T. (eds). Head injury: A family matter. Baltimore, MD: Paul H. Brookes Publishing Co., 165–77.

Kreutzer, J.S., and Wehman, P. (eds). (1990). Community integration following traumatic brain injury. Baltimore, MD: Paul H. Brookes Publishing Co.

Lerner, M.J. (1965). Evaluation of performance as a function of performer's reward and attractiveness. JPSP, 1:355–60.

Lewis, B.E. (1987). "How are families managing at home?" Architectural barriers in households of children with special needs: An issue ignored by health professionals. Children's Environments Quarterly, 4(3):36–41.

MacKenzie, E.J., Shapiro, S., and Siegel, J.H. (1988). The economic impact of traumatic injuries. Journal of the American Medical Association, 260(22):3290–96.

MacKenzie, E., Shapiro, S., Moody, M., Siegel, J., and Smith, R. (1986). Predicting post-trauma functional disability for individuals without severe brain injury. Medical Care, 24(5):377–87.

Medical-Rehabilitation Department of the American Re-Insurance Company. (1990). Guidelines for reserving traumatic brain injury. Princeton, NJ: Corporate Communications and Advertising Department, American Re-Insurance Company.

Mullins, L.L. (1989). Hate revisited: Power, envy and greed in the rehabilitation setting. Archives of Physical Medicine and Rehabilitation, 70(10):740–44.

Rappaport, M., Herrerro-Backe, C., Rappaport, M.L., and Winterfield, D.M. (1989). Head injury outcome up to ten years later. Archives of Physical Medicine and Rehabilitation, 70(12):885-92.

Robinault, I.P. (1980). Transportation and travel. In: Robinault, I.P. (Project Director). Community resources for the social adjustment of severely disabled persons: Options for involvement. New York: ICD Rehabilitation and Research Center, 107-26.

Seaton, D. (1988). Independent living: The need to recognize long-term support. Cognitive Rehabilitation, 6(1):32.

Thomas, J.P. (1988). The evolution of model systems of care in traumatic brain injury. Journal of Head Trauma Rehabilitation, 3(4):1-5.

Turnbull, H.R. III, Turnbull, A.P., Bronicki, G.J., Summers, J.A., and Roeder-Gordon, C. (1989). Disability and the family: A guide to decisions for adulthood. Baltimore, MD: Paul H. Brookes Publishing Co.

Wachter, J.F., Fawber, H.L., and Scott, M.B. (1987). Treatment aspects of vocational evaluation and placement for traumatically brain-injured adults. In: Ylvisaker, M., and Gobble, E.M.R. (eds). Community re-entry for head injured adults. Boston, MA: Little, Brown and Company, 259-300.

Whiteneck, G.G. (1987). Outcome analysis in spinal cord injury. In: Fuhrer, M.J. (ed). Rehabilitation outcomes: Analysis and measurement. Baltimore, MD: Paul H. Brookes Publishing Co., 221-31.

Willer, B., Abosch, S., and Dahmer, E. (1990). Epidemiology of disability from traumatic brain injury. In: Wood, R. Neurobehavioral sequelae of TBI. London: Taylor and Francis Ltd., 18-33.

Willer, B., Allen, K., Liss, M., and Zicht, M. (1991). Problems and coping strategies of individuals with traumatic brain injury and their spouses. Archives of Physical Medicine and Rehabilitation, 72:460-64.

Willer, B., Allen, K., Durnan, M.C., and Ferry, A. (1990). Problems and coping strategies of mothers, siblings and young adult males with traumatic brain injury. Canadian Journal of Rehabilitation, 3(3):167-73.

Williams, J.M., and Kay, T. (1991). Head injury: A family matter. Baltimore, MD: Paul H. Brookes Publishing Co.

Wood-Dauphinee, S.L., Opzoomer, M.A., Williams, J.I., Marchand, B., and Spitzer, W.O. (1988). Assessment of global function: The reintegration to normal living index. Archives of Physical Medicine and Rehabilitation, 69(8):583-90.

World Health Organization (1980). International classification of impairments, disabilities, and handicaps: A manual of classification relating to the consequences of disease (ICIDH). Geneva, Switzerland: World Health Organization.

Ylvisaker, M., and Gobble, E.M.R. (eds). (1987). Community re-entry for head injured adults. Boston, MA: Little, Brown and Company.

17

Advocacy and Support for Victims of Brain Injury and Their Families

R.G. REMPEL

"I have been gravely disappointed with the white moderate. I have almost reached the regrettable conclusion that the Negro's great stumbling block is not the White Citizen's Council-er or the Ku Klux Klanner, but the white moderate, who prefers a negative peace which is the absence of tension to a positive peace which is the presence of justice, who constantly says 'I agree with the goal you seek, but I can't agree with your methods of direct action,' who paternalistically believes that he can set the timetable for another man's freedom. . . ."

Martin Luther King

NEED FOR EFFECTIVE ADVOCACY

In 1980, our family and our immediate circle of friends were propelled into a totally foreign world. We were ill-prepared to handle the crisis. It was terrible, and for many years it would not go away. While riding his bicycle, our son, Jeremy, was struck by a passing motorist. What followed was a period of acute psychologic trauma to the family, as we attempted to secure appropriate services and resources to diminish his physical and neurobehavioral trauma and to facilitate his recovery. We drew initial comfort by our understanding that Canada was reputed to have the most developed health care system in the world.

This is neither the time nor the place to evaluate the Canadian health care system, but we found a tremendous disparity between the current practice of brain injury rehabilitation and the research and clinical literature that was readily available. One could fairly state that there existed, and continues to exist, a dearth of informed service providers (Rempel and Roberts, 1989). In fact, in our case, the need to secure opportunities for our son finally meant a career change for myself at a time that I was comfortably ensconced in the profession of my choice.

We discerned what thousands of Canadian families both before and after us have known as truth, that generally the various segments of treatment/opportunity are not readily available and frequently do not exist within Canada. It is evident as one scans the various journals, periodicals, and books, that this phenomena is not confined to Canada. Rather, it is endemic to most developed countries. This will not be startling to those who have read the numerous studies prepared for state and provincial authorities throughout North America and other continents. In Canada alone, within the province of Ontario, the Ministry of Health and the Ministry of Community and Social Services each completed comprehensive studies and reviews in 1988 that described inadequate services in every segment of the continuum of care for persons who live with the effects of varying degrees of injury to the brain. The 1989 Hearings to Determine the Status of Wellness of Ontario Residents Who Live With the Effects of Brain Injury coined the term Post Coma Abandonment (PCA) to illustrate the dearth of appropriate opportunities for this population.

"The stage in one's recovery following a traumatic brain injury when the appropriate opportunity is not available within the human services network" (Rempel and Roberts, 1989).

The failure of the network to respond results in decreased functional abilities, limited autonomy, and, ultimately, an inferior quality of life.

The above mentioned documents are representative of an abundance of literature produced within the past decade by government agencies, as they have been made to respond to the growing demands of a segment of the population who represent the victims of the number one disabler and killer of young Americans, as described by J. Everett Koop, past U.S. Surgeon General to the National Head Injury Foundation at their annual conference (December, 1988).

ADVOCATING FOR PLANNING

Advocacy means many different things to each of the sectors with a vested interest in the availability of appropriate resources for persons affected by injury to the brain and to their care givers. Those responsible for the planning of such opportunity see advocacy and the issues it raises differently. Rather than replicate existing lists of possible advocacy activity, it is appropriate to review the need for such action and to discuss workable methods of obtaining desirable outcomes that, though seemingly daunting, are, in fact, possible to obtain.

Reports, such as those just cited, very effectively document the dearth of appropriate services for this population. In contrast are the thousands of articles available through literature searches that attest to the abundance of research and clinical observation that have the capacity to substantively reduce handicapping conditions for persons who live with the effects of injury to the brain.

For individuals disabled as a result of injury to the brain this means that although the skill and knowledge exists to provide appropriate opportunities (care), to most all persons who have sustained injury to the brain, such appropriate opportunities are frequently unavailable when actually required by individuals. In some jurisdictions, the reason may be a lack of appropriate insurance coverage. However, in Canada, where the insurer is the provincial government, it is simply a result of poor health care planning with those in positions of responsibility either reneging on their trust or demonstrating an apparent disinterest in learning about and initiating the new knowledge that has emerged during the past two decades. Included in this group are also the policy makers from within both the public and private sectors of the insurance industry.

Perhaps the following statement, from an unpublished report to the Ministry of Health, presented as recently as 1991 by the chairperson of Ontario Ministry of Health, Rehabilitation Advisory Committee, provides insight into the reason for the lack of knowledge regarding rehabilitation opportunities for persons with injury to the brain:

> "... I would like to stress the importance of recognizing rehabilitation as an important and distinct component in the health care continuum, ... rehabilitation is more than a collection of isolated interventions, or the provision of assistive devices.
>
> Historically, rehabilitation has never really been identified as a discreet component within the health care continuum."

Subsequently a definition of the word rehabilitation was written by the committee to be presented for consideration by the Ministry:

> "Rehabilitation is a dynamic, goal-oriented and often time-specific process which can be recurrent for some degenerative conditions. It is aimed at enabling persons with impairments to reach an optimum mental, physical, and/or social level for the individual. Rehabilitation services are consumer-centered and delivered in an interdisciplinary environment which provides the opportunity for the individual to accommodate for a loss of function or functional limitation, and aims to facilitate social re-adjustment and independence."

If in fact the Ministries of Health have been providing dollars for rehabilitation for delivery of a product that has never been adequately defined, small wonder that we are frequently disappointed with the outcome of the service provided.

We regularly hear that families have been told that their injured spouse, sibling or child will plateau, implying that improvement will cease. It would be more appropriate for them to be introduced to the WHO model of impairment, disability, and handicap. The WHO model suggests that although little can be done to diminish impairment, new ways continue to emerge to reduce handicapping conditions. Implicit within this model is the belief that as long as there is human spirit, persons continue to change in either productive or counterproductive ways, depending upon the relative sterility of richness of their environment.

CONTINUITY OF OPPORTUNITY

It is evident that many care givers do not recognize the profound differences on the continuum of injury to the brain between the initial segment of lifesaving neurosurgical intervention and the completely and totally different issues confronting such persons as they continue to live. We regularly see and hear reports of persons with skill in one area making apparent statements of fact in areas completely removed from their field of education and professional development. In fact, when you read the transcripts of head injury court cases, you will observe that the defense frequently call neurosurgeons and neurologists and has them comment upon an individual victim's long-term outcome and community re-entry capabilities. These professionals are trained and educated to deal with impairment, not "long-term handicapping conditions." The plaintiffs' lawyer calls the experts from the field of vocational rehabilitation, physiatrists, neuropsychologists, behavior therapists and cognitive therapists. The latter work with the individual throughout the rest of her life, after she has been medically stabilized. These professionals work with disability and the conditions that handicap. The neurosurgeon works primarily with the impairment and somewhat with the disability. The physiatrist and neurologist work with the impairment and the disability. They, along with various therapists work at identifying and removing handicapping conditions. Yet the courts and the general population frequently recognize impairment and seem to defer to those people who play a vital role in saving and stabilizing life. Because they know how to save lives, the assumption is made that they can then comment upon life-long living issues. Less value is assigned to those professionals who have hands on, day-to-day experience with functional living.

I recently attended a meeting on Life-Long Living. A neurosurgeon had been asked to present his model for Community Re-entry. He regularly demonstrates a high degree of skill and knowledge working with the brain and central nervous system. However, the literature that he used to describe a Community Living Model was archaic and representative of the early attempts of the late '70's. Current literature abounds showing that Life-Long Living Programs based upon neurobehavioral rehabilitation allow persons within a broad spectrum of disability severity to function within the community.

I could be criticized for being unduly harsh if the above incident were an isolated example. Unfortunately, it is representative of the attitudes and beliefs of health care professionals as shown in the results of the Misconceptions Study developed and conducted at Louisiana State, Department of Psychology, (Gouvier, 1988) and replicated at the Research and Training Center at Buffalo (Willer, 1991). As recently as the Spring of 1991, we took that same study to a national Canadian health care conference. Forty-one percent of the respondents did not recognize that "after someone has had a head injury, it is usually harder to learn new things than it is to remember things before the injury." Twenty percent believed that "how quickly a person recovers from a head injury depends mainly how hard they work at recovering." Fifty-five percent did not recognize that "complete recovery from a severe head injury is not possible no matter how badly a person wants to recover."

TRADITIONAL MODELS OF SERVICE DELIVERY

As we began our search for answers, we discovered that although not readily available in Canada, answers based upon good research and excellent clinical experience did, in fact, exist. Unfortunately, it has generally been left to ourselves, and others like us, not only to discover this literature, but also to insist upon the inclusion of such information in the rehabilitation opportunities provided. Very few families have the will, time, strength, or corporate decision making skills necessary to insure that what is relevant, rather than what is available, becomes the rehabilitation opportunity of choice.

This is the environment into which the family and friends of the newly head injured person are thrust. Further affecting an already counterproductive experience is the wish of the family in crisis that the professionals providing care/opportunity will have the appropriate strategies to assure "hoped for" outcomes. Outcomes that are too frequently built upon the mythology of television drama and our wish-for-a-cure society. (Willer, Johnston, and Linn, 1990).

Compounding the emerging dilemma is the too frequently prevailing "fix the problem" approach to health care. Condelucci (1991) has described such traditional health care philosophy (Fig. 17.1) and he then goes on and describes a model much more appropriate for the 90's.

The institutional approach that developed throughout the first half of the 20th Century enshrined a model that saw the patient, his/her impairments, or his/her disabilities as the problem. The trained health care worker was the solution. A more appropriate model sees the handicaps imposed upon the disabled person as the problem. Attempts to diminish these same handicaps must be the solution of choice.

Medical Paradigms	
The Problem,	Person with the condition
Core of the Problem	Within the person
Action of the Paradigm	Classify, congregate, treat
Power person	Expert (doctor)
Goal of Paradigm	fix, heal, change

Figure 17.1. Medical Paradigms. From Condeluci, A.I. (1991). Interdependence, the route to community. Paul M. Deutsch Press. Reprinted with permission from Paul M. Deutsch Press.

FAILURE OF TRADITIONAL ADVOCACY

While the past three decades have seen tremendous improvement for many segments of the population requiring health care, such has not been the case for persons who have sustained injury to the brain.

History is largely an accounting of change and much is written about the agents of change. Rarely have innovators been admired or encouraged by their peers. In fact, they are often vilified. It is subsequent generations that benefit from such actions and who, then, posthumously venerate the advocate.

To proponents of the status quo, the need for change seems to be less problematic than the immediate perceived insurrection. A graphic example of such a statement is the change in status of black Americans that occurred in the early King years and continued through to the late 1980's (Branch, 1990). Though a national holiday now pays tribute to the man and his accomplishments, King's many jailings, and very death, demonstrate the hatred directed at him for his persistent challenge to the established order.

Advocacy, as defined by Webster, is a weak word meaning "asking for, . . . pleading." The definition does not include demand for an appropriate outcome. Unfortunately, survivors and their families have bought into the dictionary definition and have not insisted upon outcomes that were possible, but not readily available. In fact, in recent years advocacy has too frequently been relegated to professional people, such as lawyers, ombudspersons, case managers, social workers, and others, for whom the task has become a career choice rather than an activity resulting from a burning desire to insure necessary change. While professional advocates continue to perform functions important to the head injury community, the current sorry state of opportunity generally available to this population indicates that alternate methods of advocacy are sorely needed. It is hardly profound to indicate that effective advocacy achieves outcomes that appropriately respond to the perceived need.

ADVOCACY FOR TODAY

It should be recognized that what is needed may frequently differ from what may be desired. An informed advocate recognizes that it is not fantasy and wishful thinking that cause satisfactory outcomes; rather they are the result of implementation of activities based upon informed decision making. Such action necessitates committing oneself to acquiring the necessary skills and knowledge base and to engage in risk-taking actions that challenge, and sometimes intimidate, family, community, health care workers, civil servants, and politicians. Effective advocacy is persistent advocacy. Such activity is energy consuming and expensive, both in time spent and in dollar costs.

"Advocacy is a process in which the family and survivor learn to be proactive in decisions about the survivor and his/her needs. Successful advocacy requires understanding the processes and policies of services systems, and learning how they can be changed to fit the needs of each individual's situation. Advocacy is a cycle in which no single step is independent of the other steps. The cycle should be started as soon as possible after the injury has occurred.

[Figure 17.2] is a diagram of the advocacy cycle. Begin reading the diagram with the 'Determine Needs' box and follow the arrow through 'Research', 'Education', 'Develop Action Plan', and 'Implement Action Plan.' The diagram is in the form of a loop because even when an action plan has been implemented, new situations will arise—particularly during transitional phases—which require a re-determination of needs and re-entry into the process." (NHIF Advocating for Funds TIP (Tailored Information Packet), 1988.)

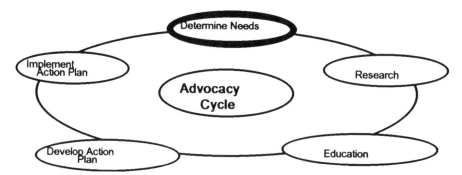

Figure 17.2. Advocacy Cycle. From N.H.I.F. Advocating for Funds TIP (Tailored Information Packet). (1988). Reprinted with permission from National Head Injury Foundation, Inc.

It is important that those who have a vested interest in the outcomes, both immediate and long-term, recognize their potential to facilitate those outcomes. Regularly, we defer to the person who appears to be in charge. When we defer decision making to authority figures, it is they who determine our direction. Unfortunately, they are then making decisions for us that are based upon their life experience, their value systems, and their wants. Appropriate decision making must take into account not only the skill and knowledge of the professional but also the life experience of the individual in question and that of each of the principal players.

Remember that though certain decisions must be made by the health care professional, many decisions can best be made by those who will have to live with the outcomes long after the professional in question has moved on to other endeavors.

ADVOCACY: AN INGREDIENT TO SUCCESSFUL LIVING

The newly disabled person unaccustomed to thinking of herself as an advocate should consider three different stages of advocacy development. It is an unfair expectation to think that you will immediately have the skills to sustain an attitude that exudes control of your life similar to or greater than the degree that you demonstrated prior to the recently experienced trauma. It will take time and effort to learn the paradigms, both superficial and real, that you inherited with your newly acquired impairment.

1. **Internal acceptance of the new and altered condition.**
   Acknowledgment that life will definitely be different, though with appropriate skill, knowledge and actions not necessarily better or worse,
2. **Commitment to changed lifestyle.**
   As a person who lives with the effects of a recently acquired disability, you, as the person with the disability or a "best friend," begin to include the newly acquired disability and learn what is necessary to successfully diminish handicapping conditions,
3. **Proactively pursuing re-directed outcomes.**
   Comfortable with your altered lifestyle, your enlightened attitude gives you confidence to focus upon new and different goals. This level empowers the person to influence and affect the attitudes and outcomes of those within their comfort zone. Such a grouping can be limited to your natural peer group or as broad as your country's national policy toward disability (Rempel and Roberts, 1989).

Most of our life we have taken orders or deferred to others and followed directions. Much of our life is spent standing in a queue. When we move out of our comfort zone we tend to defer to others who appear to have more knowledge. Especially during periods of trauma, it is natural to want to defer to authority figures. However, it is important that we insist upon participatory decision making. It truly is important that it is you who ultimately makes the choice. Having had input from informed persons with appropriate experience, skill and knowledge, you can then, with confidence, make decisions you deem to lead to the outcome of choice.

STARTING TO ADVOCATE

It is my observation that most persons, be they health care workers unhappy with the program that they are allowed to deliver or disenfranchised consumers, do not recognize the potential available to them through the implementation of appropriate advocacy strategies and the requisite follow through. This is evident with the continued existence of each of the inadequately staffed programs that are mandated to deliver appropriate service to persons who live with the effects of injury to the brain. It is further evident when one recognizes the lack of appropriate services and programs, but routinely accepts the benign attitude of federal, provincial, and local agencies and their continued lack of planning and subsequent reticence to implement appropriate opportunities for persons who live with the effects of injury to the brain. Again it is evident when injured persons, their families, friends, and health care advisors, accept psychiatric wards, jails, and sheltered workshops as acceptable opportunities for living.

Actualized advocacy must take an appropriate form for each occurrence. While the basic principles of preparedness remain constant, each of us will have different stories that reflect our interests, needs, and dreams. Our peer groups and those who either stymie or empower us will also uniquely shape each story.

When planning successful advocacy, consideration must be given to the various factors that would compel the person or agency who controls the power in the situation to initiate appropriate change. Such persons include, but are not limited to, politicians, government employees, program directors, neurosurgeons, family doctors, nurses, rehabilitation workers, social workers, and entrenched family members. The greater the knowledge of political, social, and health care paradigms, and the literature describing outcome possibilities, the more implementation options will be available to the persons developing the advocacy plan.

The letter writing campaign that was implemented to correspond to the opening of the Ontario Head Injury Association offices in 1985, is a model for effecting systemic change. A month prior to the opening, we cofounders visited each of the 11 identified support groups in the province and the few head injury programs that were supportive of our effort. Participants were encouraged to sit down with neighbors, relatives, associates at work, and anyone else whom they could muster, and guide them through, at minimum, a very simple and straightforward three sentence letter. We suggested that they write to one of the five high ranking politicians and Cabinet Ministers on a list that we provided and to copy the other four, their local politicians, and anyone else who came to mind. Letter captains were appointed as contact persons to collect the letters and we then did much of the actual mailing.

Within 2 months, in excess of 2400 letters had arrived at Queen's Park, our provincial capital. By then, our little office was inundated by political staff requesting clarification and information about services that they were convinced must exist within their constituencies, but that they could not readily identify. Overnight it established for us a database of people who had felt compelled to answer us and to either defend the status quo or to admit that it was deficient. Some responded because they were politicians who had a desire to please and hopefully do what was right. Others responded because they were health care employees who had to defend the inadequate status quo to the politicians and the media. For a variety of reasons we had a group of people who had demonstrated by their responses that they were vulnerable to our concerns. We identified those with whom we could work to alter a weak and inadequate brain injury continuum of opportunity (care). Many of these initial contacts have become an important part of our expanded network. I can identify a few who have had a tremendous influence upon our effort. This was the beginning of political action that eventually encouraged the Ministries of Health and Social Services to begin to address the shortcomings, as they related to service for persons who lived with the effects of injury to the brain, within the province of Ontario.

Since that time, we can graph the ebb and flow of political activity directed toward the development of opportunity for this population. Our records make it abundantly clear that proactive political activity occurs only during times of effective consumer action.

ADVOCATING FOR APPROPRIATE SERVICES

For many of the impairments associated with injury to the brain, the literature describing the productive result of appropriate opportunity is very clear. Once the severely injured person has been medically stabilized, the process of relearning that must occur can best be accomplished back within a community that fosters generalization of both existing knowledge and the acquisition of new skills and information. The most apparent rationale being that the physically altered brain generalizes new information very poorly. However, in 1993, a mere 75 community re-entry programs can be identified in the United States and perhaps 10 programs, with 60 residential spaces, are available throughout Canada. Even this discouraging report is unduly kind to health care planners when one recognizes that many of these community re-entry programs have rigid admission criteria that preclude persons with unresolved neurobehavioral issues from accessing their programs. Keep in mind that the impaired organ is the brain, and that the brain is responsible for the initiation of behavior. Yet it is this primary neurobehavioral function that most re-entry programs in Canada do not have the capacity to address.

I recently had opportunity to review a letter describing to a person with impaired cognition why he was no longer a candidate for a program that is designed to enhance cognitive function and to facilitate more appropriate behavioral social activity. At the time of writing the facility had never employed a person with a specialty in the neurosciences. In Canada, the few brain injury re-entry programs that do exist, controlled as they are by provincial governments, have been funded largely along the lines of the traditional group home model, staffed to minimum standards, with some minimal concessions for additional support. This facility has no person on staff with a strong neurobehavioral background, although each of the clientele would have, as a primary diagnosis, altered neurobehavioral capacities as a result of an altered neuroanatomy. Oncology patients are treated by persons who were trained in the science and practice of oncology. Obstetric patients are treated by persons with the skill and knowledge appropriate to ensure healthy outcomes to parent and child. But, persons attempting to maximize recovery following a trauma that has induced permanent damage to their neuroanatomy do not have access in their rehabilitation to persons with expertise in neurobehavioral change resulting from an altered neuroanatomy. The young adult in question has limited decision making ability. Additionally, he demonstrates difficulty in appropriate self-initiation. To his credit he has survived the past 9 years since his injury, at times living at home, at times on his own.

I am confident that the program cited does excellent work with certain clients that they admit. However, the words that damn both the program in particular, and the health care planners, is the section of the letter that reads,

> "As stated in the rules and regulations . . . physical and verbal aggression will not be tolerated. Serious and/or repeated offenses will result in suspension and possible termination from the program."

There are two injustices to consider within this example. The first is that were rehabilitation programs for persons with neurobehavioral disabilities designed upon rehabilitation principles that recognized an altered neuroanatomy, such letters would never be sent to persons whose very impairment precludes their being able to respond appropriately until they have had adequate treatment. Newly emerging behavior following loss of brain cells should never be considered aberrant or disordered. Rather, it should be anticipated as an outcome to be expected. The behavior may not be socially acceptable, and the role, then, of rehabilitation is to provide the client with the skill necessary to remove this newly acquired handicap.

The second injustice is that the government that funds, monitors, and certifies this program does not have the will to provide service and opportunity necessary which it knew would be required when the decision was made to sustain the life at roadside and in the emergency room. We have come to identify this as an issue that would not pass the scrutiny of an ethicist considering minimum standards of care/opportunity.

Sadly, it has become abundantly apparent that the existing paradigms that benignly restrict requisite opportunities, at least in Canada where the policy maker is also the insurer and the payer, will not change under current health care planning modalities. Such change will require informed, creative and persistent advocacy.

Advocacy has come to mean many things to various people. As it pertains to those of us who live with the effects of injury to the brain, it means assuring appropriate opportunity that will insure access to satisfactory living, loving, and doing (see Chapter 2) in an appropriate combination. This is all that we seek.

EXAMPLES OF PROACTIVE ADVOCACY

The past 5 years have seen various models emerge that do provide for the beginnings leading to satisfactory living, loving, and doing. Following 3 years spent gaining knowledge and establishing the network necessary for successful advocacy, in 1990 the Ontario Head Injury Association entered into local association development and support. There is no shortage of persons willing to establish support groups and community associations. However, the generally unempowered position in which many associations have found themselves mired, is testimony to the fact that acquiring a disabled family member does not automatically mean that you inherit corporate decision making skills or the understanding necessary to provide wise and necessary council. This has necessitated the ongoing development of resource materials, including topics such as running a board meeting, planning support group meetings, developing fundraising campaigns, initiating prevention initiatives, developing friendship programs, and preventing caregiver burnout.

Networks consisting of leaders within the delivery system surely do assist in the development of an advocacy initiative. One such benefit has been the Research and Training Center on Community Integration for Head Injury at SUNY at Buffalo, funded by the NIDDR in the United States. We have very directly benefitted from, and participated in, its Family Retreat Workshops. Participating families still give testimony to the quality of the experience. As importantly, these weekend retreats have allowed us to collect valuable data that have provided us with powerful information to be used as we petition both our only health care insurer, the Ontario government, and our national government.

It should be noted that the Research and Training Centers for injury to the brain came about largely because of the outstanding work of my mentor, Marilyn Spivak, and the organization she founded, the National Head Injury Foundation, in the United States. One of Marilyn's many strengths is her unmatched ability to network. In so doing, she gained the utmost respect of the people that she influenced. In the late 1980's, U.S. federal legislators were calling the NHIF, the most effective health care advocacy group in America. Networking by creating trusting relationships was the cornerstone of that success.

An additional valuable product of Research and Training Centers, has been the ever growing database of abstracted head injury journal articles, which now exceed 2500 in number and are available through the Buffalo program and various state and provincial offices. The Head Injury Glossary developed by the Institute for Rehabilitation and Research, Model Head Injury Rehabilitation System Research Project in Houston, Texas, is a valuable resource guide for the person wanting to be accurately informed.

It is these same Research and Training Centers that cooperate with five hospitals in a Model Systems program and database. Their increasing collection of data has and will continue to influence the direction of services to persons who live with the effects of injury to the brain and who can benefit from rehabilitative opportunities.

At the time of the announcement of the development of the Provincial Acquired Brain Injury program at Chedoke-McMaster in Ontario, Canada, the Minister of Health very clearly described how the advocacy work of the provincial head injury association had convinced government of the need to initiate an actual program. Since that time the provincial association has presented that ministry with research and anecdotal evidence powerful enough to sustain their attention.

Within the Ontario Head Injury Association the one most identifiable advocacy activity that provides outstanding measurable results is the Caregiver Information and Support Link (CISL). While identifying "best fit" available resources for families and health care professionals, CISL collects data valuable to our advocacy, as well as providing health care planners with accurate data required for informed decision making.

EVOLVING ADVOCACY

Over the many years since our son's injury, the conditions and issues confronting him have changed. Today, as a successful international athlete, active advocate, and very sociable person, his concerns and handicapping conditions deal with issues that include removing barriers that restrict freedom to commute about our community and across the country. As well, finding and following a satisfying career is fraught with road blocks that would make a lesser person give up. Such are the issues that he, along with his counterparts, are confronted with on a daily basis.

The barriers that handicap our son are only some of the barriers experienced by the 240 people who each month call our help line. Unfortunately, most of the callers to our provincial help line cannot be provided with simple, easy to access resources or referrals that could readily diminish their handicapping conditions. An informed service network, except for isolated pockets of appropriate skill and knowledge, does not generally exist. Even more frightening has been the lack of political will as demonstrated by the reluctance to significantly alter the status quo. Politicians have not been given ample reason to initiate adequate changes. Those who would be deemed to by the largest natural group of informed individuals, the health care community, have generally either not acquired the skill and knowledge required (Rempel and Roberts, 1989) or they are unwilling to pay the price to initiate change.

It is my observation that during this century health care became the health industry. The evolution of health care can be seen as a marriage between needed health support and inquisitive minds doing the necessary science. The continually escalating desire to cure and the subsequent need to find such cures created a rapidly developing health care industry, largely fuelled by the notion that if some is good even more should be better. This is apparent in the zeal to find new and better ways to patch up trauma victims, stabilize their life signs, provide them with a dose of physiologically based rehabilitation, and then discharge them from hospital. If, in fact, this is outcome oriented medicine, the outcome of choice appears to be the ego satisfaction of having "saved another life." For what?

Outcome oriented medicine must look at "reason to live" issues. This past summer, a young man whom I had come to know through my interest in advocacy, made the decision to terminate his life by jumping from the balcony of his fourth floor apartment. My initial reaction was one of sadness. As I thought back to his 14-year journey following the injury, my feelings changed. I have come to respect his informed choice. Of the miserable options available, known, and understood by him, his selection demonstrated insight. He picked the one he deemed most appropriate and implemented his decision. His story could be the dictionary definition of

Post Coma Abandonment, as I defined the term while writing the previously referred to report, "The Status of Wellness of Ontario Residents Who Live With the Effects of Traumatic Brain Injury." I am sure that a goodly number of well-intentioned and competent people worked to patch up the impairment resulting from the motor vehicle collision during the successful attempts to save that portion of his anatomy that could be saved. However, very little informed intervention, available as necessary, occurred in assisting him to minimize the effects of the disability resulting from his altered neuroanatomy.

Willer, et al., in Chapter 16, discusses WHO and its work defining impairment, disability, and handicap. While this work is a description of methods to diminish handicapping conditions resulting from brain injury that have been acquired, such opportunity was never readily available to our friend. If the story had ended with the observation that health care has still not come up with answers to his problems, then sadness would be an appropriate response. And we should then debate the ethics of keeping the person alive. This book is testimony that a broad variety of opportunities do exist to empower persons of all degrees of injury with the availability of handicap diminishing tools. However, the political will to provide what is decent and right has never been established, generally relegating such information to the dusty bookshelves in the back rooms of research libraries. While it is easy to criticize the leadership within all levels of the health care industry, appropriate change will only occur as leadership deems change to be in their best interest. An early step in the process of insuring change is through providing appropriate educational material. A second step is to move the subject onto the public stage for debate and to sustain the issue as an ongoing health care dilemma.

"Head Injury Hurts Forever" was our first attempt at public communication. The pamphlet attempted to justify its title. This leaflet was meaningful to very few folks. It was our first attempt to reach out, but, to my knowledge, not one person called us to say that they were going to live differently because of what they read. Nor did any politician or civil servant come forward with a commitment to help because of this very sincere effort by hurting people to communicate. No agencies or well-spirited citizens emerged to take up the fight on our behalf. This pamphlet's major benefit was to reinforce, for those of us reeling from the problems associated with acquired injury to the brain, that we were right, head injury hurts and, at that time, it seemed that it would hurt forever. (We had yet to discover that an alternative to grief is to remove what handicapping conditions you can, adjust your life's goal, and go on.)

We learned, through these early efforts, that we needed to be able to answer the questions arising from the statement "head injury hurts forever." Our first step was to visualize what we wanted. We wanted normalcy. The initial logo, a bandaged head which screamed hurt, was replaced by one that described normalcy, a complete family circle. A mission statement emerged that showed we were after reasonable things that would directly assist persons living with the effects of injury to the brain which would also diminish costs to government and society. For those who had not yet sustained such an injury, the plan was to insure their safety through prevention.

The record of the past decades shows that appropriate access to requisite opportunity is only gaining begrudging acceptance as the status quo is slowly exposed as archaic and unethical. One has only to consider the lack of will to provide appropriate rehabilitation based upon the abundant literature that has emerged from the early 1970's. It is evident that the pleading and begging of an earlier generation is not an effective catalyst for change. The mission statement created by the Ontario Head Injury Association had the answer inherent to it. Instead of pleading for leadership we needed to provide leadership. Leadership does not always have to be expensive to be good. One of the significant contributions of the Ontario Head Injury Association has been to introduce a new vocabulary into the system. Earlier we referred to the "continuum of care" as rather a "continuum of opportunity." While some may cynically view the change in words as unnecessary semantics, the word "care" conjures up an entirely different image and type of responsibility in the mind of the health worker, be she a doctor, therapist, or technician. The injured party can too readily view the care giver as the party who is "responsible to restore me to my former status." Conversely the word opportunity generates an attitude of empowerment, self-empowerment for the victim and attempting or assisting to empower in the mind of the helper.

Another example of leadership is the following mission statement with its list of proactive anticipated outcomes. It has become a standard by which health/care service efforts must now be evaluated.

Develop an environment within the province of Ontario that encourages persons who live with the effects of a traumatic brain injury to recapture, to the greatest degree possible, a most productive lifestyle.

Such a changed environment includes the development of educational, avocational, vocational and living opportunities of equal value to persons who live with the effects of a traumatic brain injury as are available to the population-at-large of the province of Ontario.

Alter the attitudes and understanding of society regarding the importance of the prevention of traumatic brain injuries.

1. Secure a reduction of 15% in the incidence of traumatic brain injuries within the province of Ontario,

2. Significantly improve the quality and availability of resources that benefit persons who live with the effects of traumatic brain injury,
3. Undertake and encourage the development of research and education initiatives as they relate to traumatic brain injury issues,
4. Assist in the development and successful operation of community associations throughout Ontario, and
5. Operate a financially secure charitable organization.

The National Head Injury Foundation in the United States, Headway in England, the Traumatic Head Injuries Network of Australia, along with the Canadian Head Injury Coalition in Canada, are representative of movements that have emerged to take issue with, and to respond to, the currently underwhelming efforts to address issues that have affordable, practical, and workable solutions. Each of these agencies are driven by a combination of consumers and health care professionals who continue to redefine the existing, mediocre paradigms specifying quality of living issues for persons who live with the effects of injury to the brain.

Perhaps the single most cogent message that these groups send, is that certain standards and rights have emerged in developed countries as minimum, ethical benchmarks. Therefore, where third parties intervene to sustain a life, the society for whom they act can no longer be allowed to regularly abandon that life to a living hell. Rather, persons who live with the effects of injury to the brain, must have the freedom to recapture a most productive lifestyle to the greatest degree possible.

References

Branch, T. (1988). Parting the waters—America in the King years, 1954-63. Simon and Schuster.

Condelucci, A.I. (1991). Interdependence, the route to community. Paul M. Deutsch Press.

Johnson, W., Willer, B., and Linn, R. (1992, unpublished). Misconceptions about brain injury among medical students. Rehabilitation Research and Training Center on Community Integration for Persons with Traumatic Brain Injury: University at Buffalo, New York.

Rempel, R.G., and Roberts, W. (1989). 1989 Hearings to determine the status of wellness of ontario residents who live with the effects of brain injury. Ontario Head Injury Association.

18

Working Together: Reflections on Fostering an Integrated Service Network for Individuals with Brain Injury

STEFFEN-MALIK HØEGH

The consequences of a brain injury are devastating both to the individual and his family. An individual with brain injury needs to learn to live with changed, and often reduced, resources and potential in the realms of physical, emotional, intellectual, and social areas.

Physical changes may be a lack of coordination, decreased vision, and pareses. Emotional reactions may include lability, depression, and anxiety. Concentration, learning, memory, and problem solving skills may be affected in the intellectual domain. Two or more of these changes directly impact on the brain-injured individual's identity and may greatly change family roles and psychosocial functions and work capacity (Prigatano, 1986; Rosenthal, 1990). Figure 18.1 conveys the complexity and severity of problems to be addressed in brain injury rehabilitation.

At this time we do not have the means to "repair" structural damage. This implies that it is exceptional to regain the premorbid level of function following a brain injury. In the process of trying to establish a "new" life, many resources and institutions are drawn on. After medical and surgical services, inpatient and outpatient rehabilitation is provided, and then community based services are utilized. In the course of recovery, individuals draw on resources ranging from support groups to sheltered work places to schools, but, in many instances, end up relying heavily on the support family members can provide. Depending on the severity of dysfunction, the process of trying to "relearn" how to live rarely takes less than 2 years from the time of the injury.

Today brain-injured individuals and their families experience gaps and lack of coordination in the services that are intended to make the arduous journey towards a normalization of their lifestyle less painful. The purpose

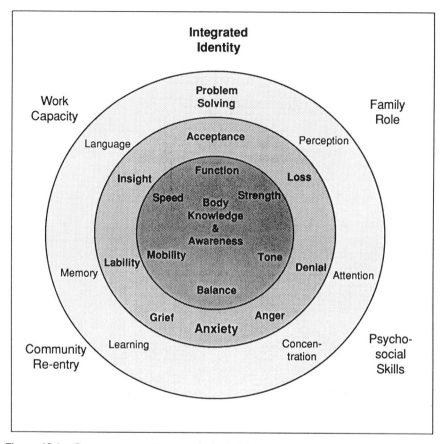

Figure 18.1. Consequences of traumatic brain injury.

of this chapter is to discuss some of the shortcomings brain-injured individuals and their families are exposed to in trying to reestablish their lives.

Suggestions as to how we can try to overcome some inconsistencies will be presented. This will hopefully inspire decision makers to work on establishing an Integrated Service Network, whereby "each piece of the puzzle" is used to build a continuum of services from the Hospital Services via Transitional Living and Out-Reach Services to Community-Based Services.

CHANGE—A MUST FOR THE CLINICAL SERVICES

The delivery of clinical services is typically linked to inpatient and outpatient settings. However, many shortcomings are currently encountered in clinical services.

When Need is Greatest—Help Seems Farthest Away

The most common experience families report is that little help and support are provided at the most crucial periods following a brain injury. There is rarely anybody to lean on in the acute phase. Few emergency rooms have trained clinicians who can address the fears family members experience in the acute phase. Everybody focuses on the injured person— little attention is paid to the life/death crises relatives go through. Family members sometimes even "sign off" organ donor certificates and later have the good fortune of seeing their loved one pull through. Issues like these are seldom dealt with until they boomerang months or years later.

Providers of clinical services display shortcomings in the phase when the injured individual is still nonoriented and confused. At our neurologic unit in Sonderborg, Denmark, we made an informal count of the number of staff and visitors a low level confused brain-injured client was exposed to over a 24-hour period. It was a surprise to many that the average number of different persons encountered amounted to the mid-twenties. I am sad to say that we, of course, had advised even the closest family to try to reduce their visits and the number of visitors they would like to bring along. I think we as providers keep clients in a state of confusion merely by the way we use uniforms that are indistinguishable, involve too many clinicians in the initial phase, and frequently change nursing staff. The most "dangerous" and disruptive situations for families and their injured relatives are changes and transitions.

Transitions

When a client is in transition from one phase in the recovery process to another, the providers are basically without a responsible "case supervisor." No matter whether the transition is from a hospital to a rehabilitation facility or from health care services to community based services, break down in communication is very likely. If the transition involves geographical change as well as shift from a for-profit to a public funded service, few societies have managed to establish a safety net that ensures continuity in the client's situation. The exporting of Canadian brain-injured individuals to rehabilitation centers in the United States is one example involving many transitions and where outcome may be adversely affected.

No matter whether you receive or provide clinical services in a for-profit or socialized health care system, the dilemma of trying to provide optimal clinical and community services under a limited financial "umbrella" exists. There are also a number of inherent problems in the organization and delivery of clinical services.

Organization of Clinical Services

Allocation and utilization of financial resources are the challenges confronting decision makers who want to provide optimal clinical and community resources for brain-injured individuals. Providing individual physiotherapy (PT), occupational therapy (OT), speech therapy (SP), recreational therapy (RT), vocational therapy (VOC), and neuropsychologic therapy (NP), has been, and still is, the standard in many rehabilitation facilities—both in for-profit companies and in the socialized health care systems. This prevalent approach to rehabilitation could be named the "Medical assembly line approach."

In the medical assembly line approach, brain-injured individuals are initially evaluated by a physician, who prescribes individual PT, OT, SP, etc. The clients start at one end of the assembly line and, with any luck, receive therapy in appropriate doses. The sequence and amount of "therapy doses" are seldom addressed and discussed. Each discipline department contributes one or more "spare parts" in trying to fix the dysfunctions. This approach results in a "piecemeal" approach lacking coordination.

The worst case scenario in this "piecemeal" approach is when patient needs are extensively assessed from each clinical discipline and each clinician establishes 5–10 goals. Treatment is initiated and progress evaluation is attempted on a weekly basis. A client who receives PT, OT, SP, RT, NP, and VOC ends up being exposed to, and imposed upon, by 6 clinicians, altogether having between 12–30 different treatment objectives. If we just try to calculate the amount of time available to address each objective—then it becomes obvious that we are left with very few minutes spread out over the week for each objective. Revision of this approach seems necessary.

The window of opportunity to provide a learning situation targeting our objective seems very slim. Add to this fragmentation, the fact that treatment needs may not be prioritized initially. This window of opportunity, to provide a learning situation, is further limited by the fact that clinicians often neglect to consult the client in establishing and prioritizing the treatment needs.

If a *clinical contract* is not established at the outset, then we have setup the patient, and ourselves, for failure, and we see clinical disciplines "pulling" the patient in different and sometimes opposing directions. A clinical contract is one way in which you align yourself with the client and make it possible to design appropriate learning situations. The development of a simple clinical contract is one of the central tasks for any rehabilitation team. When this is not done it counteracts good outcome.

The conflicting interests and "pulling" clients in opposite directions, touches on the professional self-images or caricatures we carry. In the medical assembly line approach, where therapy is "prescribed" much like medicine, we often encounter stereotype images and expectations for each discipline. Typical attribution may sound like this:

Physiotherapy deals with lower extremities;
Occupational therapy with upper extremities;
Nursing provides care;
Speech has cognitive training;
Psychology is crises and emotions;
Physician is pharmacology;
AND Tech's do all the dirty work.
(Case Management and Recreational Therapy are left out on purpose.)

Such images are stumbling stones in the creation of good learning situations. These preconceived ideas can best be changed through cotreatment and in group settings where clinicians have to rely on another professional's input and backup.

Demands on Staff

Due to the tremendous growth in numbers of rehabilitation hospitals offering brain injury rehabilitation, the need for clinical staff has surpassed the supply. The rise to more than 500 facilities at the end of the 1980's (Sandal, 1989), makes it virtually impossible to get qualified and experienced clinicians. This is especially critical when we start looking for clinical leadership in the rehabilitation facilities. It is not an unexceptional sight to see clinicians without specific neuropsychologic background trying to set standards of intervention. The generated treatment plans lack a clear focus and are unable to specify attainable goals.

In rehabilitation hospitals, the high performance demand (80%–95% productivity) and the number of meetings clinicians must attend, often exceeds what is realistically possible. Clinicians are forced to, at best, run in and out of meetings or, at worst, report for their colleagues on patients they may have never seen.

Due to cost containment, bringing down the cost of rehabilitation services is essential at any for-profit rehabilitation facility. As a consequence lower paid and less educated staff are scheduled to interact and provide the majority of training for the clients. Having licensed therapists do the evaluation, and then having assistants do the training under "supervision," is the most recent trend in staff utilization, cost containment, and overall service delivery. We do not accept that the least trained worker should do the majority of the work on any of our material possessions yet this mentality is prevalent in rehabilitation.

White- and Blue-collar in Rehabilitation

We are faced with an often overlooked conflict in providing learning opportunities for brain-injured individuals. Well educated people who are fond of literature and verbal/intellectual challenges, determine the content of training situations for brain-injured individuals who may not at all share the clinician's interests. We know that 75% of our clients tend to be young males who display sensation-seeking behavior. They end up being trained by clinicians of whom the majority are women, who on their part do not "display sensation-seeking behavior." As a consequence, clients often get bored, and of course start to act out since they may feel trapped in a situation where they are not altogether happy with the interaction and task expectancies.

Treating Too Diverse Patient Populations

Today many rehabilitation hospitals in the United States are struggling to survive (make a profit). This is sometimes done by diversifying the range of rehabilitation services provided. In doing so, the revenue must stay within limits predefined by the corporate parent. A few clinicians are expected to provide services to many and diverse diagnostic patient groups. Clearly, the focus and intensity of treatment becomes endangered. The clinical risk involved in diversifying is that specialization and the quality of rehabilitation services are diminished.

NEW DIRECTIONS IN THE DELIVERY OF CLINICAL SERVICES

To change some of the current shortcomings in the delivery of clinical services, and in trying to establish a continuum of services, it is necessary to formulate a clear and concise statement of purpose. This kind of statement can help us organize and streamline the services available and it can be used as the point of reference.

The goal of brain injury rehabilitation is to reduce handicap.

From this global statement, let us look at practical ways to make the delivery of clinical services fulfill the goal of brain injury rehabilitation. First, the simplest way to provide support will be presented. Then the product line approach, which focuses on small, decentralized self-directing units, will be described. This approach is considered to hold a lot of promise in trying to establish a continuum of clinical services.

Establish "Help Lines"

A conference at Sunass Rehab Hospital, Norway, 1990, on "Family Issues in Brain Injury Rehabilitation," made it clear to all the participants that support groups may play a much more vital and long-lasting role for the brain-injured and their families than any clinician can hope to fulfill. A first rule is to establish contact with relevant support groups. They provide information and support around the clock, unlike hospitals and rehabilitation facilities.

Each country has a number of Head Injury and Stroke groups ready to provide information and support; e.g., National Head Injury Foundation (USA); CHIF Canada; Hovedcirklen and Apopleksi Foreningen, Denmark; Highwatch, Great Britain.

Rethinking rehabilitation on a more global level involves looking at the total organization and delivery of clinical services. In recent years the "Product Line Approach" has attracted attention.

Product Line Approach

Product lines have been utilized in the automobile industry to increase product quality and ensure job appreciation and satisfaction. In health care, the product line approach is characterized by decentralization into small, self-directing and self-correcting rehabilitation teams and units where client and family needs are in focus.

At Mediplex Rehab—Bradenton, Florida, three product lines were established in the Autumn of 1991, under the guidance of this author.

A. Comprehensive Medical Rehab Line.
B. Comprehensive General Rehab Line.
C. Comprehensive Brain injury Line.

Given the appropriate number of clients a continuum of services can be organized as different programs with specified purpose, staff, and location within a given product line, i.e., Coma, Orientation, Neurobehavioral, Social Reintegration, and Work Preparation. All these programs are contained in the brain injury product line. Inherent in this product line approach is the utilization of coordinated intervention, a core staff, curricula, group-based treatment, cotreatment, and time frames. Each will be addressed in the following.

Coordinated Intervention

To utilize learning situations as effectively as possible at any stage in the process of recovery, it is necessary to coordinate efforts at many levels. Core staffs are designated to obtain coordination.

Core Staff

It is not unusual to see rehabilitation facilities just throwing every discipline at a client and hoping for the best. This practice confuses both the client and staff members with respect to their relevance. The principle of minimal sufficiency has been developed in order to involve the most relevant therapeutic disciplines at the right time in the rehabilitation process.

This guiding principle states that in the early phase of recovery, the majority of treatment needs are medical in nature, hence the primary involvement of physicians, nurses, physical therapists, and respiratory therapists. At the level of social reintegration the treatment needs, typically being nonmedical in nature, call for primary involvement of occupational therapists, speech therapists, recreational therapists, social workers, and psychologists. (See Fig. 18.2.)

Using core staff as one team makes it relatively easy to establish administrative and clinical guidelines for staff/client ratio at any stage in the recovery process.

More than anything it is crucial that teams get established and supported in their function. Only a core staff that works together for at least 12 months can hope to get a thorough knowledge of what each discipline can contribute to the rehabilitation process. Beyond that, a team needs to know its limitations and when to draw on other disciplines for advice and supervision. Inefficient meetings can also be eliminated since scheduling for a team is simple as opposed to scheduling for randomly assigned clinicians from several department. Using devoted teams will result in better quality of service due to higher involvement, more focused training, and clearer job expectations. The trend of high staff turnover in American rehabilitation facilities may also be reversed—benefiting the clients and their families.

Curriculum-Based Team Approach

The type and extent of problems following a brain injury do have a lot of similarities. Listing the shared and common observed dysfunctions is easy: reduced concentration, decreased psychomotor speed and coordination, learning difficulties, memory difficulties, changed emotional reactions, and inefficient executive functions.

Realizing these common traits in brain-injured individuals prompts the idea of dealing with these problems in a structured and group-oriented fashion. The simplest way of addressing this is through the utilization of a curriculum. **A curriculum is a structured plan, listing the sequence in which learning situations are to be provided for one or more patients at any given time in the rehabilitation process.**

The curriculum creates a progression of learning opportunities and ensures that relevant emotional and cognitive deficits are addressed in training sessions. Each specified time period within the curriculum has an identified theme that all of the therapeutic disciplines address during

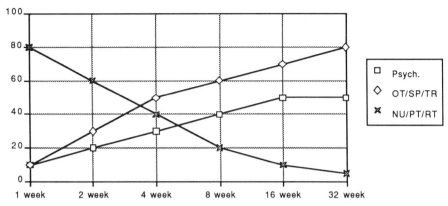

Figure 18.2. Principle of minimal sufficiency.

their group and individual sessions. For example, the theme for the third week of the Social Reintegration Module might address sequencing.

The curriculum can constitute the backbone of any rehabilitation program if developed by the clinicians who are to provide learning situations. Utilizing a team developed curriculum guarantees that the contribution of each discipline is levelled and coordinated with other activities in the curriculum.

Basically each product line must have at least one or more coherent curricula. Given the patient population, it will be possible to create a continuum of curricula. Each curriculum should have a different focus and be developed by the appropriate constellation of therapists.

A rehabilitation facility may offer several distinct curricula, each focusing on a different stage in the rehabilitation process. Each curricula can specify the learning situations on which it focuses. This is already known to some extent through terms such as Orientation Program, Neurobehavioral Program, Transitional Living Program, and Vocational Rehabilitation Program.

Through this systematic approach, an individual with brain injury will be exposed to learning situations at the time and in the sequence that is ideal. The success of a curriculum depends on the experience and creativity displayed by the clinicians, and the interaction with the brain-injured individual. This is not different from what teachers in our school systems are confronted with daily.

Ecological Learning Approach

A clear statement regarding one of the dilemmas encountered in rehabilitation is "If there is a major strand running through my comments on generalization, it is that we should not *expect* generalization to occur"

(Wilson, 1987). This implies that the learning situations we have to create together with our clients need to be real life situations or very close simulations thereof. This affects both the type of activities to be incorporated in a curriculum, but, even more, the way in which clinicians interact with their clients.

Later, I will address and discuss guidelines for activities to be incorporated in a curriculum—for the time being it is more important to dwell on the social situation we create—the milieu in which rehabilitation is provided.

Group-Oriented Treatment Approach

We are aware that every patient has different individual needs; however, there are many similar needs between patients within a given level of functioning. The group-oriented treatment approach identifies the similarities in the life situations that a brain-injured individual and his family encounters and stimulates group process in order to increase the ability to cope. Because the group process is more difficult than individual therapy, there are always two therapists to facilitate the group.

Cotreatment

Cotreatment is one of the obvious staff benefits from using a core staff and group-oriented treatment. It is possible to establish cotreatment between therapeutic disciplines, between therapists and rehabilitation nurses, and between therapist and technicians, where appropriate. Thus breaking down traditional interdisciplinary barriers.

Time Frames

Recovery from a brain injury is a lifelong learning experience. Rehabilitation can only provide time limited learning opportunities. In order to focus on the learning milieu, clearly marked time limited modules (classes) have been created. Time limits vary from module to module, due to the complexity of problems addressed in each module. For example, orientation is a relatively limited and easily defined goal for a module to address, relative to social reintegration which can be a neverending process. The time frames in each module are set partly based on the funding available for a typical patient at that level of functioning and partly based on the clinical needs. Even though it is possible to make the two meet, it is not necessarily the clinical needs that determine time frames, but more often the funding available—especially in the for-profit setting.

In trying to apply the principles from the product line approach, an inpatient and outpatient rehabilitation system was developed called "The

Functional-Modular Approach." This approach will be described as a model that can be adopted in many and diverse rehabilitation facilities.

FUNCTIONAL-MODULAR APPROACH APPLIED TO THE DELIVERY OF CLINICAL SERVICES

The Functional-Modular approach to brain injury rehabilitation was developed by the author. The goal was to establish a continuum of clinical services that could optimize brain injury rehabilitation as well as be cost competitive.

The ideas that constitute the Functional-Modular approach have evolved over the last 7 years, and draw on inspiration from David Ellis, Lance Trexler, Yehuda Ben-Yishay, George Prigatano, and, last but not least, Anne-Lise Christensen with whom I had the pleasure of working over a 2 year period.

This approach began by looking at the learning curve following a brain injury and from there developed into an elaborate rehabilitation system. Learning following brain injury usually requires more repetition due to concentration and memory disturbances. Generalization of attained knowledge is more difficult due to lack of mental flexibility and decreased problem solving skills. Hence, the learning curve following brain injury is supposed to be different from the "developmental" learning curve (Miller, 1985). The learning curve following brain injury seems to be uneven with unpredictable plateaus (Fig. 18.3).

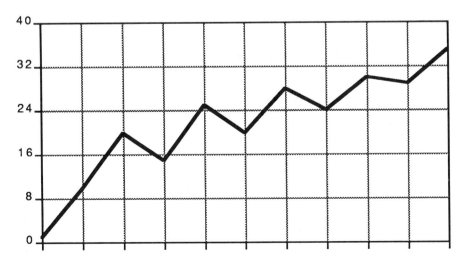

Figure 18.3. Learning curve following brain injury.

Knowledge about this learning curve makes it essential to determine the level of function for a given client before any rehabilitation activities are initiated. Once the level of function is established then, and only then, is it possible to provide appropriate group based learning situations for the client within a predefined time frame (Module). Once learning situations have been provided, reevaluation is necessary to determine whether the client has benefited from the rehabilitation provided.

Three Basic Concepts of FM

The three basis concepts—level of function; highly structured group-oriented treatment modules; and reevaluation—are the foundation on which the Functional-Modular approach has been developed. Each concept will be described.

Level of Function

The Functional-Modular approach demands constant attention to the concept of function. The term function has several connotations. Presently, function is defined as an objectively measurable entity resulting from observable behaviors. Therefore, level of function refers to discipline specific evaluation procedures that can objectify observable behaviors, for example, results of a neuropsychologic test battery, structured activity of daily living (ADL) observations, etc.

Baseline levels are established in at least the following areas: medical stability, physical capacities, emotional characteristics, cognitive abilities, personality responses, psychosocial skills, and work capacity. The baseline level of function serves the purpose of clarifying the patients rehabilitation needs. This is why the baseline must be very extensive and encompass data from every rehabilitation discipline. The procedure of using baseline level of function automatically sets the stage for outcome evaluation and program evaluation.

Once a baseline level of functioning has been established, it is important to relate it to the estimated premorbid level of functioning. This helps the client and the team to develop realistic expectations for the rehabilitation process and its outcome.

A baseline level of function needs to be established in order to clarify and thoroughly understand the specific set of symptoms (syndrome) that the patient is experiencing after brain injury. Once the syndrome has been established through an evaluation, then you can determine the most effective approaches towards establishing learning situations.

Following baseline level of function, attention must be paid to the learning situations to which clients are exposed.

Highly Structured Group-Oriented Treatment Modules

A treatment module needs to have a **"Common Denominator"** which in reality can be *clinical, objective, financial, or a combination* thereof. It focuses around a particular predefined level of dysfunctioning and entails team specialization and focused treatment approaches.

The Functional-Modular approach consists of several modules superimposed on the recovery curve. Each module makes up a portion of the sequence of a continuum of care during brain injury rehabilitation. To maximize the treatment focus, transdisciplinary module specific **curricula** are utilized. These are specific to a **time limited** stage of the brain injury rehabilitation process.

Based on the social learning approach and the need for making behaviors generalize to real life settings, most of the treatment occurs in **groups.** In fact, approximately 2/3 of treatment occurs in a group settings.

Reevaluation

Once clients are exposed to learning situations in a given module, then it is important to keep track of their progress. When a baseline level of function has been established, 4 steps will allow you to assess and monitor a client's progress and at the same time provide program evaluation:

1. Major aspects of care should be hierarchically organized. The team needs to prioritize the treatment needs of the client and then agree on the sequence in which they want to set up learning situations for a given client.
2. Indicators must be established. Before providing learning situations, the team should agree as to what they will accept as an indicator of progress.
3. Threshold (outcome expectations) should be specified for a given patient. Because indicators may vary in range, thresholds should be chosen.
4. Degree of excellence can be calculated. Knowing aspects of care, indicators, and thresholds, allow calculation of the degree of excellence for a given client as well as for a module. In this way, it is relatively simple to evaluate the program and to make appropriate changes in staffing, time frames, learning situations, or client mix.

Reevaluation allows us to identify slow-to-recover patients, quick-to-recover patients, and patients who plateau during the recovery process. Entrance and exit criteria for modules can then be stipulated.

Entrance and Exit Criteria

The presence of a curriculum to address particular levels of functioning makes it possible to establish objective, measurable entrance and exit criteria for each module.

The entrance criteria specifies the lowest common denominator of functioning necessary for benefiting from the learning opportunities in a given module.

The exit evaluation provides objective data in the form of cutoff values or pass-fail scores that are necessary to determine if the patient should repeat the module, be discharged, or admitted to the next module.

Practical Development of the Functional-Modular Approach

Initially, following brain injury, patients may be in a prolonged state of semi- or unconsciousness with lack of environmental responsiveness.

Patients emerging from coma and those suffering moderate brain injury may experience a state of confusion, disorientation, and significant emotional and cognitive dysfunction, including speech and language disturbances.

During the later stages of recovery, patients will continue to have residual deficits to varying degrees that may interfere with social and occupational functioning. During this stage the patient may also develop significant problems with regulation of behavior.

The Functional-Modular approach addresses the above mentioned stages of the recovery process following brain injury by superimposing rehabilitation modules focused in:

A. Coma recovery.
B. Orientation and mobilization.
C. Neurobehavioral disturbances.
D. Social reintegration.

After a short period it became obvious that two categories of clients needed special attention: Clients who did not emerge from coma and aphasic clients. Modules addressing these rehabilitation needs were incorporated and the full continuum of services are depicted in Figure 18.4.

The continuum of rehabilitation modules provided within the Functional-Modular approach has been arranged in a progression addressing each stage of brain injury recovery. The patient with severe brain injury would be expected to progress through the sequence of rehabilitation modules from come recovery via orientation and mobilization, to social reintegration. However, modules can be used without the necessity of movement through other modules. For example, a patient with a relatively mild brain injury can use the Social Reintegration Module without participating in the preceding modules (Fig. 18.5).

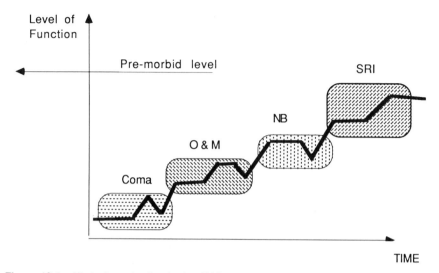

Figure 18.4. First phase in developing F-M approach.

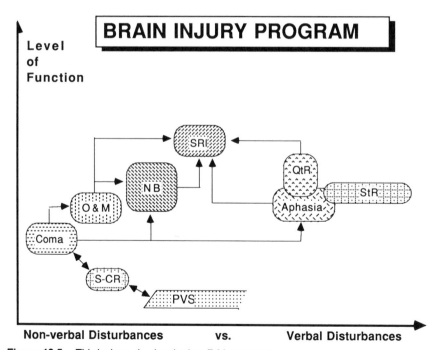

Figure 18.5. Third phase in developing F-M approach.

Rehabilitation Activities

In choosing rehabilitation activities for different programs and patient populations, a few general guidelines can be followed: structure, predictability, and control.

Structure

In organizing any rehabilitation activities for brain-injured individuals, providing structure is essential. The structure in rehabilitation activities must address two issues.

The *formal structure* emphasizes time management through modules, time frames, and daily scheduling. *Content structure* is correctly sequenced activities relevant at the appropriate phase in the recovery process, i.e., providing procedural memory learning situations for confused patients and neuropsychotherapy for clients who are working on social reintegration (Ellis and Christensen, 1989).

The apparent thing to avoid is the establishment of an isolated rehabilitation program in which setting and activities are only remotely related to the client's life situation. Extensive utilization of unsupervised computer based cognitive retraining is a good example thereof.

Predictability

For brain-injured clients to feel confident and secure, a sense of continuity and predictability is essential. Activities can, and ought to, be organized and scheduled to help clients develop the sense of immediate predictability on an hour-to-hour and a day-to-day basis.

Activities that allow performance predictability and evaluation are also invaluable—irrespective of whether the activity is geared towards physical endurance, cognitive performance, or control of emotional expression.

Control

Activities fostering self-directed behavior, self-monitoring, and, of course, responsibility are preferable. This seems to be one of the hardest things for many clinicians to grasp. Clients have to do the work.

The key task is to provide learning situations in which the *client takes charge*. Learning to do this in a social setting is one of the main points in rehabilitation. Using these three guidelines allows appropriate learning situations to constitute a curriculum linked to a specific module.

Advantages of the Functional-Modular Approach

The Functional-Modular approach has benefits for patient, clinician, organization, consumer/payer, and the rehabilitation community. Finally, it is easy to specify how to run the Functional-Modular Approach.

The treatment received in the Functional-Modular approach is specifically designed for the patient's level of functioning. The patient is given the opportunity to interact with other patients with similar needs and level of functioning, which is a good way to provide insight into problems and their solutions. The patient and his family can be provided with a precise picture of the expected length, kind, and cost of treatment. The patient will experience consistency in therapists and treatment orientation due to the team approach.

By specializing and focusing within one module, the **clinician** develops a high degree of competence and knowledge concerning a particular stage in the recovery process. They benefit from working with other professionals in a transdisciplinary approach. The clinician is able to experience "modular autonomy" in developing and carrying out treatment plans. Within the modular treatment group the clinician is able to use modelling techniques in a more realistic setting. The clinicians are able to experience a sense of "closure" as they see clients complete and graduate from their module.

The Functional-Modular approach is a highly structured management and **organizational** tool that allows:

A. Clear statement of a mission.
B. A high degree of control over resource allocation.
C. Clearly defined staff/patient ratio.
D. Per diem rate for services in each module.
E. Prediction of rehabilitation cost (minus medical expenses).

The Functional-Modular approach can easily be packaged for effective marketing. Precise knowledge of the product is available for the **consumer/payer** with respect to time frames, expenses, content, therapists involved, and expected outcome. Treatment is focused only on the areas required by the patient's identified needs.

The Functional-Modular approach introduces a new standard for delivery of rehabilitation services by shifting the rehabilitation focus *from* a medical perspective to a pedagogic process orientated approach. A change which is believed to benefit the brain-injured individual and his family.

Finally, it is easy to specify how the Functional-Modular approach can be **ruined:** Start rehabilitation without assessment and baseline of the level of function. Create a mismatch between patient characteristics and the common denominator for a module. Disregard the time frames. Do not provide feedback and neuropsychotherapy for your clients and make administrative issues more important than clinical issues. If these "guidelines" are followed, then you can be sure that extensive community based services are needed to compensate for the confusing learning situations provided in an unorganized clinical setting.

COMMUNITY RESOURCES—ORGANIZATION AND UTILIZATION

The potential need and demand for community based services has indeed been greatly underestimated. We must remember that the expected life span for a brain-injured individual is not shortened by a brain injury. This implies that brain-injured individuals will have to rely on and use community based services considerably longer than they will have utilized institutional services. Yet community based services have hitherto not attracted the attention brain injury rehabilitation has enjoyed. When clients are discharged from health care and rehabilitation facilities, they enter a domain with scattered and, some may say, undeveloped community based services.

A few guidelines are suggested for types of community services that are needed and how they are supposed to complement each other. In relation to community services, we can look at content and quality of life in relation to a few broad variables:

A. THE PUBLIC SPHERE which consists of: (a) Living situation, (b) Community reintegration, and (c) Work capacity.

The organization is not random as each area typically is funded and managed by different and separate administrations.

To supplement the previously listed dimension, we also need to look at:

B. THE PRIVATE SPHERE, which consists of: (a) Marital status, (b) Relatives and friends, and (c) Financial and legal situation.

Superimposed on the spheres are three dimensions designating the severity of injury. The dimensions are associated with type of community based services which are most likely to be utilized and with the level of independence displayed:

Severity—Level of Independence
Mild—Independent
Moderate—Semi-independent or "Transitional" and
Severe—Assisted.

The public and private spheres are fundamental indicators that help us understand the content and quality of life for a given individual (Fig. 18.6).

Work Capacity

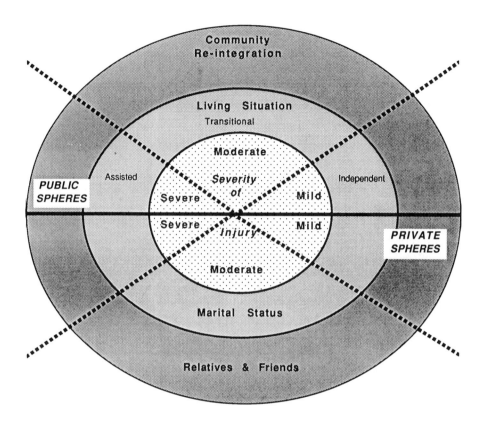

Financial & Legal
Situation

Figure 18.6. Spheres of community-based services.

The public spheres—living situation, community reintegration, and work capacity—are aspects of life closely related to an individual's socio-economic value. If a person is homeless, an outcast, and unemployed, then most industrial societies will provide some kind of social welfare program and consider it part of society's concern.

The private spheres—marital status, relatives and friends, and financial and legal status—are seldom thought of as being part of society's responsibility. Yet, these aspects of our lives are very relevant in order to obtain and gain acknowledgement, social position, and recognition. The private spheres are often overlooked when discussing community based services.

Overview of Community Based Services

To get an overview of the community based services available, it is helpful to organize these according to the different "spheres." The areas to be focused on in the public spheres are housing, recreational therapy, educational and cultural services, and work opportunities.

Housing and Living Situation

Basically, three options are available: independent, semi-independent (supervised or transitional living), and assisted living. These are closely connected to severity of injury and level of function.

The two groups that seem easiest to deal with are the clients who are capable of independent living as well as those requiring assisted living. Independent living implies return to premorbid options. Assisted living can be offered in a nursing home, residential home, sheltered housing, or as a commune/shared house/multioccupied house with adequate staffing. In parts of Denmark this has been developed for young disabled individuals. Unfortunately, sometimes brain-injured are housed with the mentally retarded. This represents a lack of both understanding and respect. At worst, the multioccupied housing sometimes develops into a "ghetto-like" environment.

A *Professional Foster Family* can be a unique alternative. For brain-injured individuals with moderate to severe dysfunctions, who need a highly structured and stable environment for years in order to develop basic routines of daily living, the professional foster family may be ideal.

For individuals who are semi-independent and where the level of function is fluctuating, problems are encountered in setting up appropriate living conditions. It is not rare to see these clients in a nursing home and as a result become more dependent rather than independent.

Long-term (1/2–2 years) transitional living and the training in ADL functions, is one of the least developed and most needed services. Many clients with a potential for independent living could attain this through appropriate transitional living programs, but funding remains the major problem enroute to independent living.

Recreational Therapy

This service is sometimes linked to either residential or nursing homes. Alternatively, it can be offered through a day center. The diversity in clients is great with respect to age and level of function. Activities are usually general in character.

Lately centers have developed in Denmark where recreational therapy

is offered selectively to individuals with an acquired brain injury. "Skodborg centret" provides specific services to approximately 10 clients over a 6–12 month period. The goal is to prevent regression and ensure that clients maintain their level of function.

Educational and Cultural Services

Special education is offered to anyone in Denmark who has a disability. The purpose of this education is to cushion the consequences of any disability irrespective of diagnosis. The focus is on teaching compensation strategies. Teaching is offered on an individual basis and in small groups with 2–6 participants. Teaching can, in principle, be offered in any subject as long as a few clients show interest in the topic.

Traditionally, education has focused on speech and language disturbances. Today new technology, i.e., computers, is being widely tested. Unfortunately, teaching compensation strategies for nonverbal cognitive dysfunctions have not been as extensively addressed.

Many cultural services overlap and serve educational purposes. Two of the most widely used services with this added function are "Folk high schools" and "Adult education associations." Folk high schools offer educational programs ranging from 1 week to more than 1 year. Only a few Folk high schools offer specialized programs for brain-injured individuals. The majority of Folk high schools serve anybody with an interest in learning and interacting with other people.

Adult education is a major contributor to stimulating learning in Denmark. Government supported day and evening programs are readily available to anyone in any subject—as long as the program can gather approximately 10–12 participants. Fewer participants may be needed if the program can be established as special education.

Many societies and associations offer meetings for people with specific diagnoses or disabilities. They focus on support, information, prevention, rehabilitation, research, and general acceptance. Most of these groups are run by family members of individuals with disabilities.

Despite all the effort put into this work, the overshadowing problems for these support groups are obviously to be able to provide services and to have impact in rural districts. Still, nonclinical networks will always be the backbone and guard dog when attention has to be drawn to the needs of individuals with brain injury and the situation of their family.

Work Opportunities

Many consider it a human right to have a job, and all are aware of the psychosocial consequences of being unemployed. Following a brain injury, the prospects of getting back to work and keeping it are indeed slim. Not only may brain-injured individuals experience change in level of function and competence, they may also have to "fight" the general unemployment situation. An unknown, living individual with brain injury must not constitute a potential "danger" to their employer with respect to creating legal or compensation problems.

Following a brain injury, getting back to employment is indeed one of the hardest tasks to be confronted. Socioeconomically, it is still debated whether or not trying to reestablish employment is cost effective. From a humanistic point of view, there is no question about the value of emphasizing nondemeaning employment for brain-injured individuals. If there is any work capacity left, it should be utilized fully.

Many rehabilitation facilities provide prevocational training, but the eventual test has to be carried out through job coaching, reeducation, work trials, work rehabilitation, or sheltered employment. Again, funding these services is getting increasingly difficult. With the unemployment rate continuing to escalate, the relevance of vocational rehabilitation is more and more debated.

An alternative question has often been raised: Is it possible to do away with many of the clinical services if elaborate work-like rehabilitation, with increasing demands, was provided as soon as clients were mobilized? Unfortunately this idea has not been tested.

Private Sphere in Relation to Community Based Services

Marital Status

In the private sphere, we find a strong relationship between severity of dysfunction after a brain injury and how burdened relatives perceive themselves to be. Changes in emotional reactions, personalty, and behavior are especially troublesome for relatives to cope with.

For married people, or people living in marriage-like conditions, changes in personality and behavior pose a direct threat to their relationship (Brooks, 1984). From research on crisis intervention, we know that death or loosing your significant other is a most stressful event, closely followed by loss of a job. Persons with brain injuries are at high risk of experiencing both these crises in addition to their change in level of function.

Relatives and Friends

The emotional fluctuation, characterized by lack of control and predictability, drive most brain-injured into social isolation. They frequently become estranged from their friends and relatives.

Adding to the complexity of problems, beyond the risk of divorce and social isolation, we find decreased income due to reduced or lost work capacity.

Financial and Legal Situation

At present, nobody takes charge and stringently investigates the possibilities for financial compensation for a brain-injured individual. This may be more pronounced in countries with socialized health care since the medical expenses are already covered. Few professionals are familiar with evaluations and procedures regarding compensation, which often results in suboptimal financial compensation. The fact that it may take years to reach a final settlement complicates matters. Legal steps are often only taken when the brain-injured individual poses a potential threat to himself or others.

Today nobody follows a brain-injured individual for the length of time necessary to resolve legal and financial matters—unless a lawyer has been hired. Clinicians providing clinical or community based services, unfortunately do not consider it part of their job to ensure optimal financial compensation for their "clinical" clients. In some instances in Denmark, insurance companies have been seen to ask the brain-injured individual to report back to them as much as 1 year after the initial contact—knowing that the client suffers from cognitive disturbances including memory problems.

Marital status, social isolation, and decreased income are seldom considered part of the public concern regarding disabilities. Yet only by addressing and working through these fundamental problems, is it possible to motivate a brain-injured individual and his family for a "new" and changed lifestyle.

Closeness and Diversity of Community Based Services

Ideally, the whole spectrum of community based services should be available to brain-injured individuals in their local areas—but several factors present this from ever being possible.

Funding, relative to establishing and maintaining a continuum of community based services, is the primary factor determining closeness, as well as diversity, of services. Next, a high degree of mobility in a population counteracts closeness and diversity of community based services. Family involvement and extensive follow-up are also increasingly difficult to ensure under these circumstances.

Some might think that the size of the population and the incidence/prevalence of brain injuries determine the extent of community based services—but this is not always the case. Political prioritization of social problems determines which services are to be provided in a socialized health care system. In Denmark, we have seen a small municipality, of approximately 11,000 inhabitants, being willing and able to provide specific and long-term services for people with brain injuries. Yet, it has been suggested that a population of at least 600,000 is necessary in order to be able to establish and maintain a full continuum of clinical and community based services (Finset, 1992). Private initiatives and/or opportunities for making a profit determine the closeness and diversity of community based services in countries with less developed socialized services.

In general, more densely populated areas are, of course, able to maintain a fair diversity of services. Living in remote and rural districts forces brain-injured individuals to move great distances in order to receive services. By moving they will be able to benefit from clinical services, but community based services are almost impossible to get incorporated in their process of recovery. Being transplanted into unfamiliar surroundings adds to the confusion of a brain-injured individual's experiences. It is not unusual to see foreign clients take weeks to adapt to American rehabilitation facilities. Of course as clients return to their native region, extraordinary measures may be needed. This trafficking results in the development of cost consuming and essentially unnecessary auxiliary programs, like "Repatriation Programs." By not providing local services, expenses are most likely to build up due to "system-failures."

A sensible alternative has been the development of "outreach programs." Rather than having clients come to the rehabilitation facilities or community based services, mobile teams show up in the brain-injured individual's home environment. This way, learning situations can be structured and tried out in familiar surroundings. So, rather than creating an artificial training environment and then hoping for generalization, onsite training is used. Mobile outreach teams make family involvement inevitable, and the team can encourage, and actually train, the brain-injured individual to access community based services. Families will not be separated and the environment will remain well known.

Outreach programs run by experienced clinicians, social workers, or teachers are bound to increase in numbers, partly due to its "common sense" function, but also because it will be a more cost effective way to provide services over an extended time span. If successful, then outreach programs will blur the present distinction between clinical and community based services—because outreach teams should be able to contain and serve both clinical and community functions.

Problems Related to the Delivery of Community Based Services

Two outstanding problems present themselves in relation to community based services. They are the lack of a unifying statement of purpose and the lack of coordination of resources and services available.

Statements of purpose for community based services range from preventing regression via dampening the effect of disability to promoting independent living. A unifying statement of purpose is most certainly needed if we want community based services to be anything but a safe-guard against regression.

It has been pointed out that community based services have to address public and private sphere dimensions in a persons life. All these aspects have to be addressed with the same perspective and set of values, since different administrations are responsible for providing community services.

The goal for community based services is *to normalize the lifestyle for a brain-injured individual and his family in both the private and the public spheres.* If this goal for community based services cannot be attained, the "quality of life" in all the above listed dimensions must be the common denominator and goal.

How to get there is the most pressing question. Today, many bits and pieces of community based services are already available in well developed societies but the coordination of resources and available services is miss-ing. Based on an extensive investigation into these matters, the counties of Denmark have come up with one very practical suggestion regarding service utilization and transition between services (Poulsen and Frich, 1991). They suggest that each county establish a "referral and visitation team." This team consists of representatives from the administrations that fund both clinical and community based services.

Traditionally, the separate administrations have been unaware of how services could and should be linked, and they have, of course, been argu-ing about funding. Different administrations have provided overlapping services in order to try to extend their territory while neglecting to pro-vide services in their own area of accountability.

The referral and visitation team would be responsible for establishing a "life care plan" identifying the clinical and community based services that could benefit clients and their family. This also involves specifying the dif-ferent types of funding required to implement the life care plan. Last, but not least, such a referral and visitation team needs to be given the author-ity to impact the rehabilitation scene through supervision, guidance, and working on "statements of purpose." This could empower the team to "dare" take responsibility for ensuring the life care plans are followed and implemented.

A number of people in the United States are already creating life care plans for insurance companies. They can specify down to the last penny the total expenses involved in providing rehabilitation and community based services, BUT they are not responsible for overseeing and taking charge if the life care plan is not implemented or when it may need revision.

The overall value in establishing a referral and visitation team that keeps track of the number of services and their quality, is that the team also will be able to point out areas in which new initiatives are needed or where services are outdated and obsolete.

A primary procedure to be developed is smooth **transition** between services, because this is the most frequent way in which clients "get lost in the system." Clients seldom realize the extent to which they may need clinical and community based services. Clinicians rarely inform them about services that a brain-injured individual may need as he leaves the hospital. This is largely due to ignorance about other services and lack of communication between service providers. Communication usually breaks down when services "belong" to different administrations; when public and private for-profit services refer to each other; or as two or more private services are "negotiating." The human suffering due to services and systems colliding, or, even worse, their ignorance of each other, ought to be one of the easiest areas to rectify.

Making somebody look at, and be responsible for, transitions is the simplest way to avoid wasting precious time in the process of recovery. Again, a referral and visitation team could oversee this. Cutting down on redundancy, making current services more efficient, and interlinking these through managed transition will most certainly benefit clients and their families. Clarifying, coordinating, and streamlining services across for-profit companies and public funded services are bound to benefit users and providers and it can not but pay off financially.

FUTURE DIRECTIONS IN CREATING AN INTEGRATED NETWORK

The most obvious way of establishing an integrated network would be if an outreach team could be "attached" to each and every brain-injured individual and his family. Then the network would refer to the "brain-injured family's network" and the task would be to reestablish and vitalize that network. This is a development to be hoped for in the future. Today, an integrated network refers only to the utilization of clinical and community based services.

It is needless to say that clinical and community based services serve common ends regardless of whether services are to be provided in a socialized or a for-profit health care system.

In trying to establish an Integrated Service Network, clear and concise statements of purpose need to be the point of reference. This holds true especially when our goal is to have different clinicians, social workers, and teachers working together through private companies and public agencies—ideally with the single purpose of normalizing the lifestyle following a brain injury.

The goal of brain injury rehabilitation (clinical services) has, therefore, become:

*To provide the brain-injured individual and his family with **learning situations** which facilitate insight into and if possible acceptance of their "new" life.*

Secondarily the aim, of course, is to bring a brain-injured individual as close to his premorbid level of function as possible.

In the delivery of health care services the product line approach holds much promise. This organizational principle, coupled with unifying statements of purpose emphasizing pedagogic learning situations, needs further exploration. The Functional-Modular approach is just one example of its application. The shift away from a medical assembly line approach also implies moving away from focusing on signs, symptoms, and diagnoses towards focusing on learning, growth, and mastering.

A change like this must involve a change in professionals involved in rehabilitation away *from* medically orientated clinicians *towards* professionals with more specific teaching and pedagogic background. With some adaptation, the product line approach and the emphasis on learning could be extended to, and serve, the goals of community based services.

The goal for community based services becomes:

To normalize the lifestyle for a brain-injured individual and his family in both the private and the public spheres.

If the goal for community based services can not be attained, then "quality of life" must be the common denominator and goal.

The two statements of purpose—one for clinical services and one for community based services—can help us to become aware of needs or clients that are not being served and helped today.

In concluding this chapter on creating an integrated network, it is necessary to draw attention to groups of clients that tend to be overlooked and who receive less than satisfying services today. In countries where rehabilitation and community based services are primarily provided by for-profit companies, we find uninsured and low income groups at high risk of not receiving adequate "learning situations" following a brain injury. In most countries, regardless of how health care is funded, we find three groups for whom services are scarce: children, teenagers, and elderly people.

The common denominator for these three groups is that they are not considered to be productive (labor power). Rehabilitation has, until today, primarily focused on "return to work" as an indicator of successful outcome of rehabilitation. It is suggested that we try to move away from "return to work" as the single most important indicator of "good" outcome of rehabilitation. This can be done by broadening our understanding of the importance of other aspects of life beyond work.

In conclusion, we must recognize that we are just at the starting point in trying to create an integrated network for brain-injured individuals. So far we have been working on bits and pieces. We still need to put these together on a larger scale. The first steps are currently being taken but much initiative and effort is still needed.

SUMMARY

This chapter has presented some of the current shortcomings of the "medical assembly line approach" to brain injury rehabilitation. As an alternative, the "product line approach" has been suggested. An example of its application, "the Functional-Modular Approach" has been described. The shift from a medical oriented framework towards understanding brain injury rehabilitation in a pedagogic context has been stressed.

An overview of community based services has been provided, and the closeness and diversity of these services discussed. In trying to establish an Integrated Service Network the need for statements of purpose have been pointed out. As a practical solution to creating a continuum of clinical and community based services, the importance of a referral and visitation team has been emphasized. Finally, future directions and needs in creating an integrated network for all brain-injured individuals and their families have been suggested.

"Whatever the problem and however severe it is, there is always something to be done which can improve matters" (Wilson, 1987).

Acknowledgments

Supported by the Institute of Brain Injury Research and Training, Mediplex Group Inc., Boston, MA 02181, USA, and Wiedener University, Chester, PA 19013, USA. It was implemented by B. Boyd, Ph.D., and staff at Mediplex Rehab—Denver.

The pretest of this approach was carried out 1987–1991 at Neuropsychological Department N50, Sonderborg Sygehus, Denmark. I am grateful for the input from the staff there, namely: E. Andersen, M. Hjort, K. Gotfredsen, and H. Philipsen.

References

Brooks, N. (ed). (1984). Closed head injury: Psychological, social, and family consequences. Oxford University Press.

Edgar, M. (1985). Recovery and management of neuropsychological impairments. John Wiley and Sons.

Ellis, D.W., and Christensen, A.L. (1989). Neuropsychological treatment after brain injury. Kluwer Academic Publishers.

Finset, A. (February, 1992). Personal communication. Vejlefjord Centre for Rehabilitation and Development.

Prigatano, G.P., et al. (1986). Neuropsychological rehabilitation after brain injury. The Johns Hopkins University Press.

Poulsen, J.G., and Frich, T. (May, 1991). Amtsrådsforeningen i Danmark, Rapport—Behandling og genoptraening af hjerneskadede. Amstrådsforeningen i Danmarks.

Rosenthal, M., et al. (1990). Rehabilitation of the adult and child with traumatic brain injury (2nd ed). F.A. Davis Company.

Sandal, M.E. (1989). Interventions in inpatient setting. In: Ellis, D.W., and Christensen, A.L. Neuropsychological treatment after brain injury. Kluwer Academic Publishers.

Wilson, B. (1987). Rehabilitation of memory. The Guildford Press.

Appendix

COMMUNITY INTEGRATION QUESTIONNAIRE

Home Integration:

1. Who usually does shopping for groceries or other necessities in your household?
2. Who usually prepares meals in your household?
3. In your home who usually does normal everyday housework?
4. Who usually cares for the children in your home?
5. Who usually plans social arrangements such as get-togethers with family and friends?

Social Integration:

6. Who usually looks after your personal finances, such as banking or paying bills?

Can you tell me approximately how many times a month you now usually participate in the following activities *outside your home*?

7. SHOPPING
8. LEISURE ACTIVITIES SUCH AS MOVIES, SPORTS, RESTAURANTS....
9. VISITING FRIENDS OR RELATIVES

10. When you participate in leisure activities do you usually do this alone or with others?
11. Do you have a best friend with whom you confide?

Integration Into Productive Activities:

12. How often do you travel outside the home?
13. Please choose the answer below that best corresponds to your current (during the past month) work situation:
    Full-time employment (more than 20 hours per week)
    Part-time employment (less than or equal to 20 hours per week)
    Not working, but actively looking for work
    Not working, not looking for work
    Not applicable, retired due to age

Volunteer job in the community
14. Please choose the answer below that best corresponds to your current (during the past month) school or training program situation:
Full-time
Part-time
Not attending school or training program
15. In the past month, how often did you engage in volunteer activities?

Index

Page numbers in italics denote figures; those followed by "t" denote tables.